A Practical Guide to Crisis Intervention

A Practical Guide to Crisis Intervention

Alan A. Cavaiola

Monmouth University

Joseph E. Colford

Georgian Court University

Lahaska Press
Houghton Mifflin Company
BOSTON   NEW YORK

Publisher, Lahaska Press: Barry Fetterolf
Senior Editor, Lahaska Press: Mary Falcon
Editorial Assistant: Lindsey Gentel
Senior Project Editor: Margaret Park Bridges
Manufacturing Coordinator: Chuck Dutton
Marketing Manager: Brenda L. Bravener-Greville

COVER IMAGE: © Hamish MacEwan / Superstock

Lahaska Press, a unique collaboration between the Houghton Mifflin College Division and Lawrence Erlbaum Associates, is dedicated to publishing books and offering services for the academic and professional counseling communities. The partnership of Lahaska Press was formed in late 1999. The name "Lahaska" is a Native American Lenape word meaning "source of much writing." The small eastern Pennsylvania town of Lahaska, named by the Lenape, is the home of the Lahaska Press editorial offices.

Printed in the U.S.A.

Library of Congress Control Number: 2001133254

ISBN: 0-618-11632-X

123456789-MP-09 08 07 06 05

CONTENTS

PREFACE

Most of us go through our daily lives with the expectation that each day will be somewhat predictable. When we leave for work or school in the morning, we know what we will do, who we will meet and talk with, and approximately when we will return home in the evening. However, we also know how fragile our expectations are and how—in an instant—our lives can be thrown into crisis and turmoil.

Crises can be personal (the death of a loved one); they can be regional (a tornado, hurricane, or some other natural disaster); or they can be national in scope (the World Trade Center and Pentagon attacks on September 11, 2001). As practicing clinical and school psychologists for many years, we (the authors) have come to appreciate how differently people react to similar types of crises. Whether it is an individual going through the personal crisis of a painful, contentious divorce, or our nation healing and rebuilding after September 11, there is a great deal of variability in how we, as human beings, respond to and cope with crises in our lives.

The Goals of This Book

Our purpose in writing this book was threefold. First, we very much wanted to write a text that would prepare third- and fourth-year undergraduates and beginning graduate students in human service fields (psychology, counseling, social work, education, nursing, criminal justice) with basic information pertaining to crisis intervention in a variety of crisis situations. We took upon ourselves the difficult task of writing a text that would be relevant to all human service providers because we noted a lack of published textbooks that had taken a broad-brush approach to crisis intervention. Some texts were oriented to particular specialties (e.g., criminal justice or psychiatric professionals); others seemed to be written for the purpose of promoting a particular crisis intervention model. Our goal was to create a text that would have practical application and relevance for students who will eventually enter into human service occupations. We strongly believe that crisis intervention coursework should be integrated into all undergraduate and graduate human service curricula. Of all the skills that students learn, crisis intervention skills will serve them best in managing a variety of situations. Crisis intervention coursework also covers information that may not be dealt with in any depth in any of the traditional human service curricula. For example, while an abnormal psychology or psychopathology course may describe the various symptoms of Posttraumatic Stress Disorder, crisis intervention coursework further describes how to effectively work with someone who has been trau-matized.

Our second purpose in writing this text was to provide students with an understanding of how crisis intervention services are actually being offered in the community. Students often complain that many of the courses they are required to take as part of their major have very little practical relevance to what they will be doing once they are working in the field. This is not the case with the crisis intervention course we developed for our school and this crisis intervention textbook. One of the assignments that we have used over the years in our undergraduate crisis intervention course is to have our students interview people in their community who provide crisis services. We have found that our students can be very creative in approaching this assignment. They interview psychiatric crisis screeners in local emergency rooms and men-tal health clinics, counselors at rape crisis centers, teachers who work with emotionally disturbed children, counselors at domestic violence shelters, county prosecutors who are involved in homicide investigations, obstetrical nurses who work with the parents of premature or very sick infants, police offi-cers who do hostage negotiation or domestic violence calls, and emergency medical technicians who provide first aid or vital emergency medical care to accident victims. All these individuals play a key role in the crisis intervention delivery system. Interestingly, with few exceptions, what these crisis interven-tionists convey to the interviewers is that they received little, if any, specific training in doing crisis intervention work and wished that they had. One female police officer told a student that the hardest thing she ever had to do was to tell parents that their nine-year-old son was killed by a drunk driver while riding his bike home from school and that she felt totally unprepared to handle such a heartbreaking task. In this textbook we provide a wide variety of crisis cases and demonstrate appropriate intervention techniques.

Our third purpose in writing this book was to give future practitioners a survey of the key elements of crisis intervention from a variety of models found in the professional literature, then boil it all down for them into one sim-ple, effective model—the Listen Assess Plan Commit (LAPC) model—that they can use in a variety of crisis situations. Through repeated exposure to the var-ied uses of this model it is our hope that the techniques will become second nature to students as they begin their work in the human service field.

The Organization of This Book

In chapter 1, we provide a framework of basic information pertaining to crisis intervention. Here we present definitions of what constitutes a crisis, various subtypes of crises, and the range of how individuals respond to crisis events. In chapter 2, we present an overview of vital crisis counseling skills that can be useful in any crisis intervention situation. We also present a description of the LAPC model, a guide that crisis workers can use at the basic level in their first intervention and at a more sophisticated level as they gain experience in their chosen field. In subsequent chapters covering a variety of crises, we provide an example of the LAPC model in use. In chapter 3, we present information regarding the crisis of child abuse and provide an overview of the various types of child abuse and how to effectively manage the crisis once it is identified. In chapter 4, domestic violence and intimate partner violence is discussed, along with useful information on how to help those in crisis due to physical battering and/or emotional abuse. In chapter 5, issues pertaining to the crises of suicide and homicide are presented, along with strategies to help save the lives of those in danger. Chapter 6 deals with issues surrounding the crises of rape and sexual assault. This chapter also presents valuable information on how to help rape victims in crisis. Chapter 7 deals with those crises that come about as a result of alcohol or substance abuse. In this chapter, we make important delineations between medical crises and crises that come about as a result of a pattern of alcohol or drug abuse. Crisis management strategies and treatment options are also discussed. In chapter 8, we present information on bereavement and the myriad losses that people experience in their daily lives. Chapters 9 and 10 deal with crises that impact the school, community, or nation as a whole. Chapter 9 specifically addresses the different types of crises that take place within our nation's schools, ranging from school violence to student or teacher deaths. This chapter presents valuable information on school crisis teams, crisis response policies, and how school administrators, staff, and teachers can play a key role in ameliorating crisis situations. Finally, chapter 10 addresses the national, state, and local community response to crises in the face of national disasters.

One of the problems with writing any crisis intervention text is deciding what to include and what to exclude. We have attempted to include information about crises that are timely and relevant to most undergraduate and graduate students. Naturally, it is impossible to include information about every type of conceivable crisis. However, we believe that students will garner enough information from this text, and will be presented with enough examples of the LAPC intervention model at work to be ready for any type of crisis situation that they may encounter in their professional lives. It also may be impossible for instructors to cover everything that we present in this text, in which case we recommend to our faculty colleagues that you have students read the first two foundation chapters, but then feel free to focus on those areas that are perhaps more relevant to your student population or more relevant to the overall goals of your department.

Acknowledgments

First we wish to thank the manuscript reviewers who offered constructive criticism and many useful suggestions: Ronald Allen, Liberty University Center for Counseling and Family Studies; Irene Ametrano, Eastern Michigan

University Department of Leadership and Counseling; Paul Ancona, Edmonds Community College Department of Human Services; Ronald Colonna, John Carroll University School of Education and Allied Studies; Noreen Glover, The University of Texas-Pan American Department of Rehabilitative Services; Teri McCartney, Adams State College Department of Psychology and Counselor Education; and Karen Neuman, Madonna University Social Work Program.

Finally, we would like to thank all the people at Houghton Mifflin and Lahaska Press who helped make this text a reality. We are especially grateful to Debby Seme who encouraged us to submit a proposal to write this text. We are also thankful to Lahaska Press Publisher Barry Fetterolf for his continuing encouragement and support throughout this project and for making this text become a reality. We are most grateful to Mary Falcon, our Senior Editor, for her astute recommendations and patience in shaping the draft manuscripts into a comprehensive, comprehendible textbook.

Alan Cavaiola
Joseph Colford

ABOUT THE AUTHORS

Alan A. Cavaiola, Ph.D., is associate professor of psychology at Monmouth University, where he developed and teaches a crisis intervention course, one of the most popular elective courses in the undergraduate psychology curriculum. Unsatisfied with available crisis intervention textbooks, Dr. Cavaiola developed his own teaching materials, which eventually became the foundation for this book. Dr. Cavaiola also has extensive experience as a clinician. Before taking his present academic position, he was clinical director of the chemical dependency treatment programs at Monmouth Medical Center. In his capacity as outpatient staff psychologist at the center, Dr. Cavaiola's responsibilities included providing crisis services to emergency room patients.

Joseph E. Colford, Ph.D., an assistant professor of psychology at Georgian Court University, has 26 years of experience in public education as a school psychologist, as well as extensive experience in a part-time clinical practice with a specialty in children, adolescents, and families. This work has provided him with a wealth of experience in crisis intervention, particularly as it impacts schools and families. Dr. Colford's years as a practitioner, combined with his experience teaching crisis intervention as an undergraduate course at Monmouth University with Dr. Cavaiola, were the motivation behind his decision to co-author this practitioner-oriented text for students interested in the field. The events of September 11 also convinced him that this textbook would be a timely addition to the libraries of the increasing numbers of undergraduates seeking to take courses in crisis intervention.

CHAPTER 1

Understanding Crisis

Brooklyn Woman Kills Daughter, 7, and Stabs a Friend, Police Say
A Brooklyn woman who the police said was high on drugs stabbed her
7-year-old daughter to death yesterday morning and critically
wounded a friend who intervened in the stabbing, according to the
authorities. They said the woman later turned a pair of scissors on herself. ... According to friends and relatives, the woman, Yolanda
Billingslea, 27, had recently lost her job at RCN, a cable television
provider, and had argued with the girl's father on Thursday night.
(Jacob Fries, July 27, 2002, *New York Times,* p. B1)

Ex-Student Frees Last of Hostages and Gives Up A former Fairfield
University student who claimed to have a bomb surrendered to police
last night after releasing the last of 24 hostages he had taken in a 7-hour
drama at the Roman Catholic School, police said. Patrick Arbelo, 24,
released the last hostage at 10:10 P.M. and gave himself up 50 minutes
later. (February 13, 2002, Associated Press)

College President Calls Suit "Unfair" The president of the
Massachusetts Institute of Technology said a wrongful death suit filed
by the family of a New Jersey student who committed suicide is "unfair
and inaccurate." President Charles Vest defended the school's handling
of the case of sophomore Elizabeth Shin in an e-mail to MIT's students,
faculty and staff. ... Shin, 19, of Livingston, NJ, died in April 2000 after
setting herself on fire in her dormitory room. (February 8, 2002, *Newark
Star Ledger,* Associated Press)

Police Seek Gunmen who Abducted, Raped Florida Waitress Police
on Wednesday were searching for two gunmen who abducted a woman
near her apartment and raped her as they drove around Central Florida.
The assailants released the woman naked on a secluded road at about
5:00 A.M. Tuesday, and she ran to a house for help, according to police
reports. (*Miami Herald,* February 14, 2002, Miami, Florida)

U.S. Attacked; President Vows to Exact Punishment for 'Evil'
Hijackers rammed jetliners into each of New York's World Trade Center
towers yesterday, toppling both in a hellish storm of ash, glass, smoke

and leaping victims, while a third jetliner crashed into the Pentagon in Virginia. ... a fourth [plane] plunged to the ground near Pittsburgh ... the military is put on highest alert ... National Guard units are called at Washington and New York ... two aircraft carriers are called to New York harbor. (Serge Schmemann, September 12, 2001, *The New York Times*, p. A1)

*P*ick up any newspaper or watch a newscast on any given day, in any city or town in the United States, and you will read or hear of people in the midst of crisis. A car accident, a domestic violence incident, a kidnapping, a school shooting, a rape, an earthquake, or a terrorist attack experienced by an entire nation—each of these situations constitutes a crisis event. Imagine being thrown into one of these situations unexpectedly, suddenly, and without forewarning. Most individuals find some means of coping in the aftermath of a crisis, relying on support and assistance from family, friends, or trusted individuals, such as clergy or family physicians. However, it is common to find many people who feel overwhelmed and immobilized, or who find that they are unable to cope, even with the assistance of well-meaning friends or family members. Some find that the coping mechanisms they have relied on in the past do not work when dealing with a new crisis.

Often when one hears the term *crisis intervention,* one may immediately think of those services that mental health professionals would ordinarily provide in a mental health clinic or other environment, such as a hospital emergency room. While psychiatrists, psychologists, psychiatric social workers, and professional counselors often provide these services, an array of other individuals also provide such services. Police officers, teachers, school counselors, college counselors, firefighters, rescue workers, community volunteers, first aid squads, nurses, physicians, clergy, funeral directors, attorneys, employee assistance counselors, human resource managers, neighbors, friends, roommates, and family members may find themselves performing crisis intervention services, sometimes without realizing it.

It seems that there are so many more crisis situations and traumatic events that occur in today's society. This perception is due, in part, to the media coverage of such events. What is clearly different today is that there are many more types of crisis service delivery systems than there were forty or fifty years ago, including hotlines; mobile emergency teams trained in crisis intervention; school intervention programs, such as student assistance programs; workplace interventions, such as employee assistance programs; and emergency room services, which include crisis services for both psychiatric emergencies and substance abuse. This chapter provides an overview of crisis intervention, definitions of crisis, various types of crises, and diagnostic considerations for people in crisis. Because it is critical to consider cultural issues when working with someone experiencing a crisis, these topics will also be discussed. In the chapters ahead, we will describe some of the service delivery systems and provide examples of how individuals provide crisis intervention services in those settings.

Defining Crisis

As Noreen Graf suggested (personal communication, August 19, 2002), a broad definition of crisis is *a predictable or unpredictable life event that an individual perceives stressful to the extent that normal coping mechanisms are insufficient.* Gerard Caplan, one of the early pioneers in the crisis intervention field, was the first to articulate what he referred to as crisis theory. In order to understand his crisis theory, it is helpful to look at how he defined *crisis.* For Caplan (1964), a crisis is "a temporary state of upset and disorganization, characterized chiefly by an individual's inability to cope with a particular situation using customary methods of problem solving, and by the potential for a radically positive or negative outcome" (p. 45). Caplan makes many assumptions, which are implicit in his definition. First, *a crisis begins with a precipitating event.* These precipitants can be specific predictable life events, such as getting married, graduating from school, moving to a new town, a planned pregnancy, and retirement, or they can be unpredictable, such as natural disasters, accidents, an untimely death of a loved one, being the victim of a crime, or other traumatic events.

The second assumption made is that a crisis state, by its very definition, is *time-limited.* According to Caplan, this means that the immediate impact of the crisis will usually last from 6 to 8 weeks, depending on the nature and intensity of the crisis. Of course, there may be long lasting effects associated with many crises. The third assumption is that *crises create a state of disequilibrium and disorganization* for the individual. Therefore, people who were once organized and went about their days with a certain degree of predictability found that they were faced with days filled with chaos, as crisis events sometimes control or dominate their lives. Another assumption Caplan explains in his crisis theory is that once the crisis event takes place, there is a *cognitive interpretation* or appraisal of the event, which accounts for the notion that not everyone reacts to a crisis in the same way. For example, being fired from a job may seem like the end of the world to one person, while for another, it can be a chance to take a few months off, do some traveling, and relax between jobs. The Greek philosopher, Epictetus once said, "It's not the events of life that make men mad, but rather the view we take of them." It is the view we take of them that implies this cognitive interpretation of crisis events. Finally, *crisis events will cause a breakdown in one's ability to cope.* The goal of crisis intervention therefore is to help people mobilize their own coping resources in an effort to restore balance or equilibrium. In developing his crisis theory,

Caplan was interested not only in identifying the crisis itself, but also in assessing individuals' ego functioning in the aftermath of crisis situations as they attempt to cope. According to Caplan, adequate ego functioning was the basis of one's mental health.

Slaikeu (1990) viewed the word *crisis* as being very rich in psychological meaning. In Chinese, the word for *crisis* is made up of two symbols that mean danger and opportunity (Wilhelm, 1967). The word therefore connotes both a time of danger, which may be physical (such as assault or a medical illness) or psychological (such as losing one's job or going through a divorce), and of opportunity (such as personal growth that results from having experienced a crisis or having come to the realization of one's inner strength). This would be the case with rape victims who come to the realization that they have survived and can use their strength to help other rape victims, or the person who experiences a job layoff and obtains training to get a better or more satisfying job. Of course, while a person is going through a crisis, the notion of opportunity probably doesn't make much sense. Often people may not realize the personal growth and self-efficacy they have achieved until months or years after crises have passed. Perhaps the old English proverb, "A smooth sea never made a skilled mariner," sums this up best.

The English word *crisis* is a derivative of the Greek word *krinein,* which means "to decide" (Lidell & Scott, 1968). This emphasizes that a crisis is a time for decision-making, a turning point, or a moment of reckoning. In some instances, these decisions will help to improve one's life. Slaikeu (1990, p. 15) notes the potential for a "radically positive or negative outcome" in the aftermath of a crisis. In a fundamental way, the direction that the outcome takes depends on the decisions the affected individuals make as part of the crisis resolution process. Often the decision reached as a result of a crisis will enable that individual to thrive. In other instances, however, these decisions may lead to a life that is negatively impacted and/or diminished in some way. To acknowledge this potential for positive or negative outcomes and the role of the individual's decisions in determining the outcome is not as simple as implying that all the person in crisis need do is to "think positively." To suggest this would be to deny the unique complexity of crisis events and the often insurmountable difficulties they pose to affected individuals.

Types of Crises

Based on the definitions presented so far, one could argue that just about any stressor could bring about a crisis situation. In order to further delineate this term, it is helpful to conceptualize crises as being grouped into four areas. According to Brammer (1985), crises can often be conceptualized to fall into three domains: (a) normal *developmental crises,* (b) *traumatic event crises,* and (c) *existential crises.* We have included a fourth domain, (d) *psychiatric crises,* because there are many instances in which a psychiatric condition can serve as the catalyst to a crisis state (e.g., a person who suffers from Bipolar Disorder may begin to experience a manic episode that results in a gambling spree). Conversely, a crisis can exacerbate an already existing psychiatric condition (e.g., a young schizophrenic adult who stops taking medication after being evicted from a boarding home).

Developmental Crises

What is unique to developmental crises is that the precipitating event of the crisis or the stimulus event is embedded in normal maturational processes (Slaikeu, 1990, p. 42). Throughout the lifespan, human beings are constantly changing; yet the normal growth process is characterized by continuity, as one passes from one stage to the next through a series of life transitions.

Erikson (1963) was one of the first developmental theorists to point out that development continues through the lifespan. What was also unique to his approach was his assertion that at each stage of development, there is a major task or conflict the individual must resolve in order to move onto the next stage. Table 1.1 summarizes Erikson's developmental stages, outlining both the transitional theme and the developmental tasks associated with each stage. It also identifies conflicts or events that could potentially precipitate a developmental crisis for an individual at each identifiable stage.

For example, according to Erikson (1963) a major task of adolescence, is identity formation. Erikson believed that by the end of the teen years healthy individuals must develop some sense of identity, including who and what kind of person one is in relationships, what one's strengths and weaknesses are, and given those insights, what one sees as future life goals and/or directions. The teenager who is unable to "find himself or herself" may wander aimlessly from job to job or from college to college feeling depressed and lonely. Stuck in a developmental crisis that Erikson refers to as "role confusion," these individuals may be unable to proceed with the later developmental tasks of young adulthood, which include establishing intimate, committed relationships and achieving occupational stability.

Midlife crisis is another example of a developmental crisis (Mayer, 1978; Levinson, 1978). This crisis may occur as men and women begin to experience various emotions of anxiety, sadness, or fear of death that occur as they contemplate their accomplishments, take stock of themselves, experience physical changes as a result of growing older, watch their children mature and leave home, or experience other major life transitions. These emotions may be exacerbated by the individual's take on specific developmental tasks. Certainly, not every man or woman experiences a crisis as they navigate these life transitions, but for some individuals the normal developmental passages do indeed precipitate crisis responses.

It should be emphasized that when individuals are experiencing what may be developmental crises, it is not always certain that they will seek professional help, nor will they necessarily identify their problems as developmental in

TABLE 1.1
Erikson's Developmental Stages with Potential Developmental Crises

Stage	Transitional Theme	Developmental Tasks	Potential Conflicts
Infancy (0–1 year)	Trust vs. mistrust	Bonding, stability	Rejection by or of caregiver
			Disruption in feeding
Toddlerhood (1–2 years)	Autonomy vs. shame and doubt	Developing independence	Conflict with caregiver
			Overprotective parenting
			Neglectful parenting
Early childhood (2–6 years)	Initiative vs. guilt	Learning motor skills and motor control	Learning cultural values
			Conflicts with parents, teachers, peers
			Entering school (preschool/kindergarten)
Middle childhood (6–12 years)	Industry vs. inferiority	Developing learning skills	Learning disabilities
		Mastery of academics	Conflicts relating to peers, and/or teachers
			Changing schools
Adolescence (12–18 years)	Identity vs. role confusion	Adjusting to puberty	Unwanted pregnancy
		Exploring relationships	Sexual identity fears
		Defining one's identity	Career indecision
		Defining one's strengths/weaknesses	Going off to college
			Peer rejection
			(Continues)

nature. Instead, they may experience frustration, anxiety, loneliness, depression, or may express other complaints. It should also be noted that developmental crises can sometimes occur simultaneously, as would be the case with a 50-year-old man or woman who is going through a divorce and also having to make decisions regarding the care of his or her elderly parents.

TABLE 1.1
Erikson's Developmental Stages with Potential Developmental Crises
(Continued)

Stage	Transitional Theme	Developmental Tasks	Potential Conflicts
Young adulthood (18–34 years)	Intimacy vs. isolation	Develop intimate relationships Settling down, starting a family Developing parenting skills Occupational development	Rejection by partner Infertility Separation/divorce Inability to parent Career problems
Middle adulthood (35–50 years)	Generativity vs. stagnation	Adjusting to middle age Adjusting to parenting Dealing with aging parents Increased productivity	Physical decline Rejection by teenager Children are rebellious Death of aging parent Midlife crisis Menopause
Maturity (50–65 years)	Generativity vs. stagnation	Adjusting to aging Prepare to retire Adjusting to grown children	Health problems Financial concerns Conflicts with children Empty nest
Old age (65–death)	Ego integrity vs. despair	Adjusting to aging Adjusting to retirement Evaluate past achievements	Health problems Financial problems Loneliness Death of friends

Note. Adapted from *Childhood & Society,* 2nd Ed., by E. H. Erikson, 1963, New York: W. W. Norton & Co.

Traumatic Event Crises

Traumatic event crises are what most people imagine a crisis to be, and each of the events reported at the beginning of this chapter were, in fact, traumatic event crises. The most distinguishing characteristic of traumatic event crises is that there is a clear external precipitating event. The traumatic event is usually an uncommon or extraordinary incident that one cannot predict or control. Unlike the developmental crises described above, traumatic event crises can occur at any time in one's development, and usually have a sudden onset, are unpredictable, have an emergent quality, and can impact more than one person (e.g., an entire state, county, or community). Examples of traumatic event crises would include natural and environmental disasters (e.g., fires, floods, earthquakes, hurricanes, tornadoes, heat waves, winter storms) and man-made disasters (e.g., train or airline crashes, nuclear and toxic waste accidents, combat, terrorist attacks, school shootings, homicide, suicide, car accidents, industrial accidents, sudden medical illnesses, domestic violence, and crimes including assaults, robberies, murders, rapes, child sexual abuse, child abuse, etc.). The ruthless destruction of human life caused by hijacked planes used as bombs at the World Trade Center and Pentagon, and the bombing of the Murrah Federal Building in Oklahoma City are examples of unpredictable traumatic emergencies that create untold suffering, leaving the survivors and surviving family members with tremendous grief as they try to rebuild their lives. The time-limited nature of such crises cannot take into account how these events will permanently scar those who are affected.

Existential Crises

An existential crisis takes place when one begins to question the meaning of life or the meaninglessness of one's existence, the lack of connectedness with other people, or the futility of one's work or profession. This type of crisis is often experienced in the wake of some particular crisis event. For example, in the aftermath of a high school student's suicide, many of her friends began to question the importance and meaning of their own day-to-day existence. The realization that one's life has been inexorably altered in profound ways by certain choices made or choices that were never available can induce a personal crisis in many individuals. This was best illustrated in the film *It's a Wonderful Life* when George Bailey experiences an existential crisis that brings him to the brink of suicide upon the realization that his lot in life cannot be changed.

Existential crises are probably the most difficult to identify because, as with developmental crises, the person experiencing this type of crisis may present with other complaints or symptoms. It is only once the crisis intervention counselor begins to scratch the surface of the presenting complaints that he or she begins to find that the individual's issues go much deeper than being upset over day-to-day hassles or annoyances.

Psychiatric Crises

As with developmental and existential crises, the triggering psychiatric crisis event may not be readily discernible. For example, a person with Bipolar Disorder who stops taking medication will often begin to re-experience the extreme mood fluctuations that represent the highs of the manic state or the lows of the depression that usually follows. This information may not be reliably conveyed to the crisis worker. Or a person with a substance use history may unintentionally overdose on painkillers, yet when that person is brought to the emergency room, he or she may appear to be stuporous or sedated and may be unable to provide an accurate account of what pills have been taken. When psychiatric crises take hold of a person, they sometimes may come on without rhyme or reason, they can be very debilitating, and they can send the person into an intense state of crisis. It is important to note that not everyone with a psychiatric condition necessarily experiences crises as part of their illness. However, when those who suffer from psychiatric conditions experience crisis situations or traumatic events, the existing conditions can often add to the feelings of devastation.

It should be noted that it is quite possible for people to experience more than one crisis at the same time. It would be helpful if crises only came along one at a time or at intervals that allowed people to resolve one crisis before having to tackle another. However, this is often not the case. Instead, it is common for people to experience multiple and rather complex crises simultaneously. Such would be the case with a woman whose husband was killed in the World Trade Center who is now faced with major decisions about whether to move, whose 8- and 10-year-old daughters are going through major grief reactions and are now failing in school as a result, whose in-laws are pressuring her to sue the U.S. government rather than accept her portion of the victim compensation funds, and who herself is naturally going through major grief reactions over the loss of her husband. Crises have no timetable, nor do they wait for people to prepare for them.

Crisis Reactions: A Continuum of Response

People who experience any of the aforementioned crises often vary in the way they respond to particular crisis events. As stated in the various definitions of *crisis*, a person in crisis usually does experience extreme upset and disorganization in functioning. One result of this disorganization is increased vulnerability; the normal defenses that may have helped the person cope in the past are no longer effective. Acute crisis reactions are debilitating and can result in extreme levels of perceived psychological distress. However, until some sense of equilibrium has been restored and crises have been constructively resolved, these individuals may feel that they are "going crazy." Many individuals in crisis will experience a fight, flight, or freeze response in the face of an immediate crisis event. The fight or flight response is that programmed, biological response that allows human beings to react in the face of imminent danger by either fighting off the danger (fight) or by fleeing (flight). An adrenalin surge and redirection of blood flow to the large muscles of the legs and arms allow the fight or flight response to occur. However, it is also natural for people to freeze in the face of imminent danger. People who have experienced car accidents will often describe a feeling of being "suspended in time" or "in slow motion" as they watch other cars collide with theirs. The freeze response is also common in rape and sexual assault victims who fear for their lives but are unable to scream, run, or fight. There are also some individuals who will not experience psychological distress in the aftermath of a crisis event. These individuals seem to have the capacity to repress the event and therefore can go about their daily lives as if nothing has happened. The ego defense mechanism of repression first described by Sigmund Freud and later elaborated upon by his daughter, Anna, allows the mind to repress the traumatic event or push it out of conscious awareness.

Individuals will exhibit various symptoms in response to crises they have experienced. *The Diagnostic and Statistical Manual of Mental Disorders,* 4th Edition *(DSM-IV-TR)* (American Psychiatric Association, 2000), presents various diagnoses that may occur in the aftermath of some of the aforementioned crisis events. Many crises will be somewhat resolved within the 6 to 8 week period and the individuals affected will attain some degree of equilibrium. However, there may also be more enduring reactions or responses to crisis events. Although the goal of crisis intervention is not to label people or to pathologize their reactions to traumas or crises, the rendering of a diagnosis does serve the purpose of conveying to other professionals that the victim of a trauma or crisis event is experiencing a particular set of symptoms or sequelae, the identification of which may become important in effectively treating that individual. For example, it is common for victims of sexual assault, such as a rape or molestation, to blame themselves for the incident. "I shouldn't have gone out to the store that night" or "I should have dressed differently" are common statements of self-blame. In the treatment of sexual abuse victims, it is important to help sexual abuse survivors relinquish these self-blaming perceptions. Hence, it is important that the diagnosis convey to other professionals some similar issues that people suffering from the same crises or trauma usually face.

The three most common diagnoses given to individuals who experience trauma or crisis events are Posttraumatic Stress Disorder (PTSD), Acute Stress Disorder, and Adjustment Disorders.

Posttraumatic Stress Disorder

As you can see from the criteria and symptoms of Posttraumatic Stress Disorder (PTSD) listed in Table 1.2, it is a rather complex diagnostic entity that encompasses thoughts, feelings, interactions with others, changes in self-concept, and changes in overall daily functioning. Trauma can have tremendous impact on the individual, whether it be the combat veteran, the rape victim, the domestic violence victim, the car accident victim, or the person who witnesses violence. A diagnosis of PTSD also lends itself more readily to *traumatic event crises,* as described in Table 1.2. Criteria A specifies that the individual must have experienced or witnessed a traumatic event in order to qualify for this diagnosis. Those who *witnessed* the horrifying scene of hijacked planes crashing into the

TABLE 1.2
Symptoms of Posttraumatic Stress Disorder

A. The person must have been exposed to a traumatic event in which both of the following are present:
1) The person experienced, witnessed or was confronted with an event or events that involved actual or threatened death or serious injury, or a threat to the physical integrity of self or others.
2) The person's response involved intense fear, helplessness, or horror. **Note:** In children, this may be expressed instead by disorganized or agitated behavior.

B. The traumatic event is persistently re-experienced in one (or more) of the following ways:
1) Recurrent and intrusive distressing recollections of the event, including images, thoughts, or perceptions. **Note:** In young children, repetitive play may occur in which aspects of the trauma are expressed.
2) Recurrent distressing dreams of the event. **Note:** In children, there may be frightening dreams without recognizable content.
3) Acting or feeling as if the traumatic event were recurring (includes a sense of reliving the experience, illusions, hallucinations and dissociative flashback episodes, including those that occur on awakening or when intoxicated). **Note:** In young children, trauma-specific reenactment may occur.
4) Intense psychological distress at exposure to internal or external cues that symbolize or resemble an aspect of the traumatic event.
5) Physiological reactivity on exposure to internal or external cues that symbolize or resemble an aspect of the traumatic event.

C. Persistent avoidance of stimuli associated with the trauma and numbing of general responsiveness (not present before the trauma), as indicated by three (or more) of the following:
1) efforts to avoid thoughts, feelings, or conversations associated with the trauma
2) efforts to avoid activities, places, or people that arouse recollections of the trauma
3) inability to recall an important aspect of the trauma
4) markedly diminished interest or participation in significant activities
5) feeling of detachment or estrangement from others
6) restricted range of affect (e.g. unable to have loving feelings)
7) sense of a foreshortened future (e.g. does not expect to have a career, marriage, children, or a normal life span)

D. Persistent symptoms of increased arousal (not present before the trauma), as indicated by two (or more) of the following:
1) difficulty falling or staying asleep
2) irritability or outbursts of anger
3) difficulty concentrating
4) hypervigilance
5) exaggerated startle response

E. Duration of the disturbance (symptoms in Criteria B, C, D) is more than one month.

(Continues)

TABLE 1.2
Symptoms of Posttraumatic Stress Disorder *(Continued)*

F.   The disturbance causes clinically significant distress or impairment in social, occupational, or other important areas of functioning.
       Specify if:
              Acute: if duration of symptoms is less than 3 months
              Chronic: if duration of symptoms is 3 months or more
              Delayed Onset: if onset of symptoms is at least 6 months after the stressor

Note. From *Desk Reference to the Diagnostic Criteria from DSM-IV-TR* (pp. 218–220), by American Psychiatric Association, 2000, Washington, DC: Author. Reprinted with permission.

World Trade Center experienced PTSD reactions, just as those who had been in the Towers at the time and *experienced* the impact of the crash, but had managed to escape, did.

Acute Stress Disorder

Individuals with acute stress disorder may experience the same severity of symptoms as the person with posttraumatic stress disorder; however, what is unique to this diagnosis is the time frame. Acute stress disorder reactions are reserved for those who experience symptoms within the first month after exposure to the traumatic event. Those who continue to experience symptoms after this time period would be diagnosed with posttraumatic stress disorder. This is why the symptoms listed for both posttraumatic stress disorder and acute stress disorder are similar.

Adjustment Disorder

It is rare that a person going through a developmental or existential crisis would meet the criteria for PTSD. For those individuals, a diagnosis of adjustment disorder would most likely characterize their symptoms. The adjustment disorder diagnosis indicates that a stressor is the catalyst to the symptomatology. These stressors might include a breakup in a relationship, a separation, a divorce, being laid off from one's job, or could emanate from various developmental events, such as going away to school, leaving home, getting married, becoming a parent, failure to attain occupational goals, or retirement. The subtypes also allow for the clinician to determine the predominant response to the stressor, for example is it depression, anxiety, acting out behavior (disturbance of conduct), or a mixed emotional or behavioral state. Again, it is important to note that individuals react quite differently to stressors.

The issue of diagnosis pertaining to crisis intervention is quite controversial. This is true especially among individuals who are victims of domestic violence

TABLE 1.3
Symptoms of Acute Stress Disorder

A. The person has been exposed to a traumatic event in which both the follow-
    ing were present:
    1) the person experienced, witnessed or was confronted with an event or
        events that involved actual or threatened death or serious injury, or a
        threat to the physical integrity of self or others
    2) the person's response involved intense fear, helplessness, or horror
B. Either while experiencing or after experiencing the distressing event, the indi-
    vidual has three (or more) of the following dissociative symptoms:
    1) a subjective sense of numbing, detachment, or absence of emotional
        responsiveness
    2) a reduction in awareness of his or her surroundings (e.g. "being in a
        daze")
    3) derealization
    4) depersonalization
    5) dissociative amnesia (i.e., inability to recall an important aspect of the
        trauma)
C. The traumatic event is persistently reexperienced in at least one of the follow-
    ing ways: recurrent images, thoughts, dreams, illusions, flashback episodes,
    or a sense of reliving the experience; or distress on exposure to reminders of
    the traumatic event.
D. Marked avoidance of stimuli that arouse recollections of the trauma (e.g.,
    thoughts, feelings, conversations, activities, places, people, etc.).
E. Marked symptoms of anxiety or increased arousal (e.g., difficulty sleeping,
    irritability, poor concentration, hypervigilance, exaggerated startle response,
    or motor restlessness).
F. The disturbance causes clinically significant distress or impairment in social,
    occupational, or other important areas of functioning or impairs the individ-
    ual's ability to pursue some necessary task, such as obtaining necessary assis-
    tance or mobilizing personal resources by telling family members about the
    traumatic experience.
G. The disturbance lasts for a minimum of 2 days and a maximum of 4 weeks
    and occurs within 4 weeks of the traumatic event.
H. The disturbance is not due to the direct physiological effects of a substance
    (e.g., a drug of abuse, a medication) or a general medical condition, is not
    better accounted for by Brief Psychotic Disorder and is not merely an exacer-
    bation of a preexisting Axis I or Axis II disorder.

Note. From *Desk Reference to the Diagnostic Criteria from DSM-IV-TR* (pp. 221–222), by
American Psychiatric Association, 2000, Washington, DC: Author. Reprinted with permission.

or rape. Many professionals who work with domestic violence and rape survivors feel that to diagnose these women is to pathologize otherwise normal reactions to horrific situations. The women's movement has made significant inroads
in this area by educating both mental health and medical professionals about the
psychological and emotional impact of victimization. Domestic violence and

TABLE 1.4
Symptoms of Adjustment Disorder

A. The development of emotional or behavioral symptoms in response to an iden-
    tifiable stressor(s) occurring within three months of the onset of the stressor(s).
B. These symptoms or behaviors are clinically significant as evidenced by either
    of the following:
    1) marked distress that is in excess of what would be expected from expo-
        sure to the stressor
    2) significant impairment in social or occupational (academic) functioning
C. The stress-related disturbance does not meet the criteria for another specific
    Axis I disorder and is not merely an exacerbation of a preexisting Axis I or
    Axis II disorder.
D. The symptoms do not represent Bereavement.
E. Once the stressor (or its consequences) has terminated, the symptoms do not
    persist for more than an additional 6 months.

> Specify if:
>
> **Acute:** the disturbance lasts less than 6 months
>
> **Chronic:** the disturbance lasts for 6 months or longer. By definition,
> symptoms cannot persist for more than 6 months after the termination of
> the stressor or its consequences. The Chronic specifier therefore applies
> when the duration of the disturbance is longer than 6 months in response
> to a chronic stressor or to a stressor that has enduring consequences.
>
> **Subtypes:**
>
> with Depressed Mood
> with Anxiety
> with Mixed Anxiety and Depressed Mood
> with Disturbance of Conduct
> with Mixed Disturbance of Emotions and Conduct
> Unspecified

Note. From *Desk Reference to the Diagnostic Criteria from DSM-IV-TR* (pp. 285–286), by
American Psychiatric Association, 2000, Washington, DC: Author. Reprinted with permission.

rape survivors may share similar symptoms with Vietnam veterans, and have
experienced similar misdiagnoses as well. They have been blamed for their reactions, been misdiagnosed with depression, or their symptoms have been blamed
on preexisting conditions or weak character. The question then arises, "Why
diagnose at all?" As indicated earlier, a diagnosis allows professionals to communicate information about an individual without developing an endless list of
potential symptoms. Diagnoses may also help survivors understand that what
they are experiencing is to be expected given the traumatic events. For example,
a rape survivor who is experiencing emotional numbing or is unable to recall
specific events of the rape may understand that this is a normal PTSD reaction to
rape trauma. This may also help significant others in her life understand that the
emotional numbing is part of the PTSD reaction and not indicative of indifference

to the traumatic event. On a practical level, a diagnosis also allows survivors of trauma to utilize their medical insurance benefits, should they decide to seek professional counseling.

Multicultural Awareness and Crisis Intervention

Whether you are a professional crisis counselor or the first police officer to arrive at the scene of a crisis event, it is of utmost importance to consider cultural, ethnic, and religious background when assessing and interpreting an individual's response to a crisis. Take for example, a person who states in a crisis interview, "I am possessed by evil spirits." At first glance, and without any prior knowledge of this individual's cultural background, the crisis counselor may begin to think that this person is suffering from some type of profound psychiatric disorder. However, what if this individual is of Native American ancestry, with a cultural heritage that is rich with tales of spirit influence? Arthur Kleinman (1991) has done extensive research into multicultural aspects of psychiatric disorders. He points to the example of a Native American from one of the Plains nations for whom hearing the voice of a deceased relative from the afterworld might be considered a normal experience. Yet if a non-Native American were to hear such "voices," he or she might be considered psychotic.

Awareness of Cultural Diversity

It is also important to understand that there is often a great deal of diversity within a particular racial group, culture, or ethnicity. For example, Spanish-speaking individuals may prefer to be called Mexican Americans, Spanish Americans, Cuban Americans, Puerto Rican Americans, Hispanics, or Latinos, depending on their country of origin. Similarly, there are some who prefer the term Black rather than African American, because these individuals may not identify with their African heritage. Native Americans represent a very diverse population composed of 554 federally recognized tribes or nations and Alaskan native villages, each with separate social organization, rituals, customs, and language. It is important for counselors to be aware of these differences and to be careful to avoid assuming that people of a particular racial, ethnic, or religious group necessarily identify with a particular cultural heritage.

Religious beliefs and culture may also influence how a particular crisis is defined or how it evolves. Examples of this are found with suicide rates. In predominantly Catholic and Muslim countries, suicide rates are lower, presumably because those religions view suicide as sinful. In Western, industrialized countries, suicide rates are higher. In Japan, suicide may be viewed as an "honorable" solution to having dishonored one's family. Kamikaze pilots during World War II considered it an honor to die for one's country. The following excerpt helps to illustrate cultural influences:

A young Japanese woman living in Los Angeles was distraught over dis-
covering that her husband was having an affair. She had no work skills,
spoke no English, and felt worthless and helpless. She became increasingly
depressed and dysfunctional. One spring day, she took her infant and four-
year-old to the beach, bought lunch, and then walked into the ocean with
the children to commit family suicide. Passersby witnessed the act and were
able to summon help. The woman survived, but both children drowned.
Although she was jailed and accused of murder, the Japanese American
community, sympathetic to her effort to resolve her dilemma through the
suicide that included her children, rallied to her support. They argued that
in traditional Japanese communities, the family is the unit, not the individual, and they called it Japanese suicide, not American murder. (Group for
the Advancement of Psychiatry, 1989)

Multicultural considerations need to be taken into account especially when
providing crisis intervention services. For example, Marilyn Aguirre-Molina
(Aguirre-Molina & Molina, 1994) describes how a counselor not familiar with
Hispanic culture can offend the head of a traditional Hispanic family, often the
father, by not asking for permission to see the identified patient, for example,
the son or daughter. By demonstrating *respecto* (respect) to elders and persons
of authority, one is being culturally sensitive to an important Hispanic value-
the importance of showing deference and obedience to elders and those in
authority (Marin & Marin, 1991). Similarly, a crisis counselor working with an
African American family must be aware of the important role of spirituality for
many in that community. Strong spiritual belief is thought to have sustained
African Americans through the horrors of slavery and racism (Robinson, Perry,
& Carey, 1995). For the counselor working with an Asian American individual
or family, awareness of the importance of the family as the unit of social and
cultural activities is important (Dana, 1993). The counselor should also be
aware that in many of the diverse Asian cultures, to look someone directly in
the eye is considered a sign of disrespect. To look away, so as to not "stare the
person down," is considered a sign of deference. Crisis counselors unaware of
this custom may misinterpret this behavior as being disrespectful, instead of as
a sign of respect.

Cultural Competence

It is important therefore, that all counselors develop a degree of *cultural competence.* According to Castro, Proescholdbell, Abeita, and Rodriquez (1999),
cultural competence refers to, "the capacity of a service provider or an organization to understand and work effectively with the cultural beliefs and practices of persons from a given ethnic/racial group" (p. 504). They concluded
that cultural competence is of utmost importance in delivering effective mental health and human services to diverse special populations. When counselors
or agencies fail to acknowledge and appreciate the important differences in
values, beliefs, and rituals, individuals from diverse populations may feel

skeptical, misunderstood, and untrusting that these counselors or agencies will be able to meet their needs (Castro, et al., 1999). Several authors have conceptualized a continuum of ability to work with members of diverse populations (Cross, Bazron, Dennis, & Isaacs, 1989; Kim, McLeod, & Shantzis, 1992; Castro, et al., 1999). At the far end of this continuum is *cultural destructiveness,* which can be defined as counselors or agencies manifesting negative attitudes towards diverse populations or considering them to be inferior to the mainstream, dominant culture. The next step along the continuum is one of *cultural blindness,* a philosophy that advocates that all people are alike and therefore should be treated equally. However, the problem with this service delivery approach is that it fails to account for cultural differences, which must be considered when helping people effectively resolve their crises. The next step along the continuum is *cultural sensitivity,* which indicates that the counselor or agency is open to acknowledging and working with issues of multicultural diversity. The next stage is *cultural competence,* which was defined earlier, followed by *cultural proficiency,* the highest level of cultural capacity, here defined as the counselor's ability to understand the nuances of cultural diversity in greater depth and to implement new and more effective service delivery approaches based upon the appreciation and understanding of these differences.

For the crisis counselor, the first step towards cultural competence and hopefully towards cultural proficiency is to avoid assuming that everyone views events and issues from the perspective of your value or belief systems. This behavior is termed *ethnocentrism,* which is the belief is that all cultures function in the same way that one's own culture does, the cultural equivalent of egocentrism. Therefore, when in doubt about particular customs, rituals, values, or belief systems, it is better to ask than to assume.

SOURCES OF CHAPTER ENRICHMENT

Print Sources

Caplan, G. (1961). *An approach to community mental health.* New York: Grune & Stratton.

Caplan, G. (1964). *Principles of preventative psychiatry.* New York: Basic Books.

Dana, R. H. (1993). *Multicultural assessment perspectives for professional psychology.* Boston: Allyn & Bacon.

Erikson, E. (1963). *Childhood and society* (2nd ed.). New York: Norton Press.

Gilliland, B. E. & James, R. K. (1997). *Crisis intervention strategies.* (3rd ed.). Pacific Grove, CA: Brooks/Cole.

Levinson, D. J. (1978). *The seasons of a man's life.* New York: Alfred A. Knopf.

Slaikeu, K. A. (1990). *Crisis intervention: A handbook for practice and research* (2nd ed.). Boston: Allyn & Bacon.

Internet Sources

Crisis: The Journal of Crisis Intervention & Suicide Prevention (http://www.hhpub .com/journals/crisis) This is a journal devoted exclusively to crisis intervention and provides an excellent example of how crisis intervention has come to be accepted as a specialized field within the human services professions.

Brief Treatment and Crisis Intervention (http://www.brief-treatment.oupjournals .org) This is also a professional journal devoted exclusively to crisis intervention and brief treatment. The journal provides up-to-date research and clinical recommendations for managing a variety of crisis situations.

Trauma Response (http://www.aaets.org) This is the journal of the American Academy of Experts in Traumatic Stress. Both the journal and the AAETS provide excellent, up-to-date information within the field of crisis intervention and traumatic stress response. The AAETS also provides specialized certifications for qualified professionals.

Journal of Traumatic Stress (http://www.wkap.nl/journalhome.htm) This is the official journal of the International Society for Traumatic Stress Studies. The journal contains excellent, up-to-date information on various empirical studies dealing with trauma resulting from domestic violence, rape, sexual assault, combat, work-related trauma, and natural disasters.

CHAPTER 2

Crisis Intervention Skills

David was a 35-year-old probation officer who was attending graduate school in the evening for a degree in counseling. He prided himself on setting and achieving goals, particularly in the area of education, as he was the first member of his immigrant family to go to college. He also kept himself in good physical condition, working out regularly at the local health club and jogging on the boardwalk along the beachfront, usually in the evening hours after work. One night while jogging, he was accosted by two young men, one of whom brandished a gun and ordered him off the boardwalk and onto a secluded part of the beach. There they threatened to kill him when they discovered that he only carried a few dollars with him when he jogged. They held the gun to his head and warned him not to leave the beach until after they were gone. David left the beach area at dawn, about 6 hours later, and returned to his apartment where he remained for the next week. A friend and coworker only learned of the attack when he called David to check on the reason for his fifth consecutive sick-day. Such absences were very atypical for David.

*I*n entertainment and media, the resolution of a crisis is usually portrayed as a rather simple affair. Consider, for example, ancient Greek and Roman trage-dians. In order to avert the demise of a protagonist in the throes of crisis, they often lowered onto the stage via a primitive mechanical crane a device intended to whisk the actor away to safety. This technique, the *deus ex machina* ("god from the machine"), typically represented the direct intervention of one of the gods. Hollywood also uses this device. The cavalry usually arrives just in time to rescue the film hero from an untimely and bloody death at the hands of the enemy. And more often than not, the fans' favorite television character usually survives the crisis of the season-ending cliffhanger to return the next year for another go at it.

Would that all crises were so easily managed, so readily dispatched!

However, without benefit of a stage prop or a screenwriter's pen, it is up to crisis workers to bring order out of the chaos of real life crises using only their training, ingenuity, and clear-headedness. In crises of all types, workers are required to help victims return to some semblance of the lives they enjoyed prior to crises. Crisis counseling requires a different set of skills than those learned in an introductory counseling course in an undergraduate program. In non-crisis counseling, clients tend to seek out treatment to resolve self-defeating patterns of behavior, to understand what lurks in the dark corners of the mind, or to comply with the urging of a spouse, supervisor, teacher, or attorney.

Crises, however, are random and unpredictable. They require more inner resources than victims can successfully muster at the time, pushing victims, reeling in the midst of chaos, to seek comfort and support. The victims are unwitting and unsuspecting participants, swept up in a rush of events not usually of their choosing, requiring them to depend on crisis counselors.

Therefore, crisis intervention techniques must match the needs of the victims. These techniques are not therapy, although they are therapeutic; they are short in duration and are designed to bring victims to a state of semi-equilibrium in the immediate aftermath of a crisis. Achieving real healing after a crisis requires therapy beyond that which the crisis counselor can provide.

The purpose of this chapter is to outline the techniques that are critical to the assessment of victims in crisis and to the intervention required to bring them to a sense of equilibrium. Group crisis intervention skills in the form of critical incident stress management is discussed in chapter 10, so the present discussion will focus on only those crisis intervention skills used when counseling a single crisis victim. This chapter will address these particular issues in four parts: physical, emotional, and cognitive responses to crisis; characteristics of effective crisis intervention; characteristics of effective crisis counselors; and effective intervention techniques. The chapter will conclude with a description of a new model of crisis intervention, the LAPC model (listen, assess, plan, commit).

Responses to Crisis

Since crisis is, by nature, a time-limited phenomenon, some victims will recover from the crisis state without the aid of outside intervention. Caplan (1964) considered the duration of a typical crisis state to be 4 to 6 weeks, although there has been some confusion regarding this timeline (Roberts, 2000). Other studies suggested that acute symptoms of stress in the majority of people exposed to severe trauma tend to subside within 3 months, and only 25% of victims eventually develop stress disorders (*New York Times*, 2001). Crisis victims are most willing to accept help during this period (Golan, 1978), and the appropriate intervention will help them emerge from it functioning at higher adaptive levels (Kanel, 1999).

Myriad factors influence crisis recovery, including the pre-crisis level of functioning, the type and intensity of the crisis encountered, and the availability of a support system. For example, the individual with a pre-existing anxiety disorder who never managed transition or change well will be at far greater risk after a crisis event than the resilient individual who has always accepted change. Similarly, the ascetic loner without a family or social group will have to cope with the crisis alone, while the victim who is surrounded by a large extended family will have access to much-needed support. Understanding the reactions of the victims of crisis enables counselors to provide appropriate interventions to meet the needs of individual victims.

Biological systems theory proposed that the rules of complementarity apply to the functioning of the living organism. That is, maintaining a steady state of functioning, a balance known as homeostasis, is one of the functions of the central nervous system; the individual is aroused to action when such action is called for and then returns to a state of equilibrium when the arousal period passes. The driver who has to activate his own emergency response system in order to swerve suddenly to avoid hitting a deer in the road will calm down before his trip is over. The tourist who must remain on alert to negotiate unknown city streets will return to a steady state once she completes her tour.

Individuals also contribute to the maintenance of their own reassuring states of equilibrium. They develop routines; cultivate templates through which they view themselves and the world; establish specific rules of order for cause-and-effect, justice, and fairness; and draw on resources from their support systems to help sustain them. Changing any one of these elements would be a source of stress for most people. However, when a sudden, random event (crisis) occurs, its victims experience a complete disruption of these established requisites for equilibrium. Crisis dislodges people from their comfort zones and makes it difficult for them to restore their balance. Senseless events throw individuals into the maelstrom, leaving them to tread water until exhaustion sets in and, it is hoped, help arrives.

According to Roberts (2000), there is a general consensus among many mental health professionals regarding the characteristics of a person in crisis. They include the following:

- perceives an event as being meaningful and threatening;
- appears unable to modify or lessen the impact of a stressful event with traditional coping methods;
- experiences increased fear, tension, and/or confusion;
- exhibits a high level of subjective discomfort; and
- proceeds rapidly to an active state of crisis—a state of disequilibrium.

The Physical Response

The physical response to crisis is one which has significant survival value for the individual. It is the same response experienced by the earliest members of humankind who had to spring to action to either run from or ward off potential predators and other impending disasters. This fight or flight reaction is the mobilization of the individual's defenses in times of threat, the body's internal device that enables it to survive another day.

When a crisis occurs, this reaction enables individuals to ready themselves for a response. Crisis victims go on alert status: pupils dilate, heart rate and blood pressure increase, digestion is inhibited, and adrenalin is secreted. The "call to arms" that the stressor sounds for the individual enables the utilization of familiar coping strategies to address the source of the stress. However, the more common stressors that lead to the mobilization of the body's defense system tend to pale in comparison to the types of crises discussed in this book. Crisis presumes a traumatic event alien to the victim, one that is beyond the range of typical experiences. Thus, the lack of familiarity with the crisis event prevents the individual from successfully employing the usual coping strategies.

The Emotional Response

Despite the state of physical arousal, victims of crisis often experience a state of frozen fright (Young, 2001), a state of shock, disorientation, and numbness. Victims are left with only the sensation that something is terribly wrong and without an understanding of the event itself or of its impact. They may suffer a psychological paralysis, an inability to react at all, for example, a parent who returns to sleep after a 3 a.m. phone call informing him of the death of his teenage son in a car accident. Roberts (2000) described the crisis victim as being anxious, confused, and helpless, as well as appearing to be disorganized, withdrawn, and apathetic. Finally, since the level of physical arousal cannot be sustained indefinitely, the individual eventually will collapse with exhaustion. Whether this exhaustion is manifested as sleep or unconsciousness, the response will serve as a break with the traumatic event (Young, 2001). The crisis victim also will experience profound sadness and grief, depending upon the level of involvement with the crisis, and will vacillate between irritability and anger, between self-blame and blaming others.

The Cognitive Response

Whereas crisis counselors can observe the physical and emotional aftermath of a crisis event, victims' belief systems, which are also shattered, are hidden from the naked eye. The standard rules of order have been violated, and the victims' understanding of how they fit into society may be forever altered (Berglas, 1985). Crisis contradicts their views about themselves and their safety in the world, particularly for crime victims. Additionally, in order to bolster their beliefs in a just world in which bad things only happen to bad people, they change their belief systems regarding the roles they played in the crisis events.

For example, if David (see the introductory case) attributed the cause of his mugging to an isolated mistake of jogging alone late at night, he might emerge from the event with some resolve, believing that he could avoid future muggings by jogging earlier in the day or in better-lit surroundings. However, if he assigned the cause of the event to a more generalized sense of personal failure or to outside events that he believed he could not control, he would recover slowly from the experience, unable to regain an expectation of safety or to trust in his own competence to provide for his safety.

Similarly, a woman's appraisal of a physical assault by her husband will, among other factors, affect how she recovers from it. Consider the following case of Gail:

> Gail was a 32-year-old woman who had been married for 3 years to Steve; both were successful business people, earning six-figure salaries each. Gail's career was on the rise due to the good fortune of her company, which she joined in its infancy, while Steve's career had stalled. In fact, it seemed that he would be a casualty of the impending downsizing of his company. Although nothing was definite in this regard, Steve assumed that the end was near. Gail, concerned about her brooding, preoccupied husband, did her best to cheer him up. One night as they were getting ready to attend a dinner party with some friends, Gail suggested that Steve wear a different color shirt than the one he had chosen. At that point, Steve stormed toward her, striking her across the face and knocking her to the floor. He stood over her and warned her not to tell him what to do again.

Will Gail blame herself for being too "bossy" by telling Steve what to wear and, therefore, blame herself and assume responsibility for the abuse? Will she consider Steve's quick temper to be indicative of his despair and resulting poor judgment in managing his own frustrations, thereby freeing herself from recriminations over the incident? The crisis counselor eventually must be able to find the answers to these types of questions to effectively intervene.

Characteristics of Effective Crisis Intervention

When Medea was rescued from the hands of a fast-approaching, vengeful Jason by a serpent-driven flying chariot (the *deus ex machina*), her crisis was avoided, and she lived to go on to other adventures. Although a neat and tidy ending, this resolution of crisis is as far removed from contemporary crisis intervention as the Greek theater is from the contemporary Broadway stage.

Crisis intervention is not about "rescue." More often than not, rescue benefits the rescuer more than the victim; rescuers make the mistake of maintaining control over the victim when control should be placed in the hands of the individual in crisis. Crisis intervention is about the foundation of the Chinese symbol for crisis: danger and opportunity.

Understanding the notion of opportunity in crisis is critical to effective crisis intervention. The crisis event drives the individual to seek help, just as hunger drives the search for food, thirst for water, and loneliness for greater connectedness with others. The search for help presents an *opportunity* to acquire more effective problem-solving skills, greater self-awareness and fulfillment, and more positive feelings of competence and self-efficacy. Effective crisis intervention should empower the individual to rise from the devastation and to resume control of daily life with a regained sense of hopefulness. In order to be effective, therefore, crisis intervention must be both empowerment-focused and flexible.

Empowerment-Focused Crisis Intervention

Young (2001) suggested that the primary goal of crisis intervention is to help victims restore control in their lives. Crisis intervention literature also presents the goal of crisis intervention to be the restoration of functioning of the individual to the level enjoyed prior to the crisis event itself. However, Fraser (1998) suggested that a counselor intervening in a crisis should assist the victim in striving for something more, and he maintained that crisis should be an opportunity to help people grow beyond their previous levels of functioning to higher, more competent levels.

In order to accomplish this latter goal, it is important for those involved in effective crisis intervention to approach a crisis event viewing victims in two ways: as *resilient* individuals and as *resourceful* individuals. Walsh (1998) refers to *resilience* as a person's ability not only to cope with and to survive traumatic experiences but also to continue to move toward greater psychological growth. Resilient people are able to draw upon their internal and external resources and to recover from adversity, perhaps stronger than before. They are not easily defeated, and they are able to integrate their crisis experiences into their belief system and learn from them. Seligman's (1990) version of resilience is based upon his notion of "learned optimism." In his model, optimistic/resilient people are able to bounce back from adversity quickly and do not hesitate to undertake other challenging, novel tasks or experiences. Consider the case of Jessie:

Jessie, a 13-year-old seventh-grader in middle school, had become lethargic in class and her performance in school had declined. One of her classroom teachers had become concerned, as Jessie was generally an outgoing, cheerful young adolescent with a wide circle of friends. The social worker who was asked to intervene with Jessie was able to uncover her secret. Although the school was aware of the car accident in which Jessie's parents had been involved a few months before, the staff did not comprehend the full impact of this event. Jessie's mother had lost a limb in the accident and suffered considerable facial scarring. Upon discharge from the hospital, she took to her bed, refusing to show herself outside the home, lest people see her disfigurement. Jessie, as a result, assumed a domestic role and undertook all household tasks: shopping, cooking, cleaning, and seeing to the general welfare of her younger brothers. She reported having no time for after-school tutorial assistance, nor for socializing with her friends. Her father became less and less available to her, as her mother believed she had lost all physical appeal and repeatedly told him to go and meet somebody else. He began to spend more and more time outside the home.

Effective crisis intervention would include viewing Jessie as a resilient individual, as she was assisting her family by assuming a new role in the family system after the car accident. Although the new role was a self-defeating one for her, it also indicated that she was able to adapt to changing circumstances; for this reason, an empowerment-focused crisis counselor would see Jessie as resilient, even prior to the intervention. This same counselor would also view David and Gail as resilient, and she would initiate intervention with the expectation that these people would emerge from their respective crises and acquire greater feelings of competence in the process.

Resourceful individuals have a variety of tools for extricating themselves from difficult situations. In effective crisis intervention, belief in the resourcefulness of the victim is essential to good practice. Counselors who entertain the rescue fantasy cannot provide effective intervention, because they believe the source of the solution lies in their hands, rather than in the hands of crisis victims. For example, the assumption that Gail will forever be stymied by her assaultive husband and that she needs a solution handed to her prevents effective crisis intervention and makes only the rescue possible. Additionally, telling Jessie and David how to exit their crises achieves little more than a short-term reprieve.

Flexible Crisis Intervention

Although in the field of geometry it may be true that the shortest distance between two points is a straight line, such a simplistic, linear view has no place in the exploration of the complexities of human behavior. A direct cause and effect analysis of the aforementioned cases might indicate that the car accident that disfigured her mother caused Jessie's depression, that the mugging incident caused David's absences from work, and that Gail's request that her husband change his attire caused the assault. Although each of these triggers had some bearing on the outcome of the crises, they were only a part of the much larger picture. Assuming a direct cause-and-effect relationship might lead a counselor to draw the conclusion that all individuals who experienced similar events would respond in similar, if not identical, ways. However, in effective crisis intervention, flexibility is essential, requiring the counselor to make a quick evaluation of the multiplicity of factors that may have influenced the reaction of the victim.

Flexibility in crisis intervention requires that counselors ask questions similar to the following:

- "What was it about Jessie and her total milieu, including all factors both internal and external to her, that resulted in her reaction to the crash?"
- "Why would David react to the mugging in the way that he did?"
- "What was it about a simple request for a clothing change that would cause Steve to assault Gail?"

COGNITIVE FACTORS   Cognitive behavior-oriented clinicians have long appreciated the role that one's cognitions play in one's emotional experiences. Between any event and the individual's emotional reaction to that event comes a cognitive mediation of the event. That is, people experience and evaluate a situation or event before assigning it meaning. Thus, as people appraise the same events in different ways, their emotional and behavioral reactions to these identical events may be drastically different. For example, in similar circumstances to Jessie's, a 10-year-old may have reacted to the crash by running away. A victim of a similar mugging to David's may have gone to work the next day to be around familiar friends and surroundings. A husband other than Steve may have reacted to Gail's request in a very benign way.

ECOLOGICAL FACTORS   Flexible crisis intervention, however, requires more than just an appreciation of the different ways in which people cognitively mediate crisis events. Crises play havoc, not only with internal (i.e., cognitions, emotions, self-efficacy beliefs, etc.) and external resources (i.e., family, friends, coworkers, etc.) of affected individuals, but also with the larger ecological systems (i.e., community, school, place of worship, etc.) (James & Gilliland, 2001). Conversely, the surrounding interdependent system within which one lives, works, and plays impacts the individual as well. For example, consider the following case of a family affected by a nationwide economic downturn that resulted in the layoffs of thousands of employees:

> Bill Bland received his pink slip after 22 years with the company. He still asserted, however, that his wife of 20 years would never have to work as long as there were children in the home; they still had two teenage sons at home. After 3 months of dwindling financial resources and a mortgage to pay with no employment possibilities, Bill started drinking heavily. His wife took a job at a local business, as much to get away from Bill's increasingly abusive behavior as to earn an income. Meanwhile, his 16-year-old son took part-time employment as well, but the night hours eventually affected his schoolwork. His relationship with his parents became quite contentious, as they fought over his failing grades. The situation reached crisis proportions when Bill, drunk again by mid-day, struck and killed an elderly woman while driving to his son's high school for a conference with the vice principal. His wife called the local crisis center when she received the call from the police.

This case illustrates the interplay between an individual and the circumstances in which he lives. The individual factors exert reciprocal influences on each other: a poor economy leads to unemployment which leads to family dysfunction which leads to the additional crisis of the woman's death. This is a system of complex interacting parts, each of which affects the others.

Bronfenbrenner (1979) articulated the complexity of the systems that are relevant to the coping behavior of individuals:

- *Microsystem*—consists of family members and the individual's immediate social group (i.e., Bill's wife, sons, and friends)
- *Exosystem*—contains the community at large, including neighborhood social networks, work-related structures, and governmental agencies (i.e., Bill's workplace, his son's school, etc.)
- *Macrosystem*—represents the largest environment that influences and, in turn, is influenced by the individual; this level includes the individual's culture and belief system, which impacts the person, his/her family, and the community as well (i.e., the economic conditions that affect Bill's income, the belief that wives should stay home and be supported by the husband, etc.)

Counselors must practice flexible crisis intervention by following the precept that no crisis takes place in a vacuum. Crisis responses cannot be understood without appreciating victims' family and social milieus, community resources, and cultural backdrops (Slaikeu, 1990), as well as the manner in which individuals, these various systems, and the environment interact with each other. To be cognizant of these multiple influences is to create a template that will guide the crisis counselor's view of the individual's response to crisis in a meaningful way.

Characteristics of Effective Crisis Counselors

Perhaps the following metaphor can best describe the role of the effective crisis counselor and the nature of crisis work:

> *Maritime Jack, the owner and captain of a 30-foot schooner, the Random Sea, awakened below deck one night to the heaving and thrashing of his ship by an unanticipated squall. Stumbling to the deck in the hopes of determining what had happened, all that was clear to Jack was that his ship had been blown far from the course he had set for his original destination; everything else was shrouded in the darkness of the night and the turbulence of the sea.*
>
> *Once on deck, Jack scurried about tending sails, checking gauges and compasses, and assessing damage to the ship's instruments in an attempt to minimize further damage and to right his course. After a seemingly unending struggle to steady the ship, Jack finally was able to do so, leaving him to ponder other more salient issues.*
>
> *He wondered to himself where his next port of call should be, where he must steer the ship for repairs and supplies. "Surely," he thought, "It may not be possible to return to the port that I left some time ago, and I may not have the necessary supplies to continue to my intended destination." It was at that time that Jack noticed in the horizon a sole beacon of light, beaming as if reassuring him that there was a harbor in which he could set anchor. Being mindful of this light throughout the rest of the storm enabled Jack to set his course accordingly. Jack then was able to put*

in at this port, one neither too distant from where he had originally embarked, nor quite the same. A safe place, nevertheless, for Jack to anchor the Random Sea for a brief respite before he set sail again.

This metaphor epitomizes the nature of crisis and crisis work: an unanticipated event disrupts the intended course of events, leaving the victim in rough waters. Throughout the course of the intervention, the victim remains captain of the ship. The role of the crisis worker is to provide the beacon of light that guides the ship to calmer waters. Were it not for the storm, Jack would not have learned to chart his course as he did, and were it not for the light, his destination would have remained unclear. Even though the beacon was not able to lead Jack back to his home port, it did beckon him to a safe place where he could drop anchor and take on those supplies that would enable him to set sail again. Those personal characteristics and professional abilities that make for an effective counselor in a more typical therapeutic setting also are essential for the crisis counselor. However, given the intensity level of crisis events, other traits are necessary as well.

TOLERANCE FOR AMBIGUITY   When chaos reigns, crisis counselors must be able to enter poorly-defined, high stress environments and wade through the morass of high emotions to conduct their work. Without a complete understanding of an event and the victim's involvement in it, the counselor must wait to hear from the victim about the experience. The counselor also must avoid the projection of a personal belief system onto the victim's experience. The crisis worker's ability to distinguish personal thoughts or feelings about the event from the actual feelings or thoughts of the victim is a critical component to crisis work. The meaning assigned to such an ambiguous event should be established by the victim rather than the counselor.

A CALM, NEUTRAL DEMEANOR   The crisis counselor must be able to maintain a calm, reassuring demeanor throughout the initial crisis session. Without this ability, the counselor would be swept away by the waves of emotion. The counselor's calm reserve in the face of the client's strong feelings will communicate to the client that it is safe to express strong emotions without overpowering or frightening the counselor. Additionally, the counselor can serve as a model of strength and serenity for the client to emulate in the face of the crisis.

TENACITY   Crisis sufferers may rebuff the best intentions of even a well-trained counselor, as recovery may be far more difficult for some than others. It may be only determination and tenacity that enable a counselor to withstand a client's intransigence, to hang in there, and to persist through the crisis until a resolution is reached.

OPTIMISM   For effective crisis intervention, the counselor must believe that people are resilient and resourceful creatures, capable of recovering from horrific events and perhaps emerging stronger than before. Otherwise, the counselor would have difficulty developing an action plan, with confidence in its success, for the client.

ADVENTURESOMENESS   Crisis work is not for the faint-hearted, but rather for the adventurous spirit. The unpredictable nature of crisis, the sense of never knowing what to expect, and the frenetic pace all necessitate this quality in a crisis counselor. If one's preferences are for a quiet sail around the local pond, then it might be a good idea to avoid rafting trips down the Colorado River during the Spring thaw. Similarly, if one is not prepared for dealing with raw emotion and uncertainty, then crisis intervention work may be something to avoid.

CAPACITY FOR EMPATHY   In addition to employing techniques learned in undergraduate or graduate schools for demonstrating empathy to a client, the crisis counselor should exhibit a capacity for openness to others, the ability to experience the world from another's point of view. Training may provide the counselor with the techniques, but only the ability and willingness to be open separates effective crisis workers from the ineffective.

FLEXIBILITY   As client needs and crisis demands shift and change over time, counselors must adapt to these changes and be flexible enough to adjust the course of the intervention.

CONFIDENCE   For crisis counselors, knowledge of oneself and a strong belief in one's ability and efficacy are critical ingredients for success. Being strong and steady in the chaos of crisis will help the counselor weather the vagaries of crisis events. Similarly, knowing oneself and understanding one's relationship to the client will help the counselor maintain realistic expectations for the intervention and maintain the client's confidence in the intervention.

LITTLE NEED TO RESCUE   Counselors who entertain a rescue fantasy invite troubles of over-involvement with clients and tend to assume ownership of clients' problems. Rescuers also tend to become involved in crisis work more for their own self-aggrandizement than for the benefit of crisis sufferers. The absence of this fantasy makes for greater clarity and objectivity in crisis work.

CAPACITY FOR LISTENING   The crisis counselor must be able to demonstrate effective listening skills. The counselor with a capacity for listening knows

- when to be passive and let the client lead the way;
- when to be active, gathering information and moving toward resolution; and
- when to seek information without being intrusive and interfering with the process.

AWARENESS OF TRAUMA INDICATORS   The counselor must be prepared to make decisions based upon observations of the client's response to crisis. Are there critical safety issues that should be addressed? Medical concerns? The counselor should be prepared to make a judgment regarding the client's response to the event by observing as well as listening.

OPENNESS TO INDIVIDUAL CRISIS REACTIONS   Individuals react differently to the same crisis event. They each bring to the experience a legacy of family relationships, learning histories, unmet and satisfied needs, and unique modes of perceiving and responding to the world. The effective crisis counselor will not approach the intervention with any preconceived notions about how the client *should* react to crisis. Rather, the counselor will come to understand individual clients by listening to their expressions of the crisis experience.

CAPACITY FOR INFORMATION MANAGEMENT   When counselors receive a flood of information, they must be able to sort through it and develop analyses pertinent to action plans. Information will appear contradictory at times, but the role of the counselor is to organize and process it.

Empathy, Genuineness, and Acceptance and Positive Regard

The work of other theorists, primarily Carkhuff (1969), Carkhuff and Berenson (1977), and Rogers (1951), actually sets the framework for the following section. Their research, as well as others', has been focused on the importance of the core conditions of empathy, respect, genuineness, and positive regard in establishing beneficial relationships and in attaining positive counseling outcomes. Individual approaches to counseling notwithstanding, these researchers have demonstrated that the presence of an empathic, involved, and genuine counselor is critical to a successful counseling relationship.

EMPATHY   Empathy is the message that counselors relay to crisis victims, indicating that they not only understand what happened but also how victims feel about it (Slaikeu, 1984, 1990). Empathy involves sharing of the victims' pain and letting them know that the counselor truly understands what it feels like to be in their situation. Counselors must be able to "walk a mile in their shoes" and to communicate this ability to victims. To understand the essential feelings and beliefs that clients express, and to be able to communicate that understanding, is the core of empathy (Carkhuff, 1969; Gladding, 1999).

There is a caveat regarding the development of empathy in crisis work, however: counselors must maintain a delicate balance between empathy and over-involvement with victims (Myer, 2001). That is, the counselor must strike a compromise in the almost dichotomous relationship between involvement and detachment in crisis work: *to feel as* the victim rather than *to be* the victim, to have a *subjective* understanding of the victim's feeling state without the *objective* experience of it. Over-involvement breeds dependence on the coun-selor and, conversely, clouds the judgment and problem-solving abilities of the counselor, who may become lost in the victims' pain.

GENUINENESS   The essence of genuineness is honesty (James & Gilliland, 2001): honesty with oneself, honesty with others. This quality is essential in any intimate interpersonal encounter, but is a particular prerequisite for the crisis counseling relationship. The genuine, honest crisis counselor is comfortable with a range of client emotions and is not threatened by them, is confident in the role of helper without having to hawk professional degrees as proof of expertise, and is not averse to self-disclosing personal information when appro-priate. The client sees honesty, consistency, and reliability in the genuine coun-selor. Although this quality has been discussed in an earlier section of this chapter as a characteristic of an effective crisis counselor, the purpose of the sec-tion to follow is to provide specific strategies for communicating genuineness to the crisis victim.

ACCEPTANCE AND POSITIVE REGARD   When the crisis counselor feels and communicates an unconditional positive regard for the client, the client will feel accepted and will move toward resolution of the crisis event. The counselor accepts all clients, regardless of differences in race, ethnicity, class, gender, size, or shape. The counselor sees only someone needful of help, some-one requiring a lifeline out of the chaos and pain of crisis. This positive regard is offered without an expectation of its reciprocity; regardless of the client's expressed feelings toward the counselor, the counselor remains steadfast in car-ing for the client.

Crisis Intervention Techniques: The LAPC Model

The purpose of this section is to provide an overview of intervention strategies and techniques designed to guide the crisis counselor through the foggy haze that usually surrounds the chaos of crisis. Despite the best intentions of people purporting to be effective counselors, crisis intervention can be all for naught unless it is guided by techniques that allow victims not only to regain some semblance of control in their lives but also to forge ahead with renewed hope and resolve. In addition to these techniques, the counselor also should be guided by a *master plan,* a frame of reference for crisis intervention that serves as a template through which the counselor's skills and techniques are applied.

Several key components of crisis intervention emerge from the common underpinnings of a number of models. Slaikeu's (1990) five-stage psychologi-cal first aid model and Roberts' (2000) seven-stage model share many common features. Central to each of these models are steps involving making contact and listening, exploring dimensions of the crisis event, securing agreement to an action plan, and providing follow-up. The goals of each of these models also are similar: providing safety, reestablishing coping mechanisms for clients, and facilitating linkages for them with other resources.

Myer (2001) stated that crisis intervention models should be simple and user-friendly, adaptable for use with many types of crises, and able to encompassing all aspects of clients' experiences. Crisis counselors should be able to utilize a straightforward model and to apply it in an effective intervention to a variety of crisis situations, such as those involving domestic violence (see Chapter 4), suicide and homicide (see Chapter 6), sexual assault (see Chapter 7), child abuse (see Chapter 3), and substance abuse (see Chapter 5). Whether a police officer called to the scene of a domestic dispute, a school counselor consoling a terrorized student after a school shooting, or a clergy member providing solace and support to a grieving family, crisis counselors require their own action plans to assist them in their work.

The following model provides a simple, straightforward plan for crisis counselors. This four-step approach incorporates the critical features of previously developed models and addresses the need for a flexible model, or template, that the practitioner can apply to multiple crisis settings. Known as the LAPC model, its steps are as follows:

> Listen: What is the victim saying? What is he or she *not* saying?
>
> Assess: What is the victim feeling? How is he or she acting? What is he or she thinking?
>
> Plan: What plans can the victim make now? Are the plans reasonable? Can they be carried out?
>
> Commit: Has the victim agreed to follow the plan? What other resources will be needed to see the plan through?

The remainder of this chapter will focus on these four stages, and particularly on those listening skills that are critical to any helping relationship. They compose an important first stage to the LAPC Model; listening begets an assessment capability that leads to a viable plan based upon the client's needs and eventually to the client's commitment to implement such a plan. Finally, family, community, or other resources are enlisted as needed to assist with this plan.

Step 1: Listen

This first step of the LAPC model accomplishes one of the goals of effective crisis intervention by communicating three important messages to victims of crisis: that they are safe, they are heard, and they are in control.

COMMUNICATE SAFETY   In the immediate aftermath of a crisis, a well-intentioned counselor can be either an intrusive or a positive presence. The numbers of people performing various functions at the crisis location can be overwhelming, leaving the victim needful of reassurances. Some simple strategies can help reassure victims.

INTRODUCE YOURSELF Regardless of an identifying name, the victim simply needs the counselor to be there, to be attentive, and to be a constant in the chaos. Nevertheless, a simple, uncomplicated introduction is essential:

> Hello. My name is John, and I am from the Brookside
> Counseling Center. I am here to listen and to learn from you
> what I can do to help.

Announcing one's name, role, and intentions will go a long way toward providing much-needed structure and support for the victim. It is essential to communicate to the individual, by a calm demeanor, the notion that perhaps order can be restored. The emphasis, however, during this introductory phase should be simplicity: the counselor should keep it simple and neither ask too many probing questions nor make any promises until he has engaged the individual in a helping and caring relationship. Delving into the crisis details prematurely also should be avoided. The relationship has not been developed yet.

ACT IMMEDIATELY AND TAKE CONTROL The assertive crisis counselor will take care of some of the details that, although seemingly small and inconsequential, can loom large for the victim in structuring and reordering the crisis. For example, the following details should be attended to:

- Keep representatives from the media away from the victim.
- Move the victim from the crisis situation to as neutral a location as can be arranged.
- State simply, "You are safe now," that is, if the assailant was indeed apprehended, if the fire was brought under control, or if the motor vehicle accident site has been secured by the police. False promises, however, should never be made regarding the individual's safety.
- Take care of other tangential distracters that weigh heavily on the individual's mind: for example, if there are children at home who may be unattended, arrange, with the victim's cooperation and input, to call a family member, friend, or other individual to provide child care. Additionally, if the victim worries that the accident will make her late for an appointment, arrange, with her permission, to call to cancel or reschedule. Securing permission for even these details serves as a way of restoring some control and authority to the individual.
- Guarantee that you will indeed be there to listen and to help, but do not promise things that you cannot control. After all, everything may *not* turn out all right. Even law enforcement officers cannot control the length of incarceration of an assailant.

BEGIN HANDING OVER SOME CONTROL TO THE VICTIM In order to restore control to the victim eventually, it is important to begin to do so at the beginning of the process, albeit in small, relatively benign steps. The victim is able to make decisions and to exert some influence over even those minor issues that are part and parcel of the intervention relationship, particularly immediately following the crisis event itself. Asking questions similar to the ones listed below can allow for some decision-making on the victim's part:

- Where would you like me to sit/stand?
- What name would you like me to call you?
- Would you like me to get you something before we talk?
- Would you prefer if we sat/stood over there instead?
- Is there anyone you would like me to call at this time?

In addition to the need to feel safe, crisis victims, particularly victims of physical or sexual abuse, also have a need to control their own boundaries. That is, once their sense of safety and security has been breached and their physical space violated, they require some control over these very issues in their relationships with crisis counselors. They need to know that their preferences are important and that they do not have to respond in any way other than how they wish (Schmookler, 1996). And in cases of physical or sexual assault, victims have to feel that they will be able to control who may touch them, if anyone at all, during the course of the crisis work. Victims also must know that they are entitled to give permission to the crisis worker to do almost anything: discuss the crisis details, talk at all, or ask any questions.

Finally, the calm demeanor of the crisis counselor communicates to the victim a sense of detachment, of neutrality, of a proverbial "blank slate" onto which the victim may place any thought or emotion experienced as a result of the crisis. Doing so lets the victim know that it is alright to express, without being judged, these thoughts and emotions, regardless of their intensity level or their content. The counselor, despite the strong feelings that the victim's own story creates, must remain a staid, nonjudgmental individual who allows the victim to control the amount and the content of the feelings expressed.

COMMUNICATE THE MESSAGE THAT THE VICTIM IS HEARD   Once safety has been assured as much as possible in the wake of a crisis, the primary goal of the crisis counselor is to *listen*. The pitfalls that often get in the way of the simple process of listening, however, are varied. Myer (2001) discussed several of the more common missteps of over-zealous crisis counselors who interfere with the recovery process of victims by intervening with well-intentioned, albeit counter-productive attempts at helping.

He decried those crisis counselors who offer premature suggestions before listening fully to victims' stories. For example, 15-year-old Angela, in the aftermath of a failed suicide attempt, rebuffed the counselor's repeated suggestion that she confide in her parents about her secret pregnancy as a way of resolving this hidden dilemma. If he were a more attentive listener, however, he may have learned eventually that Angela feared that her stepfather was the father of her child after several years of sexual abuse in the home, thus her inability to disclose her secret to them. Angela undoubtedly heard similar advice from her friends; now she just needs to tell her story to someone more adept at listening to her.

A second pitfall that results in ineffective crisis intervention is the tendency to ask for too many details (Myer, 2001). Detective Joe Friday, an earnest, clue-obsessed investigator from the old *Dragnet* television series, would doggedly pursue the crime scene witnesses, wanting only to uncover "the facts, ma'am, just the facts" about the crime. However, crisis intervention is not a crime scene interrogation designed to gather facts in the manner of a Joe Friday. Rather, it is the beginning of a helping relationship that requires a good listener who can allow the victim to lead the way and to control the direction that the intervention takes.

The crisis counselor as information-gatherer would leave Angela bereft of support. This same counselor also would stymie Jessie in her aimless search for hopefulness in the midst of her family crisis. Questions related to the time and location of the car accident, the nature and extent of her mother's injuries, and her recent failing report card grades would miss the mark and would result in the continuation of Jessie's emotional malaise. An interrogation would communicate to her that the counselor was more interested in minutia, in facts that were of concern to others but, not to Jessie, and that her feelings of despair were only of secondary importance.

Although there will be a time when the crisis counselor will require specific information about the crisis event, there are ways in which to gather it. Suggestions for collecting information that clients may choose to minimize or to leave out altogether are included later in this chapter. However, the following section will discuss those strategies and techniques designed to help the crisis counselor create a supportive emotional climate conducive to a helping relationship and to the growth of the individual in crisis.

Putting Empathy, Genuineness, and Acceptance Into Practice

Attending and listening skills are the cornerstones for the counselor in communicating to crisis victims that they are truly the focus of the intervention and that they indeed have been heard. These techniques include attending, listening, and questioning.

ATTENDING   Attending to another's words and actions is a nonverbal technique. It requires presenting oneself as attentive by looking and acting the part. Body posture, facial expression, and proximity to the client are only a few elements that communicate attention. Words can only suggest the condition of attentiveness, but they cannot produce it. Nonverbal behaviors often betray the meaning of words, so it is crucial that one practice attending behaviors rather than attending statements or phrases. For example, the crisis counselor who professes unyielding attention to the client yet sits in profile to the client belies the words. Similarly, the counselor who utters all the reassuring key phrases to the client, yet furtively glances at the clock on the wall or at other activities around them presents as less than sincere in the verbalized claims of attentiveness. The crisis counselor demonstrates attention by engaging in the following nonverbal behaviors (Greenstone & Leviton, 1993; Kanel, 1999; James & Gilliland, 2001):

- establishing and maintaining eye contact with the client;
- nodding one's head in acceptance of key elements of the client's verbalizations;
- maintaining close physical proximity to the client, as long as the counselor does not invade the client's space (the counselor should also remember to get the client's permission regarding how close to sit or stand to her without being threatening);
- leaning forward in the direction of the client and facing him or her;
- maintaining an open stance (no crossed legs, folded arms across the chest, or closed fists);
- unbuttoning one's coat or avoiding formal attire, if possible, which is better suited to a wedding reception than to a crisis counseling interaction; and
- demonstrating an appropriate range of facial expressions, for example, a smile to reassure and to relax the client, a serious expression to show commitment.

Crisis counselors can display attentiveness to clients by being mindful of the above nonverbal behaviors. Even though it takes practice and some self-reflection in order to master the skill of attending, over-learning the above skills may be just as contra-indicated as avoiding them altogether. The rigid application of eye contact, for example, may present as a stare, invoking a feeling of discomfort in clients rather than comfort, while the open stance practiced to the extreme may give a counselor a slovenly appearance. An over-learned nod may be more reminiscent of one of those perpetually-nodding bobble-head dolls than an attentive counselor.

In addition to practicing these skills prior to applying them, it is essential that counselors also monitor the reactions of clients during interventions and are attentive to their impact. Does the client lean back as the counselor leans forward? Does the client avert his or her eyes at the counselor's steady gaze? Does the client's rather formal predilections cause unease with a counselor determined to be very casual? If so, then it would be quite important for the counselor to modify his or her nonverbal behavior to keep the client engaged.

More importantly, are there cultural considerations that would account for the clients' unexpected responses to the attending behaviors listed above? That is, should the counselor interpret reactions to those nonverbal indicators of attention (i.e., eye contact) differently for non-European-Americans? Is physical closeness unsettling for some cultures? Questions such as these require the attention of the counselor. Just as individuals respond differently to crisis events, so too do different cultural and ethnic groups respond in their own unique ways. Although it is beyond the scope of the present discussion, it is incumbent upon the crisis counselor to develop an awareness and an understanding of cultural values as they pertain to the business of this textbook.

LISTENING   The primary technique for identifying and clarifying a client's feelings and emotions is active listening (Roberts, 2000). Slaikeu (1984, 1990) presents the following definition of active listening:

> In active listening, the therapist attends carefully, both physically and psychologically, to the messages transmitted by the client. The therapist communicates understanding and empathy by reformulating and summarizing the client's explicit statements, by attending to and commenting on the client's nonverbal or paraverbal signals, and by guiding the client toward an expansion of the issues addressed. It is important to allow the client to direct the flow of the conversation and to avoid critical or judgmental statements. (p. 295)

The specific techniques that compose active listening are varied, and they encompass many of those nonverbal strategies already discussed in the previous section. In fact, to separate verbal from nonverbal active listening behaviors is to create an almost artificial dichotomy between these two intricately entwined sets of skills. They do not stand alone, since the true empathic listener demonstrates congruence in words and actions when interacting with a crisis victim. For example, the look of disinterest on the counselor's face belies all those well-chosen empathic words and statements that are key to active listening, just as a fleeting eye contact betrays the professed interest in the client.

Listening is an active process that combines a repertoire of not only the aforementioned nonverbal techniques but also the following verbal ones. The purpose of these verbal techniques is to communicate understanding to clients and encourage communication.

Clarifying   Eliciting more information about previous statements is the purpose of clarification. This technique is essential in dealing with the rush of emotions and the resulting cascade of verbalizations regarding the crisis experience. It enables the counselor to place into better perspective the meaning that the event had for the victim and to clear up any confusion or ambiguity in the victim's statements. The actual experience of the death of a sibling in a car accident, for example, may conjure up common images of loss, but the more personal symbolic meaning (i.e., feelings of guilt over not being able to protect the younger sibling) may elude the crisis worker who doesn't clarify the victim's description of the crisis aftermath. If the crisis worker and the client are essentially talking about two different experiences of the crisis, then little will be achieved with this intervention. Clarifying also supports a problem-solving approach to crisis intervention. The problem-solving approach will be discussed later in the chapter.

The two most common clarification techniques, particularly in the early stages of crisis intervention, are *paraphrasing* and *verifying*. Counselors use paraphrasing to highlight the factual content of what they are hearing, rather than the emotional content, which may be premature immediately after the crisis. When paraphrasing, counselors use the clients' own words and phrases to summarize what they said; new or equivalent words are to be avoided at this point, as in the following example:

> Client: I keep hearing my wife scream as the fire raced through her office building. I wasn't even there, but I just keep imagining it over and over again. I can't concentrate at work, and I can't sleep.
>
> Crisis worker: In other words, ever since your wife died in the fire, you keep hearing her screams and can't seem to concentrate or to sleep.
>
> Client: I just can't imagine what life is going to be like without her. I am just so lonely and my days all seem so long.
>
> Crisis worker: Without her, you are so lonely that your days seem to be very long.

Lanceley (1999) suggested that paraphrasing in the client's own words keeps the client from being on the defensive and demonstrates that the listener has heard and has understood the client's story. Other benefits of paraphrasing include creating empathy and rapport, clarifying content, and highlighting issues for the client.

Unlike paraphrasing, which is a simple restatement of what was heard, *verifying* involves actually questioning what the client said in order to ensure that the statements are understood. The following exchange is an example of verifying:

> Client: I'm 48 years old and I just read that people my age have a real hard time finding employment, once they are downsized out of a job.
>
> Crisis worker: Are you saying that you are worried about not being able to find another job?
>
> Client: This is the second time in 7 years that my home has been destroyed by a tornado. My family wants me to move, but I've lived my whole life here. All my friends and family are here.
>
> Crisis worker: Are you thinking that your family wants you to leave your hometown and relocate someplace else?

When using this clarification technique, the counselor should avoid making an inferential leap regarding what the client said. It is important to remember that the purpose of this step is simply to communicate an understanding of what was said, not to interpret the content of the message being given.

Reflecting/Mirroring   Using this technique, the counselor uses the client's own words and phrases to direct the session to the emotional responses to the crisis situation. Reflecting is essentially a statement rephrasing the emotional content of the session, and is a powerful tool in creating an empathic environment

(Kanel, 1999). The crisis counselor does not interpret, but rather points out the affective state seen or heard in the client's own statements. The counselor can maintain a sense of congruence by using the client's own words, although assigning an affective label to the client's verbalizations may also be essential. The counselor, however, must exercise caution in doing so; assigning a label to the client's emotional state that does not reflect the reality can make the client defensive or simply frustrated. Following are some examples:

> Client: This is so typical for me! Five years of nothing but rotten luck, and now this!
>
> Crisis worker: Sounds like you've had quite a run of bad luck, even before today's accident.

> Client: I can't face her any more. I mean, I love her, but I'm at a loss as to how to avoid the constant fights we have.
>
> Crisis worker: You seem confused when you try to figure out how to love each other without fighting.

Summarizing   Another important indicator that a crisis counselor is truly hearing what the victim has to say is the ability to summarize—to encapsulate in a simple, verifiable statement—all that the victim has said during the crisis interview. The essence of summarizing is distilling into one or two meaningful and accurate sentences all that has been said.

In order to accomplish this technique, the counselor must combine in summary fashion the facts of the crisis (as perceived by the victim) with the feeling state expressed by the victim. Successful summarization of this material should lead to the development of a working definition of the problem attendant to the crisis situation and, ultimately, to an intervention plan for the victim. Some examples of summarizing statements:

> In other words, you are feeling not only tremendous grief over your husband's death, but also a lot of guilt, since you had a fight just before he left and said some unkind things to him. If you knew he was going to be killed in a car accident on the way to work, you wouldn't have said those things.
>
> So, your home has just been lost to the twister, and being new to the area yourself, your entire family is still back East. You are frightened and are feeling all alone with this situation.
>
> You thought that if you kept what your father has been doing to you a secret, he would leave your younger sister alone. Now that you've found out that he has started doing it to her, you're feeling very angry, and you want to do something to stop him.

If the counselor's summarizing statements truly depict the victim's experience of the crisis, then the counselor will be able to move the victim to the next level of crisis intervention: defining the problem and developing an intervention plan. However, if they do not, the victim may feel little validation of his or her crisis experience and may be unable to move forward toward some sense of resolution. The crisis counselor must understand that summarization of the crisis should be from the *victim's* vantage point, *not* the counselor's.

Using "I" Messages   Messages that communicate to the client the impact that he or she is having on the crisis counselor are called *"I" messages*. The "I" in the message is the counselor, and the message is what "I" think/feel/wish regarding the explanation of the crisis experience by the client. Additionally, referring to "I" allows the counselor to exercise some referent power with the client; the use of "I" messages allows the counselor to communicate to the client that they may share common experiences, thus enabling treatment to continue unimpeded.

"I" messages are better alternatives to "you" messages, which tend to be more threatening and can put the victim "on the hot seat" to account for feelings or reactions to the crisis. "I" messages, according to James and Gilliland (2001), "are probably more important in crisis intervention than in other kinds of therapy because of the directive stance the crisis worker often has to take with clients who are immobile and in disequilibrium" (p. 49). Nevertheless, such statements still should be used sparingly, since their overuse would make the counselor, rather than the client, the focus of treatment.

Appropriate "I" messages are as follows:

I agree that it is very confusing to try to understand all that has happened.

I know how difficult it is to talk about all of these things, and I applaud you for taking such a big step.

I need you to agree to take the steps that we talked about today.

Managing Silence   A skill that eludes many counselors is the ability to manage silence. Silence makes many people uncomfortable, since it represents the absence of communication. They then respond to this absence with some attempt to fill the void; they find words, whether well-chosen or not, to generate some discussion of the event with the client, to give advice, or simply to comment on the content of the client's crisis description.

However, it is critical for the crisis worker to view silence as just another form of communication, not its absence, similar to other forms of nonverbal communication. Counselors generally should be silent themselves, although always observing the behavior (silent and otherwise) in clients, with a particular emphasis on what clients do *not* say.

Questioning   The quality of the questions put to a crisis victim can make the difference between encouraging communication and thwarting it. The purpose of questioning during a crisis interview is twofold: to elicit information and to provide a forum for the client to speak openly and freely with the counselor. Knowing how to question and the types of questions to use in an interview are important skills for the crisis counselor.

One of the cardinal rules for counselors is to avoid the use of "why" questions. Such questions take on an accusatory tone and imply blame or responsibility where none actually exists. "Why" questions only reinforce and encourage self-blame, particularly in the case of a crisis victim who harbors some sense of guilt over an imagined role played in the crisis situation. For example, the father of a young child killed in a car accident on the way to school blames himself for the death, since he decided against keeping her home from school that day despite a slight head cold. Asking "why" he sent his daughter to school can only immerse the grieving father in tremendous guilt and can suggest that the counselor may also view him as blame-worthy. Communication, under these circumstances, is thwarted, leaving an individual in pain without the support of a counselor now perceived as accusatory. Crisis sufferers do not want to defend their actions related to the crisis.

There are at least two distinct types of appropriate questions, and each has a place in a crisis interview: closed questions and open questions. *Closed questions* enable the counselor to collect factual information related to the crisis victim and to the crisis itself. They ask for specific data that the counselor then will organize and utilize to formulate the best possible plan for assisting the client. However, care must be taken so that these questions are not perceived as an interrogation rather than a crisis interview. Gathering factual information is important in any such encounter, but too much data collection will easily put a client on the defensive at a time when the counselor really wants him the client at ease. In short, a search for too many details will miss the overall emotional picture the client wants to paint, leaving the client frustrated and convinced that the counselor has little interest in helping. Similarly, the counselor should also consider the pacing of these questions; rapid-fire questioning allows little time for reflection before responding and will shut down communication and increase, rather than decrease, the client's level of agitation.

Overuse of closed questions also creates another pitfall: the tendency to forestalling the development of a true helping relationship by allowing the client to respond "yes" or "no" only. The information gathered by these types of questions prevents a more thorough exploration of the feelings and thoughts related to the crisis. However, there is a place for closed questions that require communication of specific information, provided that they are used sparingly. Examples of appropriate closed questions include:

- How many years had you been married at the time of his death?
- Was it before or after your job relocation that you were assaulted?
- Who first told you that your son was missing?

Examples of closed questions to be avoided include:

- Are you worried that your son is still missing?
- Did you try to tell him that you didn't want to have sex that night?
- Have you ever tried to talk to your mother about these feelings?

Whereas closed questions result in specific responses, *open-ended questions* do not limit the client to a carefully circumscribed response set; there are no counselor-imposed dichotomies to frame the client's responses. Rather, these types of questions are designed to elicit feelings, thoughts, and perceptions of those events that brought the client to the counselor in the first place. The counselor, equipped with the right questions, is less an interviewer than a facilitator. The client, unencumbered by the counselor's restrictions, responds with a genuine disclosure of the crisis experience. Examples of appropriate open-ended questions include

- Could you tell me more about what happened after he entered your apartment with you?
- What were you thinking about just before you picked up the knife to cut your wrists?
- How did you feel when your teacher told you about the man with the gun in school?

Step 2: Assess

The second step of the LAPC model involves an assessment by the crisis counselor of all the verbal and nonverbal communication received from the client during the listening stage. Body language speaks volumes, but it can be far more difficult to interpret than the words actually spoken by the client. If the counselor reads the body language as being out of synch with the expressed verbal message describing the client's feeling state, then the counselor must question the verbal message further. Using the listening techniques described above, being open, accessible to the client, and committed fully to hearing the client's words, will enable the counselor to make an informed assessment of the client, which will lead to the third and fourth step in the LAPC model.

Although assessment is an ongoing and dynamic process that changes throughout the course of an intervention, the crisis counselor must assess the client across several dimensions in order to understand the impact of the crisis event on the client.

Emotions—Is the client inconsolable? sad? hopeless? anxious? angry?

Behavior—Is the client agitated? pacing the room? sluggish or slow? wanting to leave? wanting to linger?

Thoughts—How does the client interpret the crisis? What is its meaning for the client? Is the client hopeful or hopeless about the outcome? How devastating is it for the client? the client's future? How does the client judge his or her ability to cope?

Support system—How large a family or friendship network does the client have? Is the client alone and solitary, or social with many friends? Who can be called upon to assist the client at this time?

Answers to the above questions will guide the counselor in determining the direction to be taken in the next two steps of LAPC.

Step 3: Plan

The ultimate goal in crisis intervention is actually two-fold: first, assist the client in recovering from the emotional impact in the immediate aftermath of the crisis, then impart to the client via a plan a sense of hope and empowerment. This two-part approach includes a return to some state of equilibrium and a plan to help maintain this balance long after the crisis has passed. Of course, this plan requires a skilled crisis counselor who is able to strike a balance between several competing counselor and client needs. These needs include:

Counselor		Client
Need to be active	vs.	Need for autonomy
Need to model hopefulness	vs.	Need to grieve first
Need to help with problem	vs.	Need to retain ownership of problem
Need to express universality of crisis	vs.	Need to communicate individuality of crisis experience
Need for short-term treatment	vs.	Possible need for long-term work

Balancing these two sets of needs can be accomplished within the context of crisis intervention. Most individuals possess a reservoir of problem-solving inner resources that will aid their recovery. Crisis victims tend to be more resilient and resourceful than they originally thought they were, and it is the work of crisis counselors to enable them to tap these inner resources to move forward. People solve problems on their own every day, and although these problems rarely reach crisis proportions, the strategies that are used to solve them can also be applied to larger, seemingly insurmountable problems. The crisis counselor's job, in effect, is to help the client apply innate problem-solving skills to more crisis-specific dilemmas.

COMMUNICATING THE MESSAGE THAT THE CLIENT IS IN CONTROL
The assumption that the individual in crisis is resourceful enough to generate multiple solutions is one of the cornerstones of effective crisis intervention. The function of the counselor is not to change people, but rather to serve as a catalyst for victims to discover and to utilize their own resources. There is an expectation that people haven't yet identified those skills that they already possess and that they have all they need to help solve their problems (Roberts, 2000). Even though familiar coping methods may fail the person in crisis, an expectation of victim resourcefulness would lead the crisis counselor to elicit from the individual other, perhaps less familiar, solutions to the crisis situation. Following is the case of Nicole, which will illustrate this key element of crisis intervention.

Nicole was a recent widow as a result of the September 11 attacks on the World Trade Center. Several weeks after the death of her husband, she acknowledged to a crisis counselor's queries that she experienced all the signs of depression: sleep and appetite disturbances, a sense of helplessness and hopelessness, frequent crying episodes, and an inability to mobilize her own inner resources to return to work and, even more significantly, to leave the house altogether. She explained to the counselor during the initial interview that she had experienced a similar episode as an adolescent when, in the aftermath of a car accident in which she was wounded psychologically rather than physically, she remained housebound for 2 whole years. The initial crisis interview concluded with the following exchange:

Counselor: What was it that enabled you, after 2 whole years, to leave the house?

Nicole: It was the church; I went back to church for the first time in a while.

Counselor: Tell me what it was that drew you to the church for help.

Nicole: It was because I remembered that, as a girl, I always felt safe in church. I remembered that, whenever I was in church, there was nothing to fear.

Once Nicole suggested that her support in times of great distress, as evidenced by her past history, was the church, a key component of the counselor's intervention plan involved her return to church. Plans were made to initiate contact with a priest from a neighboring parish and to seek him out for support. It was Nicole, with the assistance of the counselor, who devised this plan; she had known this priest in the past and had always considered him to be a soothing and spiritual man. Thus, her plan was set in motion, and she eventually made contact with him.

The plan chosen for Nicole certainly would not necessarily be the plan chosen for other crisis victims. It was specific to Nicole and to her needs. More importantly, it utilized Nicole's own resources, her own ideas. She enlisted her recollection of what helped her emerge from trauma in the past and applied it to the present. In doing so, she began to shed the cloak of grief and to don that of empowerment; this outcome exhibits the essence of crisis intervention that capitalizes on a client's strengths and inner resources to put her back into control.

Step 4: Commit

In this final step in LAPC, the client, either through the facilitative or directive stance of the counselor, agrees to commit to a plan of action to help alleviate the strains of the crisis and to regain some level of equilibrium. Even though several different plans may be discussed along with the advantages and disadvantages of each, a specific plan that is appealing to the client and that he or she believes can be enacted is chosen. Additionally, follow-up becomes a component of this commitment. Once the client agrees to enact the plan, the client also commits to ongoing follow-up with the counselor or with some other member of the support system.

The content and protocol for this follow-up, of course, will depend on the needs of the crisis client. For some, follow-up may be with a medical professional (for medication, possible hospitalization, etc.) or a mental health professional (for ongoing counseling, etc.), while for others, follow-up may be a somewhat less formal arrangement for the client (returning to work, maintaining telephone contact only with the crisis counselor, etc.). Nicole (see above), for example, committed to accessing her local priest, while her involvement with a sizable group of friends and community members also contributed greatly to her recovery.

It is important to note that there is a problem-solving component to the planning stage. One action plan is chosen by the client for implementation. However, the counselor and the client also may discuss several others before deciding on the most viable one. One of the advantages of the fourth LAPC step is that it also affords the client the ability to follow up with the counselor or with another member of the support system to choose another plan, should the initial one not result in a successful outcome. Commitment to the plan as well as to the follow-up are equally important in step four.

SOURCES OF CHAPTER ENRICHMENT

Print Sources

Baxter, S., & Stewart, W. (1998). *Death and the adolescent: A resource handbook for bereavement support groups in schools.* Toronto: University of Toronto Press.

Heegaard, E. (1993). *The drawing our feelings series facilitator's guide for leading grief support groups.* Chapmanville, WV: Woodland Press.

James, B. (1990). *Treating traumatized children: New insights and creative interventions.* New York: Simon & Schuster.

Prout, H.T., & Brown, D. (Eds.). *Counseling and psychotherapy with children and adolescents: Theory and practice for school and clinical settings.* Indianapolis, IN: John Wiley & Sons.

Schaefer, D., & Lyons, C. (1993). *How do we tell the children? Helping children two to teen cope when someone dies.* New York: Newmarket Press.

Thompson, C., Rudolph, L., & Henderson, D. (2004). *Counseling children* (6th ed.). Belmont, CA: Brooks/Cole-Thomson Learning.

Vernon, A. (2002). *What works with children: A handbook of individual counseling techniques.* Dallas, TX: Research Press.

Webb, N. (Ed.). (2002). *Helping bereaved children: A handbook for practitioners* (2nd ed.). New York: Guilford Press.

Internet Sources

American Counseling Association (http://www.counseling.org) ACA is the world's largest association exclusively representing professional counselors in various practice settings.

National Association of School Psychologists (http://nasponline.org) NASP provides a range of resources for school psychologists and interested professionals who work with children. It addresses issues related to all facets of the psychosocial needs of children by providing resources and advocacy.

American Psychological Association (http://www.apa.org) The APA presents psychologists in the United States and is considered the largest association of psychologists worldwide.

American School Counselor Association (http://www.schoolcounselor.org) Devoted to the academic, personal/social, and career development of children, the ASCA provides professional development, advocacy, and resources for approximately 14,000 professional school counselors.

National Mental Health Association (http://www.nmha.org) NMHA is the country's oldest and largest nonprofit organization addressing all aspects of mental health issues.

National Association of Social Workers (http://www.naswdc.org) The largest membership organization of social workers in the world, NASW provides a range of resources for working with all ages, including children.

CHAPTER 3

Child Abuse and Neglect

Just several days into the new year, with the last strains of Auld Lang Syne still heard faintly in the distance, a resident of an apartment building in the middle of a congested east coast urban setting made a grisly discovery. He found two brothers, ages 7 and 4, malnourished and mal-treated, huddling in the basement of the building as if held there as prisoners. Starving and covered with signs of abuse and neglect, the boys were an appalling sight for thousands of newspaper readers the next day. The next day, investigating further, police found the mummi-fied remains of the 7-year-old's twin brother in a storage bin in one of the basement closets. The surviving boys spent the next two months in the hospital before being placed in a group home. The 4-year-old recoiled the first time a caregiver attempted to give him a bath, because his former bathtub had been the site of frequent scaldings. Just a short time after entering the group home, the older brother went to school for the very first time.

*T*he opening vignette illustrates one of the more horrific examples of child abuse and neglect. Headlines such as the ones that followed this story tend to thrust the plight of child victims of abuse and neglect into the public conscious-ness. Television talk shows, media, and politicians rally to the cause of protect-ing children. These high profile cases serve to emphasize the importance, at least for the moment, of child protective services (CPS) continuing to exercise its responsibility to protect children, and of adults being mindful of the impact of abuse of their own or of others' children. However, the abuse suffered by countless other children whose agonies do not make front-page news cries out for the constant vigilance of all who encounter children in their jobs, their com-munities, and their places of worship.

This chapter will address the more typical examples of child abuse and neg-lect and the manner in which these cases usually come to the attention of child care professionals. Although less sensationalized than broader-based traumatic events, such as school shootings, the effects of child abuse and neglect constitute a "prevalent and insidious crisis" (Webster & Browning, 2002). This crisis affects not just the almost one million victims of child abuse and neglect each year, but subsequent generations of children who will be abused or neglected by parents or caregivers who suffered the same fate in their own childhoods. Approximately one-third of abused and neglected children will continue this cycle of abuse with the next generation of children (Kaufman & Ziegler, 1987; Oliver, 1993), making it grow exponentially as a crisis among the young.

The purpose of this chapter is to explore a number of issues pertinent to the crisis of child abuse and neglect. Throughout the chapter, the word *abuse* will refer to both physical and sexual abuse, unless otherwise noted.

Definitional Issues

One of the complicating factors in the study of child abuse and neglect has been the difficulty in developing a useful, clear, and acceptable definition of what constitutes child abuse and neglect (Clark & Clark, 2001). The absence of a definition makes reporting, researching, and preventing these social ills all the more difficult. For example, incidence rates (see next section) can be established only as they relate to the standards applied.

In October of 1996, the most recently amended version of the Federal Child Abuse Prevention and Treatment Act (CAPTA; Public Law 104–235), originally enacted in 1974, expanded its initial definition of child abuse and neglect. It provided minimum standards and required that all states incorporate them into their own statutory definitions. Since each state had its own legal definition of child abuse and neglect, the following CAPTA definition served to standardize the definitions to some degree:

> The term "child abuse and neglect" means, at a minimum, any recent act or failure to act, on the part of a parent or caretaker (including any employee of a residential facility or any staff person providing out-of-home care who is responsible for the child's welfare), which results in death, serious physical or emotional harm, sexual abuse or exploitation, or an act or failure to act which presents an imminent risk of serious harm. (The term "child" means a person under the age of 18, unless the child protection law of the state in which the child resides specifies a younger age for cases not involving sexual abuse.)

This definition only specifies parents and caregivers as potential perpetrators of child maltreatment; abuse at the hands of other persons known to the child or of strangers constitutes child assault. Regardless of this distinction, both forms of abusive behavior are crimes against children (Rein, Jacobs, & Quiram, 2001). An additional expansion of this definition made an attempt to include "intent" as well, but it offered no guidance as to how to classify cases of abuse or neglect based on intent (Clark & Clark, 2001).

CAPTA also presents minimum guidelines for state definitions of child sexual abuse. They include the following:

> The employment, use, persuasion, inducement, enticement, or coercion of any child to engage in, or assist any other person to engage in, any sexually

explicit conduct or simulation of such for the purpose of producing a visual depiction of such conduct; or the rape, and in cases of caretaker or inter-familial relationships, statutory rape, molestation, prostitution, or other form of sexual exploitation of other children, or incest with children.

Despite these minimum requirements for defining child abuse and neglect, states still vary in their definitions. Some states define child abuse and neglect as a single concept, while others provide separate definitions and categories for physical abuse, sexual abuse, neglect, and/or emotional abuse. Although all states include sexual abuse in their definitions, some refer to it in general terms only, while still others refer to specific acts as sexual abuse. Neglect often is described as the deprivation of food, clothing, shelter, or medical care, but some states differentiate the failure to provide these essentials for no apparent financial reason from the same state of deprivation due to financial hardship.

Even the federal government uses different standards to define abuse and neglect in its periodic nationwide studies. The National Center on Child Abuse and Neglect (NCCAN) was established by CAPTA in 1974 and operates under the aegis of the U.S. Department of Health and Human Services. It is the primary federal agency responsible for assisting states and communities in the identification, prevention, and treatment of child abuse and neglect. Among NCCAN's major activities, besides providing funding for research in this area, are the coordination of the National Clearinghouse on Child Abuse and Neglect Information and the National Incidence Study of Child Abuse and Neglect (NIS). This latter research work is conducted periodically under federal mandate, and its findings constitute the single most comprehensive source of information about the incidence of child abuse and neglect in the United States.

The U.S. Department of Health and Human Services has conducted three studies to date. The third study (NIS-3) utilized two sets of standardized definitions of child abuse and neglect, the *Harm Standard (HS)* and the *Endangerment Standard (ES)*. Under the Harm Standard, children were identified included in the study as victims of maltreatment only if they had already experienced harm from abuse or neglect. This standard is a relatively stringent one, since the harm must be demonstrable in order to qualify as abuse or neglect. The Endangerment Standard, however, is considered a more lenient standard, as it included all children who meet the Harm Standard as well as children considered to be at risk by a non-CPS agency or children whose maltreatment was indicated via a CPS investigation.

Thus, even incidence rates vary according to the definitional standard utilized. For example, under the Harm Standard definition, the total number of abused and neglected children was two-thirds higher in the 1993 NIS-3 than in the previous 1986 NIS-2. Using the broader definition of the Endangerment Standard, however, the incidence of abuse and neglect nearly doubled, while sexual abuse more than doubled. Additionally, physical neglect and emotional abuse and neglect were more than two-and-a-half times their NIS-2 levels.

Another factor that obfuscates the definitional dilemma regarding these terms is the lack of a universal standard or definition of optimal parenting.

Some sociocultural biases favor the use of corporal punishment as an appropriate parenting strategy. Withholding medical treatment within the context of certain religious beliefs contraindicates adherence to some hard-and-fast definition of abuse and neglect, at least for those groups. Therefore, some researchers (Finkelhor & Korbin, 1988) suggest a definition that could indeed be applied across cultures and that should be able to satisfy two objectives:

1. It should distinguish child abuse from other social, economic, and health problems.
2. It should be flexible enough to apply to different situations across different social and cultural contexts.

Although considered a general term, child abuse and neglect presumes a wide range of acts of commission and omission that are carried out by a child's caregiver and that lead to death, a variety of physical injuries, illnesses, or emotional distress (Clark & Clark, 2001). These core components tend to appear in most other definitions of child abuse and neglect. For example, Wolfe (1987) defines abuse as an act of commission by caregivers or parents that is characterized by the infliction of overt physical violence, while the National Committee to Prevent Child Abuse defines it as a non-accidental injury or pattern of injury to a child. Compounding the issue are the "internal" injuries caused by emotional abuse, a condition more difficult to identify than physical abuse, which is visibly betrayed by bruises and other overt indicators (Romeo, 2000).

Despite the aforementioned definitional issues, it is important for the purposes of this chapter to have a working definition as a frame of reference. Most researchers in the area of child abuse and neglect have developed their own definitions, which tend to be fairly reflective of NCCAN's classification of the various forms of maltreatment. Thus, the following list of NCCAN's six major types of maltreatment will serve as a guide for a working definition:

1. *Physical abuse:* Acts of commission that result in physical harm, including death, to a child.
2. *Sexual abuse:* Acts of inclusion, including intrusion or penetration, molestation with genital contact, or other forms of sexual acts, in which children are used to provide sexual gratification for a perpetrator.
3. *Emotional abuse:* Acts of commission that include confinement, verbal or emotional abuse, or other types of abuse, such as withholding sleep, food, or shelter.
4. *Physical neglect:* Acts of omission that involve refusal to provide health care, delay in providing health care, abandonment, expulsion of a child from a home, inadequate supervision, failure to meet food and clothing needs, and conspicuous failure to protect a child from hazards or danger.
5. *Educational neglect:* Acts of omission and commission that include permitting chronic truancy, failure to enroll a child in school, and inattention to specific education needs.

6. *Emotional neglect:* Acts of omission that involve failing to meet the nurturing and affection needs of a child, exposing a child to chronic or severe spouse abuse, allowing or permitting a child to use alcohol or controlled substances, encouraging the child to engage in maladaptive behavior, refusal to provide psychological care, delays in providing psychological care, and other inattention to the child's psychological needs.

At this point, it is important to note the even greater difficulties in defining *neglect.* The primary distinction made between abuse and neglect lies in the distinction between the commission of a behavior (abuse) and the omission of a behavior (neglect) (Paget, 1997). The great difficulty, therefore, is in finding the best way to document a behavioral omission. How is the omission judged to be intentional? Is the omission due to poverty or to neglect? Do actual harm and the threat of harm constitute neglect (Paget, 1997)? These questions, albeit unanswered until suspected cases of abuse or neglect are investigated, are for consideration only and illustrate the ambiguous nature of these definitions.

Incidence of Child Abuse and Neglect

The third and most recent National Incidence Study of Child Abuse and Neglect (NIS-3), conducted by the U.S. Department of Health and Human Services in 1996, provides data that document a rise in abuse and neglect cases since the previous study (NIS-2), completed in 1986 (see Table 3.1). The differences observed between the HS (Harm Standard) and the ES (Endangerment Standard) are due to a comparison between a fairly stringent standard defining abuse and neglect (HS) and one which utilizes a broader standard (ES) (see previous section for discussion). However, regardless of the standard used, the NIS-3 results demonstrated an alarming increase in the number of abused and neglected children.

TABLE 3.1
National Incidence Study of Child Abuse and Neglect

		NIS-2	NIS-3	% Increase
Number abused	HS	931,000	1,553,800	67%
or neglected	ES	1,424,400	2,815,600	98%
Number abused	HS	269,700	381,700	42%
	ES	311,500	614,100	97%
Number neglected	HS	167,800	338,900	102%
(physically)	ES	507,700	1,335,100	163%
Number neglected	HS	49,200	212,800	333%
(emotionally)	ES	203,000	585,100	188%
Number sexually	HS	119,200	217,700	83%
abused	ES	133,600	300,200	125%

Note. Data for NIS-2 are from U.S. Department of Health and Human Services, 1986, Washington, DC. Data for NIS-3 are from U.S. Department of Health and Human Services, 1996, Washington, DC.

Other reports (Child Health USA, 2002, U.S. Department of Health and Human Services) indicated that in 2000, there were approximately 879,000 children who were victims of abuse or neglect, equivalent to a rate of 12.2 per 1,000 children under the age of 18, a slight increase from the 11.8 victims per 1,000 children in 1999. Seventy-nine percent of the perpetrators were the parents of the victims. According to this report, approximately 63% of all victims suffered neglect, 19% physical abuse, 10% sexual abuse, 8% psychological maltreatment, and 17% suffered other forms of maltreatment.

Victimization rates declined as age increased. That is, the highest victimization rate of 15.7 per 1,000 was found in the youngest age group (birth to 3 years old), with the smallest victimization rate of 5.7 per 1,000 found in the 16- to 17-year-old bracket. Child fatalities were associated more often with neglect (35%) than with any other form of maltreatment. Among the 1,200 children who died from abuse or neglect in 2000, about 44% were younger than 1 year of age, while children younger than 6 years old accounted for 85%.

Male and female victimization rates were reported to be similar (11.2 and 12.8 per 1,000, respectively). However, the rate for sexual abuse was more than four times higher for females than for males (0.4 males versus 1.7 females per 1,000). Although the percentage of all victims who were white (51%) outnumbered that of African-American victims (25%), African-American children suffered the highest victimization rate (20.7 per 1,000 versus 8.5 per 1,000 for whites). The victimization rate for Hispanic children (10.6 per 1,000) was lower than the national rate of 12.9 per 1,000.

According to the National Child Abuse Statistics compiled by the United States Department of Health and Human Services (June 2000), three children die each day in the United States due to abuse and neglect. The number of deaths due to abuse and neglect is larger than childhood deaths attributable to choking, suffocation, and other traumas, such as falling, car accidents, and residential fires. These statistics, however, may be only a minimal estimate of the problem, because the data include only those victims known to the protective service agencies that track abuse and neglect in the home. Approximately three million reports each year of child abuse and neglect pale in comparison to the actual incidence; estimates place the actual number at three times the reported number.

Among those serving time in the nation's prisons, there was a higher incidence of reported child abuse than in the general population. More than a third of the women in the nation's prisons reported abuse as children, compared to 12% to 17% of women in the general population. For males, the statistic is about 14% reporting abuse as children, compared to 5% to 8% of the general population.

Approximately three-fifths of the perpetrators of child maltreatment are females, with 41% of them under 30 years of age. Eighty-seven percent of all victims were maltreated by at least one parent; the most common pattern of maltreatment was a child victimized by a female parent acting alone (44%).

The vast numbers of abused and neglected children in this country continue to exact an awful price: childhoods lost and damaged beyond repair, children living nightmares day after day, and an entire society left with a legacy of adults abused as children. The adult survivors frequently continue the cycle by abusing their own children and are commonly added to the roles of drug and alcohol treatment centers, mental health centers, and prisons. Using data derived from the U.S. Department of Health and Human Services, the U.S. Department of Justice, and the U.S. Census Bureau, researchers of the national tragedy of child abuse and neglect were able to estimate the financial costs of abuse and neglect in this country. Table 3.2 shows a breakdown of their estimated total costs, based upon this data.

Factors Contributing to Child Abuse and Neglect

The factors that contribute to abuse and neglect are very complex and interactive. To pinpoint a single cause of the phenomenon of abuse is to oversimplify the multiple factors that are associated with it. Many issues that are implicated in the tragedy have a more correlational, rather than causal, link to abuse and neglect. The multidimensional nature of the problem is rooted in psychological, social, family, community, and societal factors.

TABLE 3.2
The Financial Cost of Child Abuse and Neglect in the United States

Hospitalization—565,000 children suffered serious physical harm from abuse; this figure is an estimate of the medical costs incurred by physical injury, such as fractures, dislocations, and other injuries requiring treatment in a medical facility.	**Estimated Cost:** $6,205,395,000
Chronic Health Problems—Thirty percent of maltreated children have chronic health problems.	**Estimated Cost:** $2,987,957,400
Mental Health Needs—Mental health needs includes counseling needs related to trauma, Post-Traumatic Stress Disorder, and other mental health issues. However, only one in five maltreated children receive counseling.	**Estimated Cost:** $425,110,400
Child Welfare System Needs—The costs in this category include protection, advocacy, foster care, and other requirements of the child welfare system.	**Estimated Cost:** $14,400,000,000
Law Enforcement—These costs reflect the calculations for police services for cases of neglect and abuse.	**Estimated Cost:** $24,709,800
Judicial System—These costs include court actions pertinent to these cases.	**Estimated Cost:** $341,174,702
Total Costs For All Abuse and Neglect-Related Care:	$24,384,347,302

A single-factor model of abuse and neglect cannot reliably identify abusive parents. For example, the psychiatric model, which focuses on the pathology of the perpetrators, and the sociological model, which emphasizes societal ills such as unemployment, have been proposed to explain the occurrence of child maltreatment. However, these models have failed to provide a sufficient explanation for the problem. This failure has given rise to a broader ecological framework that acknowledges the contributions of individual, family, community, and cultural factors in explaining the phenomenon (Horton, 1995).

The following section will explore some of the explanations for the high incidence of these social ills, highlighting the conclusions from the comprehensive NIS-3 study as well as explanations posited by other writers in the field. NIS-3 data indicated that the incidence of child maltreatment varied, in part, as a function of the income, structure, and size of the family.

Family Income

Family income proved to be significantly related to the incidence rates of abuse and neglect in nearly every category of maltreatment, according to NIS-3. Children in families with annual incomes less than $15,000 were

- more than 22 times more likely to experience some form of maltreatment,
- almost 16 times more likely to be physically abused,
- more than 44 times more likely to be neglected,
- almost 18 times more likely to be sexually abused,
- more than 13 times more likely to be emotionally abused,
- nearly 56 times more likely to be educationally neglected,
- 60 times more likely to die from maltreatment,
- more than 22 times more likely to be seriously injured by maltreatment, and
- more than 31 times more likely to be considered endangered, although not yet injured.

Contributing to the income factor are related issues of unemployment and socioeconomic status, which account in part for low income. An earlier National Family Violence Survey (1975) found that rates of child abuse were significantly higher in families with an unemployed father than in those that have a father who is employed full-time. A later version of the survey (1985), however, did not replicate this finding, although it did find that wives of unemployed husbands had a higher rate of abuse than wives of employed husbands.

Other researchers (Straus & Stewart, 1999; Straus & Smith, 1990) proposed that blue-collar parents from lower income brackets contribute to the higher incidence of child abuse because they tend to be more authoritarian in their child-rearing practices, are more likely to use physical punishment, and have a lesser understanding of child psychology. Workers in lower income brackets also face greater job stress, as they tend to have less control over their employment situations and fewer coping resources to address these problems. Additionally, they have more children, a risk factor for abuse, and tend to live in areas of high violence.

Family Structure

NIS-3 data also indicated that children of single parents were at higher risk of phys-ical abuse and neglect, and that they also were over-represented among the ranks of the seriously injured, the moderately injured, and the endangered. Compared with children living with both parents, children in single-parent families had

- a 77% greater chance of being physically abused,
- a 165% greater risk of being physically neglected,
- a 64% greater chance of experiencing emotional neglect,
- three times the risk of experiencing educational neglect,
- an 80% greater risk of suffering serious injury due to abuse or neglect,
- a 90% greater risk of receiving moderate injury, and
- twice the risk of being endangered.

Children living with only a father as the single parent were almost twice as likely to be abused as those living with only a mother. The multiple responsi-bilities and the stresses and strains of being a single parent contribute to this stress-induced abusive tendency, particularly if a social support network is not available to the single parent. The presence of two adults in the household, however, does not always mitigate the occurrence of child abuse or neglect. If one of the adults in the home is an unrelated man, generally the boyfriend of the mother, chances that the child will be assaulted increase greatly.

Even programs designed to assist children in need have yielded some unin-tended consequences. For example, children placed in foster care are twice as likely to be abused as children who live with their biological parents. This fact led to the family preservation movement, which began in the early 1980s. However, critics of the movement question the rationale behind it. Through the Adoption Assistance and Child Welfare Act of 1980, states were eligible for fed-eral funding for their foster care systems only if they made "reasonable efforts" to keep children within families and to reunify families as soon as possible after a child's removal to foster care. As a result, critics alleged, at-risk children were left in dysfunctional and potentially explosive family situations without proper long-term support. Dire cases with children requiring removal generally did not result in removal as often as they should have.

Family Size

The incidence of child maltreatment was related to the number of dependent children in the family (NIS-3). Incidence rates were highest for children in the largest families (four or more children), intermediate for "only" children, and lowest in families with two or three children.

Other Factors

NIS-3 data also indicated that children who experienced moderate harm through maltreatment were significantly fewer in larger urban counties than in other smaller ones. This factor was unclear, however, since it may have reflected only the anonymity of children in larger urban areas and the resulting unlikelihood that their maltreatment would come to the attention of community professionals.

Another important contributory factor to child abuse and neglect is drug and alcohol abuse among parents. Parents who abuse these substances are almost three times more likely to physically or sexually abuse their children; neglect by drug and alcohol abusers is also four times more likely. Domestic violence also contributes significantly to abuse. In fact, child abuse can often be a reflection of other forms of family conflict (Rein, Jacobs, & Quiram, 2001). Physical and verbal aggression between spouses increases the likelihood that a child in the home will be abused as well, as studies (Appel & Holden, 1998) have documented the relatively high co-occurrence rates of spousal abuse and child abuse. A parental history of abuse and neglect predisposes mothers and fathers to abuse their own children as well.

Researchers (Ammerman & Patz, 1996) also contended that an issue that has received little attention as a contributor to child abuse and neglect is the characteristics of the child. That is, certain child characteristics generate stress in the family and challenge already compromised parental coping skills; these characteristics may contribute in an interactive way to the overall risk of physical abuse (Ammerman, 2000). For example, childhood behavioral disorders, such as attention-deficit/hyperactivity disorder (ADHD), and the difficulties managing this condition can combine with other pre-existing risk factors (parental history of abuse, parental social isolation, and lack of social resources) to create fertile ground for abuse and neglect. A single mother with a hyperactive or severely autistic 10-year-old who lives hundreds of miles from her own family and who makes a meager hourly wage will be at high risk of abusing her child. Child factors may not have a causal link with abuse, but they can contribute to its occurrence and its maintenance, given the interactive influences of other factors.

Types of Abuse

Child abuse cuts across all social, economic, cultural, and ethnic lines. It is considered the least discovered of all crimes and is among the least likely to be prosecuted. Here we look at four types of abuse, as well as their symptoms or warning signs.

Physical Abuse

Physical abuse includes a variety of acts when they are continuous or extreme or if they are done intentionally to harm a child. The following list of offenses is not all-inclusive, as it does not cover the entire range of assaultive behaviors of a child abuser:

- hitting or slapping,
- throwing,
- kicking,
- choking,
- shaking (shaken baby syndrome),
- beating with an object,
- burning with a match, cigarette, stove, or other hot object,
- scalding with hot water,
- tying up,
- starving or failing to provide food,
- holding under water,
- breaking a limb,
- grabbing and twisting a body part, and
- pulling hair out.

Physical Neglect

Physical neglect includes acts that interfere with a child's growth and development:

- not providing adequate housing,
- not providing adequate clothing for the weather,
- locking a child in a closet or room,
- leaving a child alone for an extended period of time or in the care of an inappropriate caregiver,
- not providing adequate medical care if a child is sick or injured, and
- placing a child in a physically dangerous situation.

Sexual Abuse

Sexual abuse involves the following elements:

- fondling or touching a child's sex organs,
- making a child touch someone else's sex organs,
- having sex with a child (oral, anal, vaginal),
- showing a child pornographic material,
- showing sex organs to a child,
- forcing a child to undress inappropriately,
- forcing a child to have sex with someone,
- making a child pose or perform for pictures or videos, and
- telling a child sexualized stories.

Emotional Abuse

Emotional abuse is far more difficult to substantiate, but is considered just as damaging. A few examples include

- continuous ignoring,
- terrorizing or blaming,
- belittling, and
- making a child feel worthless or incompetent.

Symptoms and Warning Signs

Identifying an abused child is not always an easy task; the signs and symptoms may not be evident at first. The very nature of childhood can leave many children with bruises, scratches, and other abrasions from time to time; these signs of childhood exuberance are particularly true for more boisterous and active children. Therefore, none of these signs necessarily constitute an indication of child abuse or neglect. Additional clues or red flags are usually present to raise suspicion; counselors can determine whether abuse is occurring only through thorough investigation.

Some of the most obvious signs of physical abuse are recurring bruises, black eyes, or broken bones, but there are many signs that are less obvious. All children respond differently to abuse. Although there is no specific formula for identifying abuse and avoiding false positives (i.e., the incorrect identification of abuse or neglect when it has not actually occurred), there are numerous signs or symptoms, some of them very discreet, that warrant investigation by adults who observe them. Table 3.3 lists signs and symptoms provided by the National Clearinghouse on Child Abuse and Neglect Information (2003) that may signal the presence of neglect or of physical or sexual abuse. While there are many clues that may lead to a determination of child abuse or neglect, children respond to abuse in highly individualized ways (see following section). Very similar forms or instances of abuse often elicit different responses from different children. Therefore, people investigating possible abuse should look for a pattern of more than just one of the signs listed in Table 3.3.

Abused children often display behavioral extremes: crying often or not at all, being excessively fearful or fearless in the presence of adult authority figures, and being aggressive and destructive or passive and withdrawn. Additionally, some abused or neglected children become quite wary of physical contact, particularly when initiated by an adult, while others hunger for affection. Regression to age-inappropriate behaviors can also be a primary sign of abuse or neglect; a return to thumb-sucking, bed-wetting, clinging, and other developmentally young behaviors may be evident throughout the course of the maltreatment. It should be noted that children who have witnessed abuse but were not the direct victims can also display some of the

TABLE 3.3
Signs of Abuse or Neglect

Physical Signs

- Has unexplained burns, bites, bruises, broken bones, or black eyes
- Has fading bruises or other marks noticeable after an absence from school
- Reports injury by a parent or another adult caregiver
- Is frequently absent from school
- Lacks needed medical or dental care, immunizations, or glasses
- Is consistently dirty and has severe body odor
- Lacks sufficient clothing for the weather
- States that there is no one home to provide care
- Has not received help for physical or medical problems brought to the parent's attention
- Has difficulty walking or sitting
- Becomes pregnant or contracts a venereal disease, particularly if under the age of 14

Behavioral Signs

- Seems frightened of the parents and protests or cries when it is time to go home
- Shrinks at the approach of adults
- Begs or steals food or money
- Abuses alcohol or other drugs
- Shows sudden changes in behavior or school performance
- Has learning problems (or difficulty concentrating) that cannot be attributed to specific physical or psychological causes
- Is always watchful, as if waiting for something bad to happen
- Is overly compliant, passive, or withdrawn
- Comes to school or to other activities early, stays late, and does not want to go home
- Suddenly refuses to change for gym or to participate in physical activities
- Reports nightmares or bedwetting
- Demonstrates bizarre, sophisticated, or unusual sexual knowledge or behavior
- Reports sexual abuse by a parent or another adult caregiver

(Continues)

above-mentioned behaviors. The stress caused by certain situations, such as parental separation or divorce or other domestic problems, could also trigger some of these behaviors.

Psychological and Behavioral Consequences of Abuse

Many researchers have documented a plethora of negative psychological and behavioral outcomes for child victims of abuse and neglect (Webster & Browning,

TABLE 3.3
Signs of Abuse or Neglect *(Continued)*

Parent-Related Signs

- Shows little concern for the child
- Provides little supervision
- Denies the existence of—or blames the child for—the child's problems at school or at home
- Asks teachers or other caretakers to use harsh physical discipline if the child misbehaves
- Sees the child as extremely bad, worthless, or burdensome
- Demands a level of physical or academic performance the child cannot achieve
- Looks primarily to the child for care, attention, and satisfaction of emotional needs
- Offers conflicting, unconvincing, or no explanation for the child's injury
- Describes the child as "evil," or in some other very negative way
- Uses harsh physical discipline with the child
- Has a history of abuse as a child
- Is unduly protective of the child or severely limits the child's contact with other children, especially of the opposite sex (possible sexual abuse indicator)
- Is secretive and isolated (possible sexual abuse indicator)
- Is jealous or controlling with family members (possible sexual abuse indicator)

Note. From U.S. Department of Health and Human Services, National Clearinghouse on Child Abuse and Neglect Information, 2003. Available at http://nccanch.acf.hhs.gov/.

2002). In adulthood, symptoms of Post-Traumatic Stress Disorder and major depression are not uncommon (Silverman, Reinherz, & Giaconia, 1996), while other psychiatric disorders, such as Multiple Personality Disorder and Borderline Personality Disorder, have been linked to continuous exposure to abuse and neglect (Rivera, 1991). Additional psychological consequences for children included:

- high levels of anxiety, anger, and depression;
- increase in nightmares;
- sudden unexplainable fears;
- somatic complaints, such as stomach aches and headaches;
- increased fearfulness, edginess, and a heightened startle response;
- heightened wariness and fearfulness of adults, particularly those of the same gender as the abuser;
- depressive symptomotology, such as sadness and social withdrawal;
- suicidal ideation;
- increased irritability;
- flattened affect, or numbing to the abuse pattern; and
- feelings of guilt and shame, especially for victims of sexual abuse.

There are also behavioral consequences of abuse and neglect, such as

- developmental delays;
- regressive behavior, such as thumb sucking, clinging, enuresis, encopresis;
- disruptive classroom behavior;
- decline in academic performance;
- increase in grade retentions and discipline referrals;
- socialization problems with peers (fighting, bullying smaller or more vulnerable children);
- self-destructive behavior;
- school truancy or running away; and
- suicide (completed and attempted).

These indicators of the aftermath of abuse and neglect are identifiable and observable in children. Teachers, childcare workers, and community members are able to make judgments based on these behaviors, as they are easily observed in the classroom, day care center, and neighborhood. But there are other, possibly more insidious consequences of abuse and neglect that fall below the radar screen and beyond the watchful eye of a benevolent adult.

Ongoing abuse and neglect also compromise children's abilities to develop meaningful and healthy relationships from childhood to adulthood. They have difficulty holding on to close friendships (Oates, 1996) and trusting others (Varia, Abidin, & Dass, 1996). They also have considerable difficulty with adult relationships and with maintaining appropriate levels of intimacy with others (Gilmartin, 1994). Additionally, abused and neglected children tend to possess extremely low levels of self-esteem (Loos & Alexander, 1997) and feel both self-hatred and self-blame for the abuse itself (Oates, 1996; Gilmartin, 1994). Abused and neglected children will also tend to abuse their own children or their spouses (Gilmartin, 1994). It is these covert sequelae to ongoing abuse and neglect that constitute the silent pain, the hidden agony, that taints a life, perhaps forever. Seemingly functional to the passive observer, these individuals can struggle with legacies of abuse, surviving only by sacrificing parts of themselves in the process.

Mitigating Factors

Despite the difficult aftermath of abuse, there are several factors that can heavily influence the impact abuse and neglect will have on a particular child (Tower, 1999). For example, the age at which the child experiences the abuse is a critical determinant of the outcome for the child. The younger children are at the time of abuse, the more vulnerable they are to long-term damage (Webster & Browning, 2002), although the quality of the relationships they have with primary caregivers both before and after the abuse affects their recoveries.

The relational proximity of the abuser to the victim also plays a critical role in the abuse aftermath for a child. That is, the more distant the relationship is between the perpetrator and victim, the lesser the impact on the child; abuse at the hands of a stranger has a somewhat less devastating impact than that perpetrated by a parent or by some other trusted adult serving as a caregiver for the child. The closer the abuser is to the child, the more difficult the aftermath.

Other mitigating factors are the extensive nature of the abuse and its duration. That is, if the abuse involved physical violence resulting in injury, or if it was chronic and occurred over a long period of time, the likelihood of long-term damage would be greater than it would be if the abuse were less severe and of shorter duration. The reactions of family members to the victim's reports of abuse also are critical to the aftermath for a child. Those who respond to reports of abuse in a helpful way can greatly minimize the abuse aftermath. However, if the child perceives caregivers to be doubtful of the disclosure, the psychological damage can be significantly increased, compounded not only by the child's sense of betrayal from the perpetrator, but also from those adults who fail to fulfill their protective roles.

Finally, the inner psychological resources of the child have a great impact on recovery from abuse. Factors such as the child's level of self-esteem, the security of supportive relationships, and other resiliency factors all play a large role in the ability to resist the adverse sequelae of child abuse and neglect. Without these qualities buffering the child from the potentially devastating impact of abuse and neglect, the emotional aftermath could be far direr.

Reporting Suspected Abuse

Every state, including the District of Columbia, has statutes specifying the procedures for reporting suspected child abuse or neglect. When CAPTA was first enacted in 1974, it included a requirement that every state provide such guidelines in order to receive federal funding to assist child victims. Additionally, each state also was required to provide some form of immunity from liability for people who "in good faith" report suspected instances of abuse or neglect; this protection is from both civil and criminal liability. On the other hand, however, there are civil and criminal penalties for failure to report.

Each state designates specific agencies to receive and to investigate these reports. Typically, this responsibility belongs to child protective services (CPS) within a state's department of social services, department of human resources, or division of family and child services (The Administration for Children and Families, U.S. DHHS, 2002). Many states provide an in-state toll-free number for reporting suspected abuse. However, the nationwide number for the Childhelp USA National Child Abuse Hotline, available 24 hours a day, seven days a week, is

1-800-4-A-CHILD (1-800-422-4453; TDD 1-800-2-A-CHILD)

Mandatory reporters of child abuse and neglect and the circumstances under which they are to report typically vary from state to state. Although a mandatory reporter is one who is required by law to do so, any person can make a report. Mandatory reporting laws generally affect all professionals working with children. However, many states simply list "any person or institution" as mandatory reporters, and others add "any other person" to more specific lists of professionals and childcare workers. Those individuals usually designated as mandatory reporters include physicians, nurses, hospital personnel, and dentists; medical examiners; coroners; mental health professionals and social workers; school personnel; law enforcement officials; and child care providers.

The circumstances under which a person is required to report suspected abuse also differ from state to state, even though many state laws simply use phrases such as "reason to believe," "reasonable cause to believe," or "reasonable cause to suspect" (that abuse has taken place). When an individual makes a report, the information required generally includes the name and address of the child, the child's parents or other persons responsible for the child's care, the child's age, the nature and extent of the injuries, and other relevant information requested by the investigator.

The Child Welfare Act required that abuse be reported as soon as it is known or suspected. However, proof is not required to make such a report; the report is simply a request for an investigation into a suspected case of maltreatment (Lowenthal, 2001). It is not the responsibility of the reporter to investigate, but rather to refer the suspicion to those who have been charged by the state with conducting these investigations. Individuals who observe any one or any combination of signs or symptoms listed previously in this chapter are obligated to report.

School personnel were the predominant reporters of suspected abuse (NIS-3), being responsible for recognizing 50% to 60% of the children who suffered maltreatment. Other important sources were hospitals, police departments, social service agencies, and the general public; day care centers also have become an important source. In general, more than half of all child abuse and neglect reports were made by professionals, with the remaining referrals coming from nonprofessionals (i.e., community or family members).

Disclosure of Abuse

Typically the kindly attention of a childcare worker, teacher, or someone else who spends many hours with children results in the observation of a blackened eye, recurring bruises, or a mysterious broken bone that precipitates a report to the local CPS unit about a case of possible maltreatment. Although the individual is only required to report and not to investigate the signs, a child may confirm suspicions by disclosing the actual abuse events to someone serving in any of the above capacities.

There are several types of disclosure of child abuse. *Direct disclosure* refers to children actually reporting the incidents themselves. A child seeks out the aid of a teacher, guidance counselor, or neighbor to report being hit or touched improperly. *Indirect disclosure* occurs when a child offers hints, but does not state directly that abuse occurred. He may show his teacher a big bruise on his back, but not make any direct reference to an assault of any kind. However, if the child has a special bond with the teacher, there will be a certain expectation or hope on his part that the teacher will indeed want to know more about the bruise. Thus, the child absolves himself of the responsibility of betraying the abusing parent's trust by allowing the teacher to initiate a report of the abuse.

A child offers a *disclosure with conditions* when she states that she is willing to admit the abuse as long as there is a guarantee that the person who committed the abuse won't get into trouble. There often is an element of self-blame applied, as the child expresses some behavior of her own that may have precipitated and justified the abuse, thereby mitigating the seriousness of the perpetrator's offense. A *disguised disclosure* is a child's report that she has a "friend" who is being abused, or that something has been happening to a classmate. Children who make disguised disclosures make the incident of abuse appear to be happening to someone else. Finally, a *third party disclosure* is made when another person reports that he witnessed abuse happening to someone he knows.

Intervening After a Report of Abuse

Once disclosure of abuse has been made, a crisis worker should first provide a very safe atmosphere and assure the child that he or she will be protected by the counselor and by the other individuals who will be called as well (Kanel, 1999). The worker also should use standard interview procedures, including basic listening skills (see chapter 2 for discussion), to facilitate an understanding of what the child is trying to express (Horton & Cruise, 1997). If the recipient of the disclosure is uncomfortable with intervening, it is critical that he or she escort the child to someone on site who has such training. For example, the gym teacher who observes a series of welts on the legs of a boy in the locker room while changing should make sure that the child sees a counselor, school psychologist, or school social worker to conduct the proper interview. However, if such a discovery is not made in a setting with support staff around, then a phone call to the appropriate state-authorized CPS department should be made immediately.

Although there is variability in interview types and interviewers' styles, there are some key themes or guidelines that should be followed in all child interviews on the issue of maltreatment. Generally, children should be made to feel as comfortable as possible. Children also should be assured that they are not in trouble and that they have done nothing wrong. They often feel as if they are responsible for their own maltreatment and for inviting trouble into the family structure. Therefore, assuring children that they are not at fault and that they could not have prevented the abuse from happening is important. Horton (1995) offered some important elements of the child interview pertaining to maltreatment. She suggested that specific points be adhered to when conducting such an interview:

1. Be clear about the limits of confidentiality.
2. Respect the child's privacy.

3. Begin the interview with informal conversation.
4. Maintain a calm demeanor.
5. Use good listening and child-oriented communication skills.
6. Validate the child's feelings.
7. Avoid questions that imply blame or guilt.
8. Tell the child what will happen next.

These guidelines are discussed in detail in the following sections.

Be Clear About the Limits of Confidentiality

It is ill-advised to promise children that their disclosures will be kept in confidence, as "secrets" between them and the crisis worker. Using developmentally appropriate terms, the crisis worker must be clear about these limits with a child, particularly with younger children who feel helpless and vulnerable around the abuser and who fear retribution.

The crisis counselor should make it clear to the child that secrets cannot be kept if such secrets involve information pertaining to harm at the hands of another person, particularly an adult, on a child. In such cases, the child should know that disclosing this "secret" will result in stopping the abuse and securing assistance from other people to keep the child safe. Being honest in this way with a child, although unsettling as it may be at the time, may eventually lead to trust of the crisis worker and to comfort with the disclosure. The crisis worker should explain in very candid and child-friendly terms the appropriateness of disclosure, as well as the child's right to safety.

Respect the Child's Privacy

Considering the shame, embarrassment, and confusion that accompany the experience of abuse, privacy issues should be respected at all times, and the interview should be conducted in a private setting. Particularly in large settings, such as schools with hundreds of other children around, children might be inclined to deny abuse if they thought that others would learn of the content of an interview. Strangers in school buildings, such as social workers, usually attract interest regarding the purpose of their presence. Securing a private room for an interview is an important first step.

Ideally, in an era when children learn from an early age not to accompany unfamiliar adults to another location, the staff member designated to interview suspected child victims of abuse should be familiar to the child. If not, however, another staff member (teacher, counselor, or administrator, if in a school setting) who is known to the child should serve as a support and should accompany the child for all or part of the interview. Keeping the interview as private as possible while also supporting the child is critical to eliciting the information being sought.

Begin the Interview with Informal Conversation

The interview should begin with general, informal, and nonthreatening subjects before addressing topics related to the suspected abuse. It is very important to maintain an informal tone throughout the interview. For example, if a child is brought to the interview room wearing a sports-related sweatshirt, then a brief, informal conversation about that team or sport might be in order. Even topics such as the weather or a popular television show would suffice as introductory icebreakers to begin an interview.

An air of informality during the initial stage of an interview can go a long way toward easing a nervous child into a more relaxed state, especially if the interviewer called into the situation is a stranger to the child. Picking up cues (a T-shirt logo) allows the interviewer insight into a child's interests or personality style, making it a little easier to communicate on an appropriate and comfortable level. This informal approach, however, would be contraindicated if the child was obviously very upset or agitated. At these times, the crisis worker should address the emotional upset instead and leave the chitchat to another time.

Another way to establish an informal tone in the early stages of an interview is to avoid formal trappings such as clipboards and notepads, as they lend themselves to a more official atmosphere of interrogation and could frighten the child. As the child becomes more comfortable and begins to disclose the abuse to the interviewer, however, it would be appropriate to introduce some note-taking. In a very practical sense, the interviewer's notes provide documentation of the disclosure, which is essential for reporting the abuse to the proper agency. The crisis worker can introduce the whole process of note-taking very easily by explaining to the child that she has to write things down to help her remember them later.

Maintain a Calm Demeanor

Be careful to inhibit any reactions of extreme disgust, anger, or shock in order to avoid alarming the child, particularly in cases of child sexual abuse. If the child senses that the interviewer is the least bit squeamish about the details being shared, then the child will cease disclosing additional details, and the interview would be seriously compromised. The child would also begin to personalize the sense of disgust exhibited by the interviewer, resulting in feelings of shame and self-blame. Keeping a steady, nonjudgmental approach to the interview process is key. Recoiling at the explicit details of abuse puts children on the alert and could lead to premature termination of disclosures.

Use Good Listening and Child-Oriented Communication Skills

Attend carefully to what the child is saying, while at the same time noting those nonverbal cues that the child is sending. It is essential that the interviewer not interrupt the child while he or she is speaking, nor ask too many questions in rapid-fire succession in the manner of a formal interrogation. Children require time to process the information requested and to compose a truthful, if at first guarded, response. The crisis worker must be prepared to allow this time for the child to tell the story at his or her own pace. The crisis worker also must be able to tolerate periods of silence during such a trying interview.

Open-ended questions rather than closed-ended ones should be the primary type utilized (for a discussion of the two question types, see chapter 2). The former (i.e., Can you tell me what happened next? What did your father say to you when he took out his belt?) facilitates disclosure more than the latter. Closed-ended questions that can be answered either "yes" or "no" tend to be barriers to communication and can shut down the flow of information. They may also lead the child, rather than let the child lead through disclosure. Fact-seeking closed-ended questions also have their place in such an interview, but they are more appropriate for the end of the interview when information simply has to be clarified (i.e., What is the name of the teacher you first told about this?).

Validate the Child's Feelings

Rather than making random guesses at how a child feels about the reported abuse or telling the child how to feel, the crisis worker is best advised to validate how the child feels by reflecting back to the child those feelings that are apparent in the verbal and nonverbal statements. Children, like adults, bring to their experiences of trauma their own personal histories, their personality attributes, differing levels of resilience, and their own ways of perceiving and experiencing the world. Since the contexts in which children live vary from child to child, it is best for the crisis worker not to make assumptions about what the child must be feeling, but rather to make observations that serve as feedback to the child. Responding to tears or to awkward silences with comments such as, "I know how hard it is to talk about it when you're so sad" can go a long way toward reassuring a child unsure of making a disclosure.

Avoid Questions That Imply Blame or Guilt

In addition to avoiding the use of too many closed-ended questions (see above), the crisis worker also should avoid questions that imply blame or guilt for the child or for behavior during the course of the abuse. Abused children typically are awash in feelings of guilt and self-blame, so all attempts should be made to avoid exacerbating these feelings with poorly worded questions. The use of "why" questions, which tend to require children to justify their actions, is a surefire way of implying guilt. Questions such as "Why didn't you just leave when he came into your room?" (i.e., "It's your fault."), "Why did you wait so long to tell me about this?" (i.e., "Stupid, don't you know you could have gotten help sooner?"), and "Where was your mother when all this was going on?" (i.e., "It's her fault, too, you know!") can easily put children on the defensive by changing the context in which they view abuse, their role in it, or the roles of other people, particularly family members.

In most cases of abuse, the child is quite conflicted over giving up family secrets, angering a parent via the disclosure, or betraying the parents by talking about something that "could get them in trouble." It is typical for the child victim to continue to love the abuser but to want the abuse to stop without losing the relationship with them. Perpetrators also use coercion and threats to keep their victims silent. Therefore, definite steps must be taken to *provide reassurance to the child,* letting the child know that he or she is doing the right thing, despite any or all of the above concerns.

First, it is important that children know that their crisis workers believe them. Despite false allegations that can emerge, particularly in bitter custody disputes or as a result of Parental Alienation Syndrome (Gardner, 1987), it is far more likely that the child is disclosing an actual abuse event. The crisis worker also should communicate to the child the fact that his or her actions were courageous and that the disclosure was a very important step toward remedying the situation. However, it also is just as important that the crisis worker not make promises that he or she may not be able to keep. Reassurances to the child are not guarantees that everything will be fine after the disclosure. In reality, the advocacy and protective resources of CPS will be enacted, but this protocol still does not offer a guarantee that the abuse will cease. The most appropriate "guarantee" to the child should be that he or she did the right thing by disclosing, that the crisis worker will be there to help, and that he or she will not be abandoned.

Tell the Child What Will Happen Next

Finally, when the interview is over, the crisis worker should explain to the child what the next steps in the process will entail. Without making false promises or blind predictions as to what will definitely happen as a result of the disclosure, the crisis worker should simply offer a truthful, objective explanation of what typically happens in the instance of reported child maltreatment. This explanation should include information about the involvement of a CPS individual (i.e., counselor, social worker), that individual's role in interviewing the child and other family members, and the possible outcomes from the disclosure. The child's questions regarding the possible involvement of law enforcement with the abuser, the impact on the child ("Will they take me out of my house?"), and a variety of other developmentally appropriate concerns must be answered in truthful, objective terms, depending upon the elements of the disclosure. Generally, the messages that should be communicated clearly to the child through this process are simple:

- Children are entitled to be safe and not to be hurt.
- Children shouldn't have to be afraid to go home.
- Adults, even parents, are not permitted to hurt children.
- Abuse is not the child's fault.
- A child will not get into trouble for telling someone about abuse.
- Hitting is not the right way for parents to punish bad behavior.
- There are ways that counselors and other people can help parents so that they will stop doing hurtful things.
- The goal of the involvement of CPS is to help the family.

Documentation of the crisis worker's interview is essential. Although formalized note-taking should be avoided (see previous discussion) throughout the interview, even sketchy notes that can be expanded by the crisis worker after the interview should be kept. CPS will require some degree of detail regarding what already has been disclosed, and accurate notes will facilitate their investigation of the disclosure. The call to CPS should not be delayed once the crisis worker has intervened. If an untrained individual discovers a case of abuse or even has reason to suspect it in the absence of a trained counseling professional, he or she must make the report of the discovery or suspicion directly to CPS.

Crisis Intervention Case Example

Billy was a second grader who had several very disruptive tantrums in school; he would throw himself on the floor, flailing about as he rolled back and forth. After the second such tantrum in as many days, the classroom teacher sought out the counselor for a consultation. The teacher described the circumstances surrounding the tantrums: Billy generally would act in this way until she called for the school principal. Once the principal was able to escort Billy to her office, she then called Billy's mother to come and take him home. However, the teacher noted, as soon as Billy saw his mother enter the principal's office, he stopped his sobbing immediately. The counselor made a visit to Billy's home and learned that Billy's cocaine-addicted father, unemployed again, was beating Billy's mother. Billy, a regular target of his father's violence, had apparently learned that the best way to keep his mother safe was to behave in such a way that she would be summoned to school, thus escaping her husband's wrath, if only for a few hours.

The LAPC model of crisis intervention provides a template for evaluating this case and incorporates the recommendations discussed in this chapter. Refer to the LAPC worksheet that a counselor working with Billy may have completed for an analysis of Billy's case.

LISTEN	ASSESS	PLAN	COMMIT

Name: *Billy* Age *7*

LISTEN

What is the client saying about the crisis? *Billy fears for his own safety as well as that of his mother. Out of depression and terror, he devised a plan, albeit maladaptive, to keep his mother safe and to draw in other resources to help with the crisis.*

What happened? *Physical abuse of multiple family members.*

When did it happen? *Repeatedly when father abuses drugs.*

What type of crisis was it? (Traumatic event, Developmental, Psychiatric, Existential?) *Traumatic event (continuing) and psychiatric.*

Did the client mention anything that indicated danger? *Yes. Billy feared for his safety and his mother's.*

Other relevant information about the crisis? *Younger sister is another silent victim in this family.*

ASSESS

Feelings: Is the client's predominant emotional state one of:

Anger *Yes*   Sadness *Yes*   Hopelessness *Yes*

Anxiety *Yes*   Panic *Yes*   Numbness *Yes*

Suicidal? If yes, complete lethality assessment/suicide: *No*

Homicidal? If yes, complete lethality assessment/violence: *No*

Acting: Is the client's behavior:

Active/Restless *Yes*   Consistent with mood *Yes*

Passive/withdrawn *No*   Good eye contact *No*

Thinking: Is the client:

Logical/making sense *Yes*   Coherent/expressing self well *Yes*

Insightful *No*   Focused on topic *Yes*

Evasive/changing subject *Yes*

Other: Any medical problems? *No*

Physical limitations? *No*

Hospitalizations? *No*

Need for Hospitalization? *Hospitalization for family may be needed due to the abuse and for father for addiction.*

(Continues)

PLAN

What needs to be done now? *CPS notified to provide safety for mother and children. Father removed from home. Police notified. Domestic violence shelter called.*

What alternative plans have been discussed? *Temporary residence set up with relative or CPS-arranged shelter.*

Are these plans reasonable? *Yes*

Can they be carried out? *Yes, using other community resources.*

COMMIT

Which plan of action has the client chosen? *Remain in home with father removed via restraining order.*

Are there resources/support to implement the plan? *Yes*

Is the client motivated to implement the plan? *Yes*

What other resources/support may be needed?

Friend *Yes*   Family member *Yes*

Neighbor *Yes*   Mental health provider *Yes*

Public agency (law enforcement, child protective services, social services) *Yes*

Medical (hospitalization, medication) *Yes*

SOURCES OF CHAPTER ENRICHMENT

Print Sources

Crosson-Tower, C. (2001). *Understanding child abuse and neglect* (5th ed.). New York: Allyn & Bacon.

Garbarino, J. & Eckenrode, J. (1998). *Understanding abusive families: An ecological approach to theory and practice.* New York: Jossey-Bass.

Hefler, M., Kempe, R., & Krugman, R. (1999). *The battered child* (5th ed.). Chicago: University of Chicago Press.

Kincaid, J. (1998). *Erotic innocence: The culture of child molesting.* Durham, SC: Duke University Press.

Lowenthal, B. (2001). *Abuse and neglect: The educator's guide to the identification and prevention of child abuse.* Baltimore: Paul H. Brookes Publishing.

Pelzer, D. (1995). *A child called "it": One child's courage to survive.* Deerfield Beach, FL: Health Communications.

Pelzer, D. (1997) *The lost boy: A foster child's search for the love of a family.* Deerfield Beach, FL: Health Communications.

Pelzer, D. (1999). *A man named Dave: A story of triumph and forgiveness*. New York: Dutton.

Somers, S. (1992). *Wednesday's children: Adult survivors of abuse speak out*. New York: Putnam/Healing Vision Publishing.

Internet Sources

National Clearinghouse on Child Abuse and Neglect Information (http://nccanch.acf .hhs.gov/) This site provides access for professionals and others who are seeking information on child abuse and neglect. The Clearinghouse is a service of the Children's Bureau of the Department of Health and Human Services.

Childhelp USA (http://www.childhelpusa.org) A non-profit resource for the treatment and prevention of child abuse, it is one of the oldest and largest national non-profit organizations devoted to these topics. It provides the national child abuse hot line.

Prevent Child Abuse America (http://www.childabuse.org) This group is devoted to building awareness of child abuse and neglect and providing education as well. It is at the forefront of providing leadership to promote and implement prevention efforts.

Child Abuse Prevention Network (http://www.child-abuse.com) The network is another non-profit organization providing prevention, intervention, and therapy services to physically and sexually abused children.

CHAPTER 4

Intimate Partner Violence and Domestic Violence

John and Marie have been married for the past thirteen years. Almost from the beginning of their relationship, John was very critical of Marie. If she made an error in the checkbook, he would call her "stupid" or "retarded." Or he would constantly criticize her appearance. If she tried to look nice for John, he would accuse her of being a "slut." When she put on weight after having their first child, John would refer to her as "the mother cow" or say she looked like "a Mack truck." At first, the name-calling was confined to the home, but John soon began to call Marie names in public or around friends and family members. He would get very jealous if she spent time on the phone with her mother or sister and would go into a rage if she spent any time talking with her girlfriends. John also had threatened to cut the phone line and to take Marie's checkbook and credit cards away from her. Marie felt like a prisoner within her own home and felt that John was constantly beating her down with his temper tantrums and criticisms.

Tiffany and Nick have been living together for three years. They dated for about six months before moving in together, to which Tiffany's mother very much objected. She felt that Nick was "no good" and that there was something about him that she just didn't like. Tiffany felt that no matter who she went out with, he wouldn't be good enough in her mother's eyes. Tiffany and Nick often got into heated arguments, usually about his spending time with friends down at the local sports bar. She felt he was drinking too much and spending too much money on sports gambling. Whenever she confronted Nick, he would go into a tirade and storm around the house, sometimes breaking things. In one of these arguments, Nick punched Tiffany, giving her a black eye, and then stormed out of the house to "cool off." He came back a few hours later with flowers for Tiffany, telling her he was sorry and that it wouldn't happen again. Unfortunately, four weeks later, Nick's teams lost and he lost a lot of money. When he came home Tiffany was angry with him, as they had planned to go over to her mother's house for dinner. She told Nick to pack his things. Instead, he started turning over furniture and then beat Tiffany up, yelling, "No one is going to tell me what to do!"

E ach of the cases described on the previous page represents a different aspect of intimate partner violence or domestic violence. The case of Tiffany and Nick illustrates the physical violence that most people associate with domestic abuse. John and Marie's relationship is illustrative of the devastating impact of verbal and emotional abuse, which often accompanies physical battering and can be just as damaging as physical abuse. One client described this most accurately by stating, "At least when I got physically beat by my boyfriend, I knew when the beating would be over, but the yelling, screaming, verbal abuse, and threats were never ending." Furthermore, emotional abuse is often the precursor to physical abuse.

The terms *intimate partner violence* and *domestic violence* are often used interchangeably. Although domestic violence had been the preferred term, it was limiting in that it was often associated with physical abuse between married individuals. Intimate partner violence is more inclusive, taking into account nonmarital partner violence—in dating relationships, couples that live together, violence between siblings, violence between parents and adult sons or daughters, and violence in gay and lesbian love relationships. Although the majority of intimate partner violence involves male against female aggression, there are many instances of female abusers. Usually, these cases go unreported because men are reluctant and often embarrassed to report these incidents to the police. Violence can also erupt between roommates as in male-to-male or female-to-female violence.

In this chapter, various terms associated with intimate partner violence/domestic violence will be defined and statistics that describe the prevalence of domestic violence in the United States will be presented. Theories of domestic violence, including explanations for the prevalence of intimate partner violence in our country, will also be presented, as will the psychological characteristics that are common to batterers and their victims. Finally, various types of interventions for both batterers and their victims will be discussed.

Scope of the Problem

Domestic violence, specifically spousal or partner abuse, is a major societal problem in the United States. Estimates (U.S. Department of Justice, 1998) indicate that from 1993 through 1996, there was a decline in the number of violent victimizations by an intimate partner. However, on average from 1992 through 1996, it is estimated that 960,000 violent victimizations of women occurred each year. Estimates of the American Medical Association (1991) suggest that domestic violence injures more women than car accidents, muggings, and rapes combined. The problem of intimate violence has immense proportions with far-reaching implications that have been well documented in past and current literature (Dutton, 1996, 1998; Jacobson & Gottman, 1998; Walker, 1994a, 2000). Not only is there often lasting psychological damage to the victim (Herman, 1997; Miller, 1994; van der Kolk, McFarlane, & Weisaeth, 1996), but rates of recidivism suggest ongoing unresolved problems for both batterers and their victims (Lachkar, 1998; Simpson and Rholes, 1998; Stosny, 1995). Furthermore, intimate partner violence can have serious effects on children, both in terms of immediate concurrent emotional problems and in terms of "sleeper effects," replicating modeled violence in future relationships (Dutton 1995; Smith & Williams, 1992). The societal costs are tremendous when one considers the medical costs, judicial costs, time spent by police officers in providing initial intervention, the need for battered women's shelters, counseling programs, and similar related expenses.

Retaliatory violence—when battered partners seek to stop the abuse through violent measures—is also common. This type of violence was the subject of *The Burning Bed* (1995), a movie based on the true story of Francine Hughes who, after suffering repeated instances of severe physical abuse by her husband, finally killed him by pouring kerosene on his bed and setting him on fire (Edwards, 1989).

Often the terms *battering, abuse,* and *assault* are misused interchangeably. Battering is most frequently used to denote forms of physical violence, such as actual injuries, but also can include the coercive control that so often entraps the victim of battering in the relationship. Young and Long (1998) define *battering* as

> a pattern of behavior in which one person establishes power and control over another person through fear and intimidation, often including the threat or use of violence. Battering occurs when batterers believe they are entitled to control their partners. Battering includes emotional abuse, economic abuse, sexual abuse, manipulation of children, exercise of male privilege, intimidation, isolation, and a variety of other behaviors designed to maintain fear, intimidation, and power. (p. 188)

The term *abuse* includes physical violence, such as hitting, punching, kicking, and slapping, but also includes both emotional and verbal abuse. In contrast, *assault* is a legal term for which there are usually two subtypes: simple assault and aggravated assault. Assault is defined as the intentional inflicting of injury on another person (U.S. Department of Justice, 2000). As indicated previously, assault is the most common form of intimate partner violence, but other forms of partner violence include rape, sexual assault, robbery, and verbal threats to inflict harm on the other person, all of which are criminal offenses. It is especially noteworthy that only about half of the incidents of intimate partner violence get reported to the police.

In instances of physical battery, the abused partner may seek a temporary restraining order (TRO) against the batterer. Most states have laws that allow for temporary restraining orders. Once a judge issues a TRO, the batterer must leave the premises where the victim resides and cannot have any face-to-face, written, or phone contact with the victim. Many abuse victims worry that requesting a TRO will lead to retaliation by the batterer, which unfortunately does happen. In most states, however, if a police officer witnesses signs of physical abuse (such as a black eye, bruises, etc.), he or she can make an arrest and a TRO would then be issued by the municipal court judge. (There has been a great deal of controversy over whether police should have the right to make an arrest if the victim does not wish to make a formal complaint.) Once a TRO is issued however, the battered partner must appear before a judge, at which point the restraining order is made permanent or the complainant may decided to drop or vacate the restraining order. Prior research suggests that there are few demographic differences between those victims who drop restraining orders versus those who make them permanent (Klein, 1996). The exception is that having requested restraining orders in the past is a predictor of those who elect to make a restraining order permanent.

Once a permanent restraining order is granted by the court, the batterer will then usually be referred to a treatment program for batterers (either inpatient or outpatient). Stark (1996) noted that when offender arrest is combined with treatment, batterers were 10 times less likely to be recidivists. Dutton (1996) found similar results in his research. This suggests that treatment combined with legal mandate can be effective in preventing future instances of intimate partner violence. While legal sanctions, such as restraining orders, are necessary, they do not provide batterers with strategies for changing their behavior, nor are they a guarantee that batterers won't become abusive again in the future.

Emotional and verbal abuse is an important aspect of intimate partner violence that often gets overlooked. Prior research has shown that emotional abuse is always part of the physical abuse cycle, whether as part of the escalation stage (Campbell, 1993; Jacobson & Gottman, 1998) or as a replacement for physical abuse when the abuser wants to avoid re-arrest (upon realization that arrests are not made for verbal abusive). It has been hypothesized that many offenders initiate control over their victims first through verbal or emotional means (psychological abuse), which can take many forms. Examples include such behaviors as intimidation (e.g., screaming at or insulting the victim, shaming the victim in public), terrorizing (e.g., harassing the victim at work), and controlling the victim's freedom (e.g., preventing the victim from going to work, stopping the victim from using the car or the phone) (Evans, 1992). Verbal and emotional abuse are powerful domination tactics because they carry the threat of physical violence (Jacobson & Gottman, 1998). Emotional abuse is undoubtedly a potent form of battering, perhaps being more devastating in some instances than physical abuse, leaving invisible bruises and scars while "eating away at ... self esteem, sucking the lifeblood of ... selfhood, painfully diminishing, then devouring it" (Lachkar, 1998, p. xi).

The Battered Woman

The research literature indicates that there are some characteristics common to women who are victimized by verbal, emotional, or physical abuse. We feel it is important to discuss these characteristics because in crisis intervention situations, intimate partner abuse is not always readily identified and many battered women are too afraid to discuss the battering with the crisis counselor. Therefore, it is important that counselors know how to identify individuals that may be at risk of experiencing abuse. We are sensitive to the fact, however, that in discussing common characteristics it is important not to stereotype women who have been battered. The danger in creating a stereotype is that crisis intervention professionals may miss the battering that created the crisis. For example, if counselors think of battering as occurring more frequently in lower socioeconomic status relationships, then they may miss identifying abuse in higher socioeconomic status relationships.

As indicated previously, one of the most common characteristics found in battered women was that they grew up in homes where they were abused physically or sexually by their parents or their parents' significant others (Walker, 2000). In keeping with Learning Theory, Walker hypothesized that these women "learned" that when someone loves you they have the right to physically hurt you. Sixty-seven percent of Walker's sample had been physically abused, while 48% had been victims of childhood sexual abuse.

Rosewater (1982; 1985a; 1985b) concluded that it could be quite easy to misdiagnose a battered woman as having a psychiatric disorder, thereby missing the fact that the symptoms she is presenting are brought about by trying to cope with the trauma of abuse. Walker (1994a) also warned mental health professionals to refrain from rendering a Personality Disorder diagnosis on a battered woman until she has been in therapy for a minimum of at least six months. What was surprising in Walker's (2000) study of battered women utilizing other psychological measures is that they did not demonstrate consistent patterns of low self-esteem, depression, or an external locus of control (i.e., feeling that they are not in control of their own destiny, or are being controlled by luck, chance, or other external factors). Walker (2000) concluded "... our sample of battered women was not consistent in demonstrating the negative cognition and moods we would have expected" (p. 112). She points out that the impact of trauma can often be affected by the time of the trauma, by the victim's own coping resources and resilience, her level of stress response, and whether she receives any support from friends, family, and the community.

Kanel (1999) identified three components to the battered woman's syndrome that are similar to those described by Walker (2000):

1. *Posttraumatic Stress Disorder symptoms.* Because violence is traumatic and outside of the range of normal human experience, the woman begins to develop several symptoms of PTSD. The trauma of intimate partner abuse may result in nightmares, numbing of feelings, avoidance of situations or any conflict that may be associated with victimization trauma, detachment, loss of interest, increased anxiety, and difficulty falling asleep.

2. *Learned helplessness.* This develops as a result of attempting to leave or escape the abuse, but having no success. Here, the abused partner learns to survive rather than try to escape the battering.

3. *Self-destructive coping response to violence.* The abused partner, believing that there are no alternatives, may begin to act self-destructively by abusing drugs or alcohol or attempting suicide.

For someone who has not worked with battered partners or has not experienced physical, emotional, verbal, or psychological abuse, the question often arises, "Why does she stay in the relationship? Why doesn't she just leave?" To an outside observer, leaving may seem like a simple, rational, and reasonable thing to do; however, for the victim who is caught in the web of intimate partner violence, leaving may be anything but simple, rational, or reasonable. The explanations as to why abused partners stay have been implied thus far. For example, a woman who is experiencing the impact of PTSD symptoms or is experiencing learned helplessness feels immobilized, depressed, numb, hopeless, and helpless, and is not in any emotional condition to leave the relationship. Another important factor is that batterers are often quite adept at convincing their partners that they are worthless and that no one else would want them and at striping them of their dignity, their sense of self-worth, and self-esteem. Intimate partner violence is, in effect, brainwashing. In militaristic terms, in order to brainwash captured prisoners, you must constantly exert total control over their lives, threatening to kill them one minute, while treating them kindly or benevolently the next. The prisoners never know what to expect and they never know how their captors will act towards them. Prisoners often break under the strain of unpredictability. So, too, do abused partners experience the same unpredictability from their battering companions.

There are many other reasons why women stay. The following are some of the reasons offered by Kanel (1999):

- religious beliefs forbid her from leaving the marriage ('til death do us part);
- the children need a father;
- fear of retaliation or that he'll kill the children, pets, or other family members;
- lack of financial resources (no transportation, no money, no place to live);
- hopes that he will change;
- insecurity and feeling unable to take care of herself;
- fears of being alone; and
- influences by pro-family societal messages (keep the family together at all costs).

Denial can certainly be added to this list, as many abused partners will stay while rationalizing that the abuse is "not that bad," or that the abuser will change eventually.

Characteristics Common to Batterers

With regard to the psychological profile of men who are abusers, prior research in this area has suggested that these perpetrators tend to be a rather heterogeneous group. However, the research literature suggests that there appear to be particular subtypes of batterers sharing common characteristics. In some of the initial attempts to determine whether subtypes of male batterers exist, Hamberger and Hastings (1986) administered the Millon Clinical Multiaxial Inventory to 99 men in treatment for wife assault. They found three subtypes.

1. *Schizoid/borderline.* This type of batterer is described as being moody and sensitive to any interpersonal criticism, having a "Jekyll and Hyde" type of personality—cool and calm one minute, angry and full of rage the next. (These descriptions seem to coincide with what the *DSM IV* refers to as a Borderline Personality Disorder.)

2. *Narcissistic/antisocial.* This type of batterer is described as being very self-centered, out for himself, and cold and calculating in his violence towards his partner. The narcissistic/antisocial's violence is described as being more "instrumental" in nature, meaning that he uses intimidation, threats, and violence in a calculated way, not as impulsively as some batterers.

3. *Passive-dependent/compulsive.* Described as being passive, but also rigid and tense, the passive-dependent/compulsive tends to want things his way, and only his way. Yet because of their dependency they tend to be insecure and jealous.

From an extensive research project with severely violent couples, Jacobson and Gottman (1998) discovered that not only are personality disorders critical to understanding differences in batterers, but that these correlate with physiological differences. These researchers identified two abusive styles: the "cobra" and the "pitbull." Cobras show evidence of antisocial, criminal traits, which are generally also evident in other settings and relationships, not only manifested in the intimate relationship. Furthermore, cobras tend to act in a more sadistic way. Physiologically they become calmer as their violence escalates, similar to a cobra that focuses with clear attention on its victim before striking. This appears to relate to their cold, remorseless, and independent styles. This type of abuser was well-portrayed in the movie, *Sleeping With the Enemy,* in which the husband played a cold, calculating batterer.

Pitbulls, on the other hand, manifest less severe violent tendencies, which tend to manifest only in the intimate partner relationship. Physiologically, their biological markers, such as blood pressure, escalate as their violence does. Psychologically, they tend to be more insecure and dependent, fearing abandonment; when they become calm, they will usually express remorse. The name "pitbull" is derived from the idea that these abusers may always be "in your face"—yelling, screaming, and making threatening gestures. However, they may not always act viciously. As with the animal, pitbulls may attack only when they feel most threatened, insecure, or when they feel cornered (Jacobson & Gottman, 1998).

Prior literature indicates that male batterers tend to manifest Axis II personality disorders, perhaps more often than Axis I clinical disorders. Those

Axis II personality disorders most often found in abusive men are Narcissistic Personality Disorder (Hamberger & Hastings, 1986), Antisocial Personality Disorder (Bernard & Bernard, 1984), and Borderline Personality Disorder (Hamberger & Hastings, 1986). Table 4.1 lists some of the common characteristics of various types of male batterers.

Anger styles (experiential and expressive) in both the perpetrators and victims of violence need to be a critical focus of study and treatment (Kassinove,

TABLE 4.1
Common Characteristics of Batterers

Characteristics of the Overcontrolled Batterer

- Flat affect of constantly cheerful persona
- Attempts to ingratiate the therapist
- Tries to *avoid* conflict
- High masked dependency
- High social desirability
- Overlap of violence and alcohol abuse
- Some drunk driving arrests
- Lists "irritations" in anger diary
- Chronic resentment
- Attachment: preoccupied
- MCMI: avoidant, dependent, passive-aggressive

Characteristics of Impulsive/Undercontrolled Batterers

- Cyclical "phases"
- High levels of jealousy
- Violence predominantly/exclusively in intimate relationship
- High levels of depression, dysphoria, anxiety-based rage
- Ambivalence towards wife/partner
- Attachment: fearful/angry
- MCMI: Borderline

Characteristics of the Instrumental/Undercontrolled Batterer

- Violent inside and outside the home
- History of antisocial behavior (car theft, burglary, violence)
- High acceptance of violence
- Negative attitudes of violence (macho)
- Usually victimized by extreme physical abuse as a child
- Low empathy
- Associations with criminal marginal subculture
- Attachment: dismissing
- MCMI: antisocial, aggressive-sadistic

Note. From *The Abusive Personality* (pp. 9–10), by D. Dutton, 1998, New York, Guilford Press. Reprinted with permission.

1995). Much of the recent literature argues that abuser patterns relate to deficits in how anger is perceived and controlled (Eckhardt, Barbour, & Davison, 1998). In addition these deficits relate to personality/attachment variables (Dutton, 1995, 1998) and alcohol use (Richards, 1993). Similarly, anger style in the victim is central to systemic treatment models. Victim anger has been shown to relate to the paradox of the victim staying in an abusive relationship in what has been referred to as a fugue state (Evans, 1992; Lachkar, 1998; van der Kolk et al., 1996). Interestingly, PTSD has also been seen as important in the background of the perpetrator (Dutton, 1998; Stosny, 1995; van der Kolk et al., 1996).

There have also been links between spousal abuse (both emotional abuse and physical abuse) and alcoholism/drug addiction. Schuerger and Reigle (1988), for example, noted that within a sample of 250 men enrolled in a group treatment program for spouse abuse, alcoholism, drug abuse, and violence within the family of origin were highly prevalent. Fitch and Papantonio (1983) also found family of origin violence, as well as alcoholism, drug abuse, and economic stress, to be highly correlated with spousal abuse. Labell (1972) noted that 72% of abused women who sought shelter services reported that their mates had a drinking problem. In a survey of 500 cases of women calling a hotline for abused women, Lehmann and Krupp (1984) found that 55% said their husbands had become abusive after drinking. However, they went on to conclude that, although the association between domestic violence and alcoholism is clear, "most existing research supports the conclusion that alcohol abuse does not cause domestic violence."

Alcohol has also been shown to increase a man's preoccupation with control and tendency to over-interpret cues as maliciously intended, which is part of the escalation phase in abusive interactions (Campbell, 1993). Also, alcohol has been noted as an emotion-regulator, especially in the absence of healthy attachment-related working models with their affect modulation and balance deficits (Feeney & Noller, 1996). The research within this area points to the fact that men who drink or abuse drugs are certainly at higher risk to be abusive to their spouses; however, not all men who have drinking problems abuse their spouses. Also, it is important to note that there are men who are abusive to their spouses who do not have drinking problems. Therefore, although alcohol and drug abuse are correlated with partner abuse, they are not necessary pre-conditions for abuse to occur.

The Cycle of Violence

Much of the literature pertaining to partner violence points to a pattern of abuse that tends to be cyclical, rather than random or constant. The Walker Cycle Theory of Violence (Walker, 1980) indicates that there are usually three phases in the partner violence sequence: tension building, acute battering, and loving contrition.

1. *The tension-building phase.* The cycle of violence begins with a gradual escalation of tense emotions, as the batterer uses critical or demeaning

remarks, verbal abuse, name calling, and other intentionally intimidating remarks to keep his partner in her place, so to speak. During this phase, the woman may try to placate her partner, agree with him, do things that will please him, do things that will calm him down, or diffuse his anger. Some of these attempts may work momentarily; however, it will not take much for the tension to reappear, and the woman will often continue to try to ignore any hostile verbalizations or behaviors. Eventually, both out of sheer exhaustion and learned helplessness (i.e., "no matter what I try to do, I can't control his anger"), the woman will begin to withdraw from the partner. As she withdraws, he will begin to pursue her more vehemently, at which point the tension may become unbearable and will lead to an incident of battery.

2. *The acute battering phase.* In this phase, "the batterer typically unleashes a barrage of verbal and physical aggression, that can leave the woman severely shaken and injured" (Walker, 2000, pp. 126–127). It is obvious that this is the phase during which physical injuries take place and the police may be called. This is the pinnacle of the crisis. This phase ends when the battering incident has stopped. The batterer often experiences a reduction in tension and anger, a feeling of calm or relief, which unfortunately only reinforces the violent behavior. The victim is left feeling physically and emotionally bruised, battered, hopeless, and helpless.

3. *The loving contrition phase.* In the final phase of the cycle, the batterer apologizes for his behavior, promises he will never do this type of thing again, and expresses regret or guilt. In some instances, according to Dr. Walker, this phase is also accompanied by a reduction in tension.

Sometimes, however, the cycle ends not in loving contrition, but in murder. Although batterers often murder their partners in the explosive escalation of the acute battering phase, battering lethality is often at its greatest in the aftermath of an abusive incident, especially in the absence of any contrition or remorse. This might occur with "cobra" type batterers, who are incapable of experiencing true remorse. Cobras would also be least affected by the cries or pleas of their abused partners.

Multicultural Considerations

Intimate partner violence does not occur in a vacuum. There are many other factors that need to be taken into consideration when assessing a case of domestic violence. For example, it is important to examine the cultural milieu of the couple. Unfortunately, many cultures support male dominance rather than gender equality. Although in the United States there have been major strides towards gender equality, in many ways the United States is still considered to be a patriarchal culture, as evidenced by the larger proportion of men who are elected to public office or who rise to administrative posts in major corporations. In many households, men make the majority of decisions.

However, a patriarchal culture alone does not necessarily constitute a precursor to domestic violence. When women are viewed as subservient to men, as sexual objects, or as objects to be possessed, then these cultural attitudes are significant contributing factors in increased intimate partner violence.

Although intimate partner violence cuts across all socioeconomic, racial, and religious boundaries, there are some subcultures and societal attitudes that may inadvertently contribute to domestic violence. A crisis worker or police officer who is called to intervene in domestic violence disputes may be running headlong into these cultural issues. For example, in one such case, the police were called by neighbors to a home from which yelling and screaming were heard. The neighbors feared the wife was being beaten. When the police arrived at the scene, the outraged husband was at the door to confront them. He told the police that in his country of origin, women were considered "property," and that the police had neither rights nor jurisdiction to intervene. He demanded that the police leave his property immediately. The officers begged to differ with him, given that he had admitted to physically abusing his wife. In the state where this incident took place, this admission of physical abuse allowed the officers to make an arrest.

Religious factors can also play a role. In religions that consider divorce to be "sinful," an abused spouse may stay in an abusive relationship "for the sake of the children" or to avoid committing a sin. Although more contemporary clergy would not hesitate to recommend a marital separation and/or divorce, some pastoral counselors would advocate that couples try to work on saving their marriages, in spite of the abuse. As will be discussed in the next section, there are many instances in which couples counseling is highly contraindicated for abusive couples. Instead, individual treatment for both partners is considered the treatment of choice, so as not to endanger the battered spouse even further.

Crisis Intervention

Battered women may present for treatment or crisis counseling in a variety of settings. They may first be seen in criminal justice settings by judges or court personnel who may be involved with the legal aspect of the battering situation, such as when the police make an arrest or when the battered spouse applies for a restraining order for protection. Battered partners may seek assistance at a shelter for battered women and their children. Battered spouses may appear in an emergency room with broken bones, a broken nose, bruises, or similar physical trauma. They may also seek help at a mental health clinic for treatment of PTSD symptoms, some other anxiety disorder, depression, or alcohol or drug abuse. It is also possible that battered spouses may seek help from a clergy member with hopes of obtaining marital counseling to help preserve their marriages or with hopes that a priest, minister, or rabbi will admonish the batterer for the abusive behavior. Battered spouses may reach out to other family members or friends for help. They may be seeking financial help, a place to stay, or just emotional support.

Whatever the point of entry into the crisis intervention delivery system, there are certain givens that effective crisis counselors must take into consideration in any of these cases. First, it is probable that the battered woman will not identify her crisis as being one of domestic violence or intimate partner violence. Perhaps the only two exceptions to this are when the battered partner seeks a restraining order from the courts or specifically seeks assistance at a battered women's shelter. In those instances, the woman must have been victim to violent physical abuse or threat of physical harm in order to access those services. Although there may still be evidence of denial as to the nature and extent of the intimate partner abuse (e.g., the woman may still blame herself for her injuries), there is usually less likelihood that the abuse will be denied altogether.

In the other points of entry, the battered partner may deny that her injuries are the result of her partner's abusive, violent behavior. This is not unusual, because the abused partner may be fearful of being discovered. She may fear retaliation, that she will have no place to go, or that she lacks the financial means to support her children. So, it is important that crisis counselors take into account that they may be working with an abused partner who may be in denial about the abusive relationship or who may present with other symptoms that can lead the crisis counselor down the wrong path, assessing the crisis as something other than a domestic violence situation. Klingbeil and Boyd (1984), for example, developed a protocol that can be used in hospital emergency rooms, involving the triage nurse, the physician, and the crisis counselor. Each has a specific role to play. The triage nurse plays a key and vital role in determining whether the woman presenting for treatment may be an abuse victim. Medical records of prior emergency room treatment or hospitalizations are useful in determining if a cycle of violence exists, based upon the type of injuries the victim has sustained. The crisis counselor is then called and his or her role is to initially help calm the battered partner and support her in her decision to seek help. Once this is accomplished, a history of the events leading up to the crisis is taken. Although the focus is on the immediate crisis, it is important to also explore recent abuse incidents. The physician provides medical attention and also fully explains any medical procedures performed and the potential dangers of the medical injuries. The crisis counselor reiterates these dangers in an attempt to head off any denial or minimizing of the abuse that may begin at this point. Permission to take photographs will need to be obtained by either the triage nurse, the physician, or the crisis counselor. Also, if the victim is willing to press charges, the police must be called to take a statement. The next step involves ensuring the safety of the battered spouse. Here, the crisis counselor would work with the victim to determine if there is a safe house of a friend or family member where she can stay or, preferably, if she is willing to enter a battered woman's shelter. Interestingly, there were only seven emergency shelters for battered women in 1974 (Roberts, 1981); however, by 1998 there were more than 2,000 shelters and crisis intervention services for women and their children across the country (Roberts, 1998).

Another guideline for crisis specialists working in a variety of settings with intimate partner abuse victims is that the partners should not be interviewed together. This is suggested for two reasons. First, it is unlikely that the abused partner will give up much information while under the watchful, threatening eye of the abusive partner. In many instances, batterers have coached their abused partners in terms of what and what not to say. Therefore, it is better to conduct a separate interview if the abusive partner is present. The second reason, as mentioned previously, is that counselors should refrain from doing any couples or marital counseling with partners in an abusive relationship. If the batterer has not accepted responsibility for the abuse, the counseling may only serve to place the woman at higher risk for future abuse; she may say "the wrong thing" or reveal too much information. Once abuse is discovered in a relationship, it is a basic tenet of counseling *not* to treat the couple together, but rather to work with the individuals separately. The prevailing theory is that working with the couple together puts the battered partner in too much danger.

Another critical guideline is to ensure the safety of battered partner. No matter what the setting, it is imperative that the crisis worker has explored every possible alternative for ensuring that the battered partner cannot be re-victimized. This usually means that legal charges are brought against the batterer and that the abused partner has a safe place to go, preferably one that the batterer is unaware of or does not have access to. Just as locks are only effective with honest people, so too do restraining orders have their limitations if not effectively enforced. The police cannot be in all places at all times. Often, the batterer will defy a restraining order and will try to establish phone contact with his partner in order to talk her into dropping the restraining order. Although restraining orders mandate that there is to be no phone or written contact, this aspect of the court order cannot be enforced if the abused partner falls unwittingly into the trap of the abuser (e.g., "See you broke the law by taking my call, you're as guilty as I am"). Some treatment providers and those working in shelters for battered women feel that a restraining order can sometimes be a "red flag," which the batterer perceives as a challenge to his masculinity. It is important to take collaborative steps in order to help ensure the battered partner's safety. Although it is difficult to predict future violence, in order to assess the immediate danger that the battered partner may be in, it is important to take into account her partner's frequency and severity of violence, frequency of intoxication and drug use, threats to kill, threats to harm the children, his access to weapons, current stressors in his and her life, his attitudes towards violence, any reports of psychiatric impairment, his forced sexual acts against her, and her suicide threats or prior attempts (Sonkin & Durphy, 1993; Walker, 1994b). In instances where future violence appears to be imminent, the crisis counselor may need to take a stronger stance in trying to get the abused partner to a safe haven, such as a domestic violence shelter. If children are involved in the abuse, then some states mandate that child abuse be reported to the state child protective agency. If the abused partner refuses a safe haven, then a safety plan should be discussed. This will be described later in this section.

Another basic guideline of crisis counseling is that counselors should not judge, preach, or blame. Nor should they force the victim into choosing a course of action with which she cannot or will not follow through. It is important that the crisis counselor convey acceptance. Since most abused partners often understate their cases, it is also important that counselors believe what they say and that questions pertaining to the abuse not imply disbelief or a lack of understanding. The battered partner must trust the counselor and also believe that this trust will not be betrayed.

Survivor Therapy with Battered Women

Walker (1994b) outlined five states of treatment with battered woman, which she calls "survivor therapy." It should be noted that Stages I and II are often the focus of crisis intervention with battered woman, whereas Stages III, IV, and V would be addressed in ongoing treatment, usually over the course of several weeks or months. The stages are as follows.

STAGE I: ASSESSMENT AND LABELING OF THE ABUSE In Stage I, complete assessment of the abuse and of the battered woman occurs. This assessment combines both traditional methods of evaluation and data gathering, as well as educational histories, job and medical histories, and other relevant information. Open-ended questions are suggested as a means of helping to elicit information more spontaneously. Walker advocates using the "Four Incident Technique" for gathering abuse history information. Here, the battered partner is asked to recall four specific incidents: the first abusive incident or the first she can recall, the most recent incident, the worst incident or one of the worst, and a typical incident. If she has difficulty recalling a first incident, she might be asked to talk about one of the first incidents she can recall.

Other important areas of focus in gathering information would be childhood history, adult relationship history, support networks (family and friends), medical history, and alcohol and drug use history. In reviewing childhood history, for example, it is important to focus on anything that may reveal whether the victim or perpetrator experienced or witnessed abuse in their homes during childhood or adolescence. Psychological testing may provide an additional source of information as well.

Walker feels it is important that the abuse be labeled as such in order to present the reality of the situation to the battered partner. While labeling the abuse is important, Dr. Walker will refrain from criticizing or verbally denigrating the batterer. Doing so will usually elicit defense reactions from the battered partner. Walker will often ask the battered partner to describe some positive characteristics about the batterer in order to lessen the likelihood that the battered partner will defend the batterer.

STAGE II: HELPING THE WOMAN GET SAFE During this stage, a safety plan is discussed. Here the battered partner is asked to consider what she would do and where she would go should she see her mate's anger or resentment begin to escalate. The battered partner is asked to come up with a plan for getting out, including where she would go and what she would take. Some partners will keep a packed suitcase in the hall closet that they can grab in the event that they need to make a quick getaway.

STAGE III: DEALING WITH THE TRAUMA EFFECTS Counselors begin the therapeutic work of helping the partner to begin to deal emotionally with the abusive incidents in Stage III. Battered partners often blame themselves for the abusive incidents and will feel at fault for not being better lovers, partners, or spouses. The goal in this stage is to help the battered partner to begin to see how emotionally they have been impacted by the abusive incidents. It is important for the counselor to ask the battered partner about her feelings in different situations. Feelings of guilt, low self-esteem, self-deprecation, and over-responsibility are all quite common. Counseling in this stage focuses on helping the battered partner to begin to understand her feelings as a means of facilitating the healing process.

STAGE IV: DEALING WITH OTHER PSYCHOLOGICAL EFFECTS OF THE ABUSE AND UNDERLYING ISSUES In Stage IV, other psychological effects and related issues are dealt with. For example, at this juncture the counselor can begin a more in-depth exploration of family of origin issues, childhood trauma, the emotions associated with having experienced or witnessed trauma, and coping responses to these various issues. It is very important to listen for previous methods of coping, as these may provide helpful clues to assist in empowering the battered partner. Naturally, a woman who experiences a sense of learned helplessness will have more therapeutic work to do before she can begin to feel a sense of empowerment.

STAGE V: PREPARATION FOR TERMINATION In Stage V, the counselor and client begin the process of preparing for termination, which includes a summation of the work that has taken place and an exploration of future directions. It is important to remember that the majority of battered partners do not become re-involved with batterers, as was once assumed. If anything, according to Walker, these women are often sensitized to behaviors that are suggestive of battering, such as difficulty in controlling temper, alcohol or drug abuse, sexual jealousy, and a prior history of stormy or conflictual relationships.

Programs for Batterers

In the midst of an intimate partner violence crisis, the batterer is more than likely to focus his attention on issues of finances, food, and shelter, and often will place blame on the partner for his arrest. The crisis counselor who is dealing with a batterer at this point will often be dealing with his outrage concerning the arrest or having been put out of the house. He will often blame his partner for his loss of control of his temper or will accuse his partner of "pushing his buttons." The goal of the crisis intervention worker is to address the batterer's outrage and to assess whether further abuse is possible (e.g., the batterer verbalizes a plan to seek retaliation against his partner). If so, the crisis worker may need to report any threats to the police and to the potential victim.

Once the batterer is in a counseling program, the goal is to shift the focus back onto the batterer and the behaviors that resulted in the arrest. Programs for batterers are offered in prisons, jails, or as part of outpatient court-mandated programs. Many of these programs are designed to work with batterers in phases or stages. For example, the first stage usually focuses on defining and labeling the abuse. This is a necessary precursor to encouraging batterers to begin to take responsibility for their actions. This stage may take place over the course of several sessions and consists of both education on verbal, emotional, and physical abuse and experiential group process, whereby batterers are encouraged to identify and relate to the information they are receiving. The next stage would focus on breaking through or confronting areas of denial, including batterers blaming their partners or external factors for the abuse. In order for change to take place, batterers must admit that they have a problem. The third stage focuses on assisting batterers with the development of new tools and strategies for managing their anger, developing alternatives to verbal, physical, or emotional abuse.

Many programs for batterers will offer both stress management and anger management. It is interesting to note, however, that studies have not made a strong connection between external stress and battering (Hotaling & Sugarman, 1986). In anger management training, the goal is to help batterers to gain control over feelings of anger and in doing so, to refrain from acting on these feelings. The assumption is that by reducing or managing anger better or by learning assertiveness skills, batterers will be in better control of their emotions and will then be less likely to abuse their partners.

Many batterers (and unfortunately, therapists and lay people) operate on the myth that it is better to vent anger than to bottle it up. Unfortunately, venting often leads to an escalation of angry feelings, in which case, venting may not be the best alternative. On the other hand, suppressing anger is also not a very good alternative, because eventually the feelings may reach explosive proportions, very much like a cork in a champagne bottle that is constantly being shaken. The most viable alternative is assertiveness training, through which batterers may be taught to make "I" statements rather than "You did..." or "You should have..." statements. Blaming or accusations usually only result in an escalation of anger and resentments. This is where the tension building stage described previously begins to build and build.

The caveat to this approach with batterers is the uncertainty of whether the work done in the sessions will generalize to their intimate partner relationships. There are several factors that need to be considered when making this prediction: (a) Does the batterer engage in regular drug or alcohol use? (b) Does the batterer have an extensive history or past violent history towards partners and non-familial individuals? (c) Is there an absence of guilt or remorse for the battering incidents? (d) Does the batterer have any other criminal history? (e) Does the batterer exhibit sexual jealousy? If the answer to these questions is yes, then the likelihood of successful generalization is not very good. As discussed previously, most programs advocate a separate approach in treating the abused partner and the batterer, rather than to attempt some type of couples therapy.

In any of the programs described above, usually a thorough assessment at intake will be the first step. Intake may range from one to four sessions (Saunders & Hanusa, 1986). Although the bulk of the assessment usually takes place in the first session, it is common for additional information to be gathered in subsequent sessions. An assessment with a male batterer must address a number of issues. Naturally, it is important to gather a thorough description of the abuse, including the frequency, severity, and chronicity of abuse. It is also important to assess individual characteristics and environmental factors. Individual characteristics are important to assess in terms of whether the batterer being evaluated has personality characteristics that match with more severe types of batterers or recidivists, such as those described earlier in this chapter. Also, it is very important to perform a violence risk assessment. For example, risk of future violence is greatly increased when the batterer has a past history, which is indicative of ever-escalating violent behavior with intimate partners and others. The risk is further increased when alcohol and drug abuse are present or when there is a history of psychiatric disturbance, such as paranoid ideation. Naturally, when either implicit or explicit threats of violence have been verbalized or written or when the intimate partner fears that the batterer cannot maintain control of his anger, there is increased risk. The presence or availability of weapons to carry out threats of violence make for a highly risky situation. Assessing the level and type of denial is also of utmost importance in performing a risk assessment. Men who batter often minimize or rationalize their behavior (e.g., "I only hit her once" or "She only had a slight bruise" or " I only grabbed her to calm her down"). Often, the abuse was actually more severe and terrifying than the batterer is willing to admit. In the most extreme cases of denial, the batterer may outright deny that any abuse took place at all, claiming that it was all a figment of the victim's imagination or that the victim fabricated the whole incident just to get him out of the house. In other instances, the man may blame his partner (e.g., "If she hadn't gotten in my face, I wouldn't have overreacted" or "she goaded me into it"). It is also common for the batterer to place blame on external factors, such as alcohol or drug abuse or work stress. The level of denial and willingness to accept responsibility is usually predictive of success in treatment. The batterer in total denial is not a very good treatment candidate and is at high risk for recidivism. One of the goals of any treatment program is to confront this denial in such a way that the batterer can begin to accept responsibility for his actions.

Naturally, any one of the aforementioned risk factors are significant and should not be ignored. However, when several risk factors are present, the risk of violence is even greater. See Table 4.2, in which Edleson and Tolman (1992) provide a helpful outline for issues to be addressed in an assessment with a male batterer.

In conducting an assessment with a batterer, it is important that it not be conducted like an interrogation, but rather as the beginning of a working relationship between the practitioner and the client. Therefore, the clinician should not badger the client, accuse him of lying, or try to trip him up by producing third party evidence of the abuse (Edleson & Tolman, 1992). The therapeutic relationship must balance confrontation and support. At the same time, the therapist must be able to set firm limits without being punitive. The assessment information can be used to help the batterer see how dysfunctional and hurtful his behavior is to himself, his partner, and his children. However, it is also of utmost importance that any information gathered from the abused partner not be used in the assessment. This might inadvertently set up a hostile retaliation. It is for this same reason that the abused partner is not present at the time of the assessment. Instead, the information obtained from the

TABLE 4.2
Issues to Be Addressed in the Assessment of a Male Batterer

Nature of Abuse:

- frequency
- chronicity
- severity
- types (e.g. physical, psychological, sexual)
- injury inflicted
- other targets of abuse (family members, outside the family)
- violence in family of origin (observed, victim)
- type of denial
- agreement of corroborating sources

Individual Characteristics:

- behavioral deficits
- depression
- hostility
- alcohol and drugs
- sex roles and attitudes
- psychopathology
- reading level/intelligence
- language skills

Environmental Factors:

- current living situation (e.g., separated, living together)
- social network (e.g., supportive of abusive behavior)
- external stressors

(Continues)

TABLE 4.2
Issues to Be Addressed in the Assessment of a Male Batterer *(Continued)*

Likelihood of Follow-Through:

- level of remorse
- desire to reunite with partner
- involvement with criminal justice system
- effectiveness and saliency of external motivators
- match of program with client ability
- cultural sensitivity of program

Current Risk of Violence:

- increased frequency or severity of violence
- implicit or explicit threats
- client concern about ability to control himself
- use of alcohol or drugs
- availability of a weapon
- past history of abuse
- level of denial
- violence normalized in employment setting
- pronounced psychological disturbance
- recent separation
- custody decisions

Note. From *Intervention for Men Who Batter: An Ecological Approach* (p. 28), by J. L. Edleson & R. M. Tolman, 1992, Newbury Park, CA: Sage Publications, p. 28. Reprinted with permission.

abused partner is usually gathered in a separate session or by phone. Again, the information is not brought up to the batterer, as it would put the woman at risk for retaliative abuse. Stordeur and Stille (1989) even cautioned clinicians to be very careful about what they put into their case notes, because at some future point, batterers may have access to these records and might punish their partners for disclosing information about the abuse.

Once the assessment is completed a treatment contract will be offered to the batterer. There are instances when the batterer sees nothing wrong with his violent behavior or will absolutely deny that he was abusive or violent. However, since batterers are frequently mandated to treatment by the courts or by threats from their partners of ending the relationship, most will accept the treatment option, albeit reluctantly.

Initial treatment planning should include contracting with the batterer to abstain from all forms of violence, and safety and control planning (Hamberger & Barnett, 1995). Safety and control planning should include the following elements:

1. a clear statement that the sole responsibility for avoiding any form of violence rests with the batterer;

2. agreement by the batterer to adhere to any restrictions specified in the restraining order, if one is in place;

3. an evaluation of formal and informal social support networks; and

4. "time-out training" (Hamberger & Barnett, 1995).

The first item of the safety and control plan was discussed previously in this chapter. The second item may be difficult for some batterers. Many batterers view restraining orders as unnecessary and inappropriate societal intrusions into their private family matters, and will therefore not adhere to the restrictions. According to Hamberger and Barnett (1995), it is the role of the counselor to help the batterer redefine the meaning of restraining order. In other words, rather than viewing the order as an imposed societal restriction, view the order as a time-out period that allows the batterer to get his life together, without having to manage the stress of the relationship. The evaluation of support networks has also been discussed previously in this and other chapters.

The fourth and final element of the safety and control plan, time-out training, is used when a restraining order is not in place, and the batterer and abused partner may still be living together (Hamberger & Barnett, 1995). The purpose of the time-out training is to provide batterers with skills to temporarily remove themselves from an argument in order to avoid an escalation of emotional arousal, which may increase the potential for abuse. The batterer must be knowledgeable about his own internal arousal cues or the physical sensations that signal that his anger is escalating. At this juncture, he will agree to tell his partner that he is feeling uncomfortable and that he is going to take a 10 to 30 minute break. The batterers must be careful not to threaten his partner (e.g., "If you don't leave me alone, I'm going to get violent") and must also reassure his partner that he is not walking out or abandoning her. The purpose of the time-out is to provide a cooling off period, so that later on, the couple can discuss the conflict more calmly and try to work out a solution together. It is not intended to be an avoidance maneuver.

Once the batterer agrees to the aforementioned aspects of the contract, he will usually begin group treatment. For several reasons, group treatment is far superior to individual treatment. The group provides an opportunity for the batterer to hear about the experiences of other men who are experiencing the same problem. This then lessens the feeling of uniqueness or isolation. When some members of the group have broken through their denial and have taken on the attitude of "I have a problem that I need help overcoming," these members can be quite effective in confronting the denial of other group members. The role of the group counselor is to make certain that the group does not perpetuate denial or negative sexist stereotypes (e.g., "All women are money hungry," or "All women are good at inciting an argument, because they don't know when to keep their mouths shut"). These are sexist views, which can only serve to perpetuate negative sex role stereotypes and therefore perpetuate rationalizations for violence. The group counselor must be prepared to be active and directive in the approach to group facilitation. In setting group rules, for example, the counselor would make it known from the onset that sexist statements and blaming intimate partner victims for their behavior will not be allowed. When individual counseling is provided, it is usually done so only in conjunction with group treatment. The emphasis of individual therapy should be to deal with issues that coincide with those raised in the group session. However, it should be made clear to the batterer that individual sessions are not a substitute for raising issues with the other group members.

As discussed previously, couples therapy is usually contraindicated in the early stages of treatment. It may be used, however, in instances of verbal or emotional abuse, provided that the safety of the battered victim is ensured. Couples therapy would also be predicated on the supposition that the abusive partner has sufficient control of his anger to not act out violently. According to Geffner, Mantooth, and Franks (1989) and Geffner and Pagelow (1990), couples therapy would only be undertaken when the following preconditions are met: (a) both the perpetrator and the abused partner desire this type of treatment; (b) the abused partner has a safety plan and understands the potential dangers; (c) there are no custody issues if the couple is divorcing; (d) a lethality evaluation suggests a low presence of danger; (e) the therapist or counselor treating the couple is trained in both family systems and domestic violence counseling; (f) neither are abusing alcohol or drugs; (g) if there has been substance abuse in the past, then there is appropriate treatment for this issue; and (h) neither partner exhibits psychotic behavior.

Intervening With Domestic Violence Cases

At the beginning of this chapter, we presented two case histories, both of which portray some aspect of intimate partner violence. Following are detailed discussions of each case, focusing on the LAPC (listen, assess, plan, commit) intervention model described in chapter 3.

Crisis Intervention Case Example 1

As discussed previously, John and Marie illustrate a case in which verbal and psychological abuse are key elements. John displays many of the characteristics of verbally abusive men. He is threatening, intimidating, critical of Marie, and controlling. Although relationships like this often go on for years without escalating, it is also likely that they can erupt into physical violence.

Assuming that there have been no instances of physical violence and also assuming that John would not come in for counseling either with Marie or individually, it is likely that Marie would seek counseling individually. It is probable, however, that Marie would be too fearful to initiate counseling herself. So let's assume that Marie was referred for counseling by her physician, who noted symptoms of depression.

The crisis counselor would begin by cautiously exploring some of the things that Marie has been feeling depressed about. Assuming that she lists relationship problems with John as one of the difficulties she has been having, the counselor can then begin to explore the nature and extent of these problems in the *Listening* phase. Suspecting verbal abuse, the counselor could then begin to explore the types of verbal abuse, such as those put forth by Evans in *The Verbally Abusive Relationship* (1992), or to explore some of the items listed by Tolman (1989) in his assessment scale, The Psychological Maltreatment of Women Scale (e.g., "My partner prevented me from using the phone," "My partner threatened to have me committed to a mental institution," or "My partner threatened to leave me"). In the *Assessment* phase, the counselor concludes from Marie's description, that John tries to control just about every aspect of her life. Marie plays the dutiful codependent, as she tries to placate him due to the fear that his anger will explode out of control. However, no matter what Marie does, John continues to use his temper outbursts as a means of controlling and manipulating her into adhering to his every wish. Once this information is revealed, it is also important that the counselor not launch into an attack of John, as this would only alienate Marie or add to her feelings of guilt or responsibility.

Towards the end of the session, the counselor asks Marie to describe something nice about John. This is done to allow Marie an opportunity to present something positive about him or their relationship so that she doesn't feel guilty for having been critical of John. It also conveys to Marie that the counselor's goal is not to attack John. If this were the case, it is likely that Marie would not return for counseling. Working with someone in Marie's situation will be a long-term process, although the initial crisis intervention counseling is designed to get Marie to agree to continued counseling. This agreement becomes part of the *Plan,* which it is hoped that Marie will *Commit* to. The LAPC worksheet for Marie shows the form as a counselor would have filled it out after a session with Marie.

Evans (1992) suggested that it is important that women in verbally abusive relationships be aware of when they are being put down, ordered around, or yelled at and to recognize that this is abusive behavior. She also suggested that women recognize that abuse is unjust, disabling, destructive, and that abuse is not a rational, adult way of communicating with someone. Evans also recommended that women recognize that they are dealing with partners who are in some way trying to control, dominate, or establish superiority over them, and not to get caught up in the misconception that they have done something wrong to cause it. Although it is obvious that Marie is not financially irresponsible, she believes that she is to blame for John's wrath.

Crisis Intervention Case Example 2

The case example of Tiffany and Nick represents a classic illustration of physical and verbal battering. Nick represents an insecure batterer or a pitbull (Jacobson & Gottman, 1998) who constantly uses verbal and physical intimidation to "keep

LISTEN	ASSESS	PLAN	COMMIT

Name: _Marie_   Age _42_

LISTEN

What is the client saying about the crisis? _Marie states that she feels depressed because of financial stress at home._

What happened? _No particular triggering event._

When did it happen? _n/a_

What type of crisis was it (traumatic event, developmental, psychiatric, existential)? _Developmental because of problems in the marital relationship._

Did the client mention anything that indicated danger? _No, Marie denies physical abuse in the relationship, although this should be explored further in subsequent sessions._

Other relevant information about the crisis: _Marie is referred by her primary care physician and is willing to allow communication._

ASSESS

Feeling: Is the client's predominant emotional state one of:

Anger _No_	Sadness _Yes_	Hopelessness _Yes_
Anxiety _No_	Panic _No_	Numbness _No_

Suicidal? If yes, complete lethality assessment/suicide: _No_

Homicidal? If yes, complete lethality assessment/violence: _No_

Acting: Is the client's behavior:

Active/restless _No_	Consistent with mood _Yes_
Passive/withdrawn _Yes_	Good eye contact _No_

Thinking: Is the client:

Logical/making sense _Yes_	Coherent/expressing self well _Yes_
Insightful _No_	Focused on topic _Yes_
Evasive/changing subject _No_	

Other: Any medical problems? _No_

Physical limitations? _No_

Hospitalizations? _No_

Need for hospitalization? _No_

(Continues)

PLAN

What needs to be done now? *Hopefully Marie will agree to continued counseling.*

What alternative plans have been discussed? *If Marie is not agreeable to continuing with counseling then some provision should be made for follow-up even if by phone.*

Are these plans reasonable? *Yes*

Can they be carried out? *Yes*

COMMIT

Which plan of action has the client chosen? *Marie has chosen to continue with counseling.*

Are there resources/support to implement the plan? *Yes*

Is the client motivated to implement the plan? *Yes*

What other resources/support may be needed?

Friend *No*   Family member *No*

Neighbor *No*   Mental health provider *Yes*

Public agency (law enforcement, child protective services, social services) *No*

Medical (hospitalization, medication) *No*

Tiffany in her place." It is unlikely that individuals like Nick will present in treatment on their own, and when mandated into treatment by the courts, they usually will project blame for their explosive anger on their spouses or partners. It is important that the counselor gather information about Tiffany and her relationship with Nick in a nonjudgmental manner. It is also important to keep the focus on the here and now. This is not a time for exploration of prior relationships or family history. In the *Listening* phase, Tiffany explains that she finds herself constantly "walking on eggshells" in fear that something she will say or do will incite Nick's rage. Most beginning crisis counselors make the mistake of assuming that reasoning and rational explanation is all that is needed to get Tiffany to leave. Usually, women in Tiffany's situation will keep the abuse a secret from their friends and family because they don't want to hear those dreaded words, "Why don't you just leave him?" This would especially be true if Tiffany were to tell her mother about the abuse. Tiffany may feel invested in making the relationship work, or to try to prove to her mother that Nick is "not such a bad guy." As indicated previously however, there are many reasons why battered women stay in their relationships, so it is best that counselors listen for these various reasons in a nonjudgmental manner. Again, it is best to ask open-ended questions and to stifle the impulse to criticize Nick and his abusive behavior. In making an *Assessment* of the situation, the crisis counselor needs to determine the degree of danger or lethality. The four incident technique described earlier is a helpful way to gather information used to make an assessment. Once the counselor provides Tiffany with feedback about her situation and defines and labels the relationship as abusive, it is likely that she may vehemently deny that she is abused. She may also compare herself to other battered women she knows (or knows of) and rationalize that her situation is not as bad as theirs. Many women use this minimization as a rationale for not seeking help ("their situation is so much worse than mine"). It is important to reinforce that any woman who is verbally, emotionally, or physically abused should have access to counseling, no matter the type of abuse or how severe it may have been. Probably the most important part of the session will be developing a *safety plan,* as described by Walker (2000). The safety plan will include concrete steps that Tiffany can take if she sees that Nick is becoming agitated or upset. A safety plan would include things like keeping a bag of clothes packed and ready to go, stowing a set of car keys that will be readily accessible, having phone numbers and a cell phone readily available, and finally having a safe place to go, whether it be a women's shelter or a place where other protective individuals are present.

If Nick were to present for counseling whether by court referral or by encouragement by a family member, it is recommended that Nick be seen individually and not in conjoint sessions with Tiffany. In working with Nick individually (and batterers in general), there are four main goals: (a) to ensure the safety of the victimized partner, (b) to alter the batterer's attitudes towards relationship violence, (c) to increase the batterer's sense of personal responsibility rather than to project blame to the victimized partner, and (d) to learn nonviolent alternatives to dealing with conflict in order to change past behavior (Edleson & Tolman, 1992). In *assessing* Nick it would be important to determine if he matches the common characteristics of male batterers (see Table 4.1) and to address those issues listed in Table 4.2 as treatment ensues.

SOURCES OF CHAPTER ENRICHMENT

Print Sources

Dutton, D. (1996). *The domestic assault of women.* Vancouver: UBC Press.

Dutton, D. (1998). *The abusive personality.* New York: Guilford Press.

Edleson, J. L., & Tolman, R. M. (1992). *Intervention for men who batter.* Newbury Park, CA: Sage Publishers.

Jones, A. R. (1993). *When love goes wrong: What to do when you can't do anything right.* New York: Harper Trade.

Pizzey, E. (1974). *Scream quietly or the neighbors will hear.* London: Penguin Books.

Shupe, A., Stacey, W. A., & Hazlewood, L. R. (1987). *Violent men, violent couples.* Lexington, MA: Lexington Books.

Roberts, A. R. (1991). *Sheltering battered women.* New York: Springer.

Walker, L. (2000). *The battered woman syndrome* (2nd ed.). New York: Springer Publishing Co.

Internet Sources

Family Violence Prevention Fund (http://www.fvpf.org) Leading medical experts explore new methods to improve health care response to domestic violence.

Partnerships against Violence Network (http://www.pavnet.org) A "virtual library" of information about and data on youth-at-risk. The site represents data from seven different federal agencies.

National Coalition against Domestic Violence (http://www.ncadv.org) Information and referral center for public media, battered woman, agencies and organizations.

National Network to End Domestic Violence (http://www.nnedv.org) Site provides news and information for advocates about domestic violence. Get national perspectives on legislation and public policy, advocates in the news, training, conferences, and employment opportunities.

National Domestic Violence Hotline In 1996, President Clinton established a toll-free domestic violence hotline (1-800-799-SAFE). This hotline receives about 11,000 calls a month. There is also a number for those who are hearing impaired. That number is TDD 1-800-787-3224.

CHAPTER **5**

Alcohol and Drug Crises

Jennifer is a 19-year-old college sophomore who was brought to the emergency room of the local hospital last night when her roommate discovered Jennifer passed out on the couch in their dorm room with vomit all over herself and barely breathing. Her roommate recalled seeing Jen at one of the fraternity parties and said that she "was really tanked." Fortunately, the roommate had the sense to call the residence assistant, who in turn called an ambulance. At the emergency room, Jen's stomach was pumped and she was given a blood test, which revealed an extremely high blood alcohol level and the presence of marijuana and Percocet in her bloodstream. The crisis counselor was called in to see Jen the next day when she regained consciousness.

*S*ubstance use disorders can affect anyone, young or old, rich or poor, regardless of educational achievements, abilities, race, religion, or culture. Alcohol- and drug-related problems are pervasive in our society and so too are a variety of crises related to these disorders. Although we will be presenting general information pertaining to substance use disorders—information pertaining to diagnosis and models of addiction—the goal of this chapter is to provide the reader with an understanding of how alcohol and drug abuse can develop into crises. It is likely that when Jennifer set out for an evening of fun and partying, she didn't plan on ending up in an emergency room. Because alcohol and drug abuse are so widespread in American culture, it is commonplace for substance abusing individuals to present in crisis in a variety of settings, such as hospitals, schools, mental health clinics, or the court system. Naturally, not everyone who abuses alcohol or drugs will necessarily experience a crisis; therefore, the goal of this chapter is to focus on those crisis situations that may arise as a direct result of alcohol and drug use.

Alcohol and drug crises parallel the diagnostic categories found in the *Diagnostic and Statistical Manual of Mental Disorders*, 4th Edition, Text Revision *(DSM-IV-TR)* (American Psychiatric Association, 2000): *substance intoxication, substance withdrawal, substance abuse,* and *substance dependence.* Examples of crises related to *substance intoxication* would include a college student who ends up ingesting near-fatal amounts of alcohol or a young man who in a state of intox-ication from ecstasy becomes dehydrated and loses consciousness. *Substance withdrawal* crises occur when someone who has been physically addicted to a substance begins to experience withdrawal symptoms. This would include an alcoholic who begins to experience tremors and then falls to the ground in con-vulsions or a person addicted to pain medication, such as Vicodin or Oxycontin, who begins to experience sweats and extreme agitation when the drug supply is gone. A *substance abuse* crisis could be an arrest for driving while intoxicated (DWI). For anyone who has not had prior legal problems, a DWI becomes a cri-sis event, as this individual must now deal with a court appearance, financial loss due to court fees, fines, and worries over how to get back and forth to work. A person in the throes of a *substance dependence* crisis experiences life manage-ment problems because the individual is unable to stop using mood-altering chemicals and is no longer in control of daily life events. Crisis counselors can help alcoholics and addicts safely manage these crises, provided that proper assessment occurs to enable effective intervention. This chapter will focus on appropriate techniques for helping substance abusers manage these crises.

The Scope of Drug and Alcohol Problems

What is unique to substance abuse crises is that addictions can and do kill peo-ple. It is estimated that approximately 420,000 people die each year from com-plications related to smoking cigarettes (Benson & Sacco, 2000), approximately 100,000 to 200,000 die each year from complications from alcohol abuse (Lewis, 1997; Hymen & Cassem, 1995), and approximately 20,000 to 30,000 die as a result of drug use (Miller, 1999; Prater, Miller, & Zylstra, 1999). Consider the fol-lowing statistics: The indirect costs of alcoholism and drug abuse in the United States are estimated to be about $510 billion (Evans, 1998). Approximately one in five Americans is dependent on alcohol or drugs, approximately one third of all hospital beds are occupied by individuals with alcohol or drug-related ill-nesses. Until 1997, approximately half of all highway fatalities were linked to individuals who were driving under the influence of alcohol or drugs (National Highway Traffic Safety Administration [NHTSA], 1998).

Estimates indicate that 56% of domestic violence cases involve alcohol. Alcohol and drugs also figure heavily in both violent crimes, such as homi-cides, and property crimes, such as assaults and burglary. Between 2000 and 2001, the rates of alcohol use and the number of drinkers increased. Currently, almost half (48.3%) of Americans age 12 and older, or 109 million individuals, are drinkers. This estimate is roughly 5 million people greater than the number in 2000. Of the 10.1 million people ages 12 to 20 who indicated that they drink, nearly 6.8 million, or 19%, were binge drinkers and 2.1 million, or 6%, were heavy drinkers (Substance Abuse & Mental Health Services Administration [SAMHSA], 2002). In 1994, the National Comorbidity Survey (NCS) estimated that in the 15- to 54-year-old age group, 24.1% were tobacco dependent, 14.1% were alcohol dependent, and 7.5% had developed dependence on at least one controlled substance or drug (of which cannabis was the drug most often abused) (Anthony, Warner, & Kessler, 1997). Consider also the overlap between substance use disorder diagnoses with psychiatric disorders. Estimates indicate that approximately one third of psychiatric patients admitted to inpatient units have active drug or alcohol problems at the time of admission (Eisen, Grob, & Dill, 1987, 1988; Crowley, Chesluk, Dilts, & Hart, 1974; Davis, 1984; Fischer, Halikas, Baker, & Smith, 1975). Furthermore, it is estimated that this percentage is even greater in those individuals who seek outpatient psychiatric treatment at community mental health clinics.

Although substance use disorder is referred to as an "equal opportunity" disease, in that it can affect anyone, there are some patterns that deserve mention. For example, there are high rates of multiple substance abuse among young people. In some instances, this pattern may result in higher rates of psychological dependence rather than physiological dependence. Young people are also more likely to abuse inhalants and hallucinogens than are adults. Furthermore, African American youth tend to have lower rates of substance use than European American or Latino American youth (Johnston, O'Malley, & Bachman, 1995). In the elderly, prescription drug abuse is a major problem. With regards to gender differences, men tend to manifest alcohol and drug problems in their late teens and early twenties, while women in their 30s are at higher risk for developing alcohol and drug problems. Native Americans and those of Irish and English ancestry also tend to have higher rates of alcohol abuse and dependence (Rouse, 1995).

Based on these statistics, it is apparent that individuals in a wide variety of human services occupations (teachers, police officers, emergency room psychiatric screeners, family counselors, nurses, attorneys, social workers, psychologists) will have to deal with the direct or indirect impact of alcoholism or drug addiction. This is why it is important to know the facts about substance use disorders and to be able to deal with these types of crises effectively. In no other area is so much harm done by human services workers with good intentions. People in these occupations may unwittingly become enablers: the police officer who drives the DWI offender home rather than making an arrest; the teacher who ignores signs of drug abuse in one of his or her students; the doctor who continues to write prescriptions for painkillers or tranquilizers to an addicted patient year-after-year. Rather than becoming part of the solution, they become part of the problem. Indeed it is estimated that physicians miss alcoholism or other drug dependency diagnoses in approximately 60% to 70% of the cases they treat (Doweiko, 1998).

Defining Substance Use Disorders: Diagnostic Issues

What are alcoholism and drug addiction? What separates the alcoholic or addicted drug user from the recreational or social user? In order to answer these questions, it is important to explore some of the different definitions of substance use disorders.

The most widely used and accepted classification system for diagnosing alcoholism and other drug dependencies is the *DSM-IV-TR* (American Psychiatric Association, 2000). As stated previously, there are four main categories of substance use disorders: *substance dependence, substance abuse, substance intoxication,* and *substance withdrawal.* In assessing a patient who has come into an emergency room, a crisis counselor would first try to determine if that individual is currently under the influence of drugs or alcohol (intoxication) or in withdrawal from drugs or alcohol. Both of these categories relate to the person's condition at the time of evaluation. The diagnoses of dependence and abuse really have more to do with the impact that alcohol or drugs have had on a person over time. Basically, do alcohol or drugs *interfere* with the individual's ability to function on a daily basis? If so, then he or she may qualify for a diagnosis of dependence or abuse. It should also be pointed out that many chemically dependent individuals will use more than one substance at a time; for example, it is not uncommon to treat someone who is abusing both alcohol and prescription medication, as would be the case with Jennifer, described at the beginning of this chapter. It is also common for individuals to abuse marijuana and alcohol simultaneously and to experience problems related to both substances.

The Need for Diagnoses

There are several reasons for providing this information on diagnostic issues. First, there are many myths and misconceptions regarding what constitutes alcoholism or addiction. Many people labor under the misconception that a person must be physically dependent on alcohol or drugs or drink or use drugs everyday to be diagnosed as an alcoholic or drug addict. Or they think that a person must be a skid row drunk, or have lost everything as a result of drug use. Research points to the fact that most alcoholics are functional alcoholics— they go to work everyday, they have families, they go to Parent-Teacher Organization meetings, and coach Little League teams. However, although they may be functional, their drinking often interferes in their lives—their home lives, their health, or their psychological well-being.

Second, the majority of alcoholics or addicts that human services workers and crisis counselors may treat are in denial of their problems. Denial is considered to be part of the substance use disorders. The phrase often heard in Alcoholics Anonymous (A.A.) circles is "alcoholism is the disease that tells you, you don't have a disease." So, in making a diagnosis, it is not unusual for the alcoholic or addict to say, "What, me have an alcohol or drug problem? You've got to be kidding. I can stop any time I want. Besides, I know about ten other people who drink or use drugs more than I do." These are common statements of someone in denial. Therefore, it is important to have objective criteria, such as the *DSM-IV-TR* criteria, for making a diagnosis.

The third reason for covering diagnostic issues is that in doing crisis intervention work with alcoholics or addicts, the diagnosis will determine the interventions and treatment decisions most effective for the crisis. For example, if someone comes to a counseling center intoxicated or experiencing withdrawal, the crisis counselor would not send the person home and tell him or her to come back for outpatient counseling the next day. If a person is diagnosed with cannabis (marijuana) abuse, he or she would not be referred to a long-term rehabilitation center or detoxification center. Therefore, an accurate diagnosis is necessary in order to make an appropriate treatment plan. This will be discussed in more depth later in this chapter.

The *DSM-IV-TR* diagnostic categories for dependence and abuse each have their own criteria. These criteria and discussions of each are provided in the following sections (American Psychiatric Association, 2000).

Substance Dependence

Substance dependence is defined as:

A maladaptive pattern of substance use, leading to clinically significant impairment or distress, as manifested by *three or more* of the following diagnostic criteria occurring at any time in the same 12-month period:

1. Tolerance, as defined by either of the following:
   a. a need for markedly increased amounts of the substance to achieve intoxication or desired effect; and/or
   b. markedly diminished effect with continued use of the same amount of the substance.
2. Withdrawal, as manifested by either of the following:
   a. the characteristic withdrawal syndrome for the substance (refer to Criteria A and B of the criteria set for withdrawal from the specific substances); and/or
   b. the same or (closely related) substance is taken to relieve or avoid withdrawal symptoms.
3. The substance is often taken in larger amounts or over a longer period than was intended.
4. There is a persistent desire or unsuccessful efforts to cut down or control substance use.
5. A great deal of time is spent in activities necessary to obtain the substance (e.g., visiting multiple doctors or driving long distances), use the substance (e.g., chain smoking), or recover from its effects.
6. Important social, occupational or recreational activities are given up or reduced because of substance use.
7. The substance use is continued despite knowledge of having a persistent or recurrent physical or psychological problem that was likely to have been caused or exacerbated by the substance (e.g., current cocaine use despite recognition of cocaine-induced depression, or continued drinking despite recognition that an ulcer was made worse by alcohol consumption).[1]

1. From Diagnostic and Statistical Manual of Mental Disorders (4th ed., Text revision) (pp. 110–111), by American Psychiatric Association, 2000, Washington, DC: Author. Reprinted with permission.

Continuing with the example of the emergency room assessment, after determining if the client is under the influence of drugs or alcohol or is in withdrawal, the counselor would then try to determine whether or not the client manifests *physiological dependence*. Physiological dependence is characterized by an increase in tolerance to the substance (e.g., having to consume more and more of the substance to get the desired effect) or by withdrawal symptoms when the supply of the drug runs out or wears off. Individuals with physiological dependence experience physical craving along with the mental obsession to get high.

However, a patient can be diagnosed with *substance dependence* even though they are *not* physically addicted to the substance. This may sound confusing, but consider the case of a "periodic alcoholic"—someone who drinks once or twice per year, but drinks to excess, experiences blackouts, misses days from work, and gets into accidents. This person would not necessarily be physically dependent on alcohol, but does experience a loss of control (see criteria 3), might spend a great deal of time using the substance and recovering from its effects (see criteria 5), and could end up neglecting important occupational activities (see criteria 6). Another example of dependence without physical addition is a person who regularly uses marijuana. There is some debate over whether marijuana results in a physical addiction because there is no definitive withdrawal syndrome, as there is with heroin, alcohol, or prescription drugs, such as Valium. Yet many people do become dependent on marijuana; they center their lives on getting high, they cannot foresee a life without getting high, and their daily functioning is adversely impacted by their use of the substance.

The main factors in substance dependence diagnosis (also known as chemical dependency, alcoholism, or drug addiction) are that the alcohol or drug use is consistent, although not necessarily daily, and the use results in problems in life functioning or *interferes* with the person's life. Now think back to the social drinkers mentioned before. If they have an occasional beer with a pizza or a glass of wine with dinner, does their drinking interfere with their functioning? If they are truly social drinkers, one would not see interference in life functioning. They basically can take or leave alcohol. No one complains about their drinking. They don't miss time from work or school because of hangovers, they don't drive while drunk, and they don't become violent or experience extreme mood or personality changes when they drink.

Substance Abuse

Substance abuse is considered to be a less severe or less pervasive version of substance dependence in terms of its impact on the individual. The criteria for substance abuse is as follows:

   A. A maladaptive pattern of substance use leading to clinically significant impairment or distress, as manifested by one (or more) of the following, occurring within a 12-month period:
      1. Recurrent substance use resulting in a failure to fulfill major role obligations at work, school, or home (e.g., repeated absences or

> poor work performance related to substance use; substance-related absences, suspensions, or expulsions from school; neglect of children or household).
>
> 2. Recurrent substance use in situations in which it is physically hazardous (e.g., driving an automobile or operating a machine when impaired by substance use).
> 3. Recurrent substance-related legal problems (e.g., arrests for substance-related disorderly conduct).
> 4. Continued substance use despite having persistent or recurrent social or interpersonal problems caused or exacerbated by the effects of the substance (e.g., arguments with spouse about consequences of intoxication, physical fights).
>
> B. The symptoms have never met the criteria for *Substance Dependence* for this class of substance.[2]

With substance abuse, the individual is experiencing alcohol or substance-related problems; however, these problems are not of the same magnitude or intensity as would be found with substance dependence. Substance abusers are usually able to function on a day-to-day basis, and there is no evidence of either psychological or physical dependence on alcohol and/or drugs; however, these individuals do experience problems in their lives as a direct result of their alcohol or drug use and they will continue to use, in spite of knowing that alcohol or drugs are causing these problems.

Substance Intoxication and Substance Withdrawal

The following are the diagnostic criteria for Substance Intoxication:

> A. The development of a reversible substance-specific syndrome due to recent ingestion of (or exposure to) a substance. **Note:** Different substances may produce similar or identical syndromes.
> B. Clinically significant maladaptive behavioral or psychological changes that are due to the effect of the substance on the central nervous system (e.g., belligerence, mood lability, cognitive impairment, impaired judgment, impaired social or occupational functioning) and develop during or shortly after use of the substance.
> C. The symptoms are not due to a general medical condition and not better accounted for by another mental disorder.[3]

The following are the diagnostic criteria for Substance Withdrawal:

> A. The development of a substance-specific syndrome due to the cessation of (or reduction in) substance use that has been heavy or prolonged.

2. From Diagnostic and Statistical Manual of Mental Disorders (4th ed., Text revision) (pp. 114–115), by American Psychiatric Association, 2000, Washington, DC: Author. Reprinted with permission.
3. From Diagnostic and Statistical Manual of Mental Disorders (4th ed., Text revision) (pp. 115–116), by American Psychiatric Association, 2000, Washington, DC: Author. Reprinted with permission.

B. The substance-specific syndrome causes clinically significant distress or impairment in social, occupational, or other important areas of functioning.

C. The symptoms are not due to a general medical condition and not better accounted for by another mental disorder.[4]

As alluded to in the criteria, substances will either differ greatly or will be similar in the intoxication they produce. For example, alcohol, benzodiazepines (such as Valium, Librium, Xanax, Tranxene), barbiturates (such as Seconal, pentobarbitol), and opioids (such as heroin, codeine, OxyContin, Percocet, and methadone) are all central nervous system (CNS) depressants, and therefore will produce somewhat similar intoxicating effects, including slowed speech and movement, unstable gait, slowed reaction time, slowed cognitive processing or thought processes, and drowsiness. Alcohol is mistakenly thought to have an initial stimulating effect; however, this excitation which some intoxicated people report is often the result of inhibitions being anesthetized by alcohol. Stimulant drugs will produce similar effects. So, drugs such as cocaine, amphetamines ("crystal meth"), or methylphenidate (Ritalin[5]) will produce excitation, rapid speech, agitation, increased speech and movement, and a decreased need for sleep.

In substance withdrawal, the old adage, "What goes up, must come down" can be applied. In other words, substances often produce a withdrawal effect that is opposite to the primary effect. In the instance of stimulants, the withdrawal effects are usually characterized by depressive states with accompanying irritability. Nicotine, which is a stimulant, produces a depressant withdrawal effect characterized by lethargy, irritability, and craving. With the CNS depressant drugs, such as alcohol, benzodiazepines, barbiturates, and opioids, the withdrawal effect is usually one of stimulation or agitation. Of the various CNS depressants alcohol can produce the most potentially fatal withdrawal and is certainly a more dangerous withdrawal than that produced by heroin. Alcohol withdrawal effects can range from mild agitation, to tremors, to hallucinosis, the most severe form being delirium tremens (DTs). DTs are likened to an extreme form of withdrawal agitation, and many alcoholics die from cardiac or respiratory arrest as a result of extreme exhaustion due to DTs. At one time, it was estimated that 5% to 25% of those who experienced DTs would die (Lehman, Pilich, & Andrews, 1994; Schuckit, 1995). However, with improved medical care, the mortality rate from DTs has decreased to approximately 1% to 5% (Milzman & Soderstrom, 1994; Yost, 1996).

Interestingly, while many of the hallucinogenic drugs produce rather dangerous intoxication effects (phencyclidine, or PCP, being a prime example), this class of substances often produces very little withdrawal effects. For example, there are no documented instances of someone experiencing LSD withdrawal. An LSD flashback may produce an unexpected feeling of "tripping" with

---

4. From Diagnostic and Statistical Manual of Mental Disorders (4th ed., Text revision) (pp. 115–116), by American Psychiatric Association, 2000, Washington, DC: Author. Reprinted with permission.

5. When Ritalin is given to an individual with Attention Deficit Hyperactivity Disorder, it produces a paradoxical effect—it helps them to focus and slows things down—rather than producing an excitation or exhilaration effect.

accompanying visual hallucinations, such as seeing colors or "trails" (colorful afterimages), but a flashback is not a withdrawal phenomenon, as evidenced by the fact that not all LSD users experiences flashbacks.

The intoxicating effects of many substances, however, can often lead to several types of crises, such as fights, arrests, domestic violence incidents, suicide attempts and other forms of violent or extreme behavior. For example, phencyclidine (PCP) abusers are often known to become violent when under the influence of the drug. They will often become easily overwhelmed by any visual or auditory stimulation and as a result, they can become unpredictably violent. This is quite different from people who are under the influence of CNS depressants, such as Percocet or Darvon, which usually result in placid and nonreactive behavior. Contrast that to the cocaine abuser who may be experiencing "coke paranoia," a cocaine-induced psychotic-like reaction that is estimated to affect 53% to 65% of regular cocaine users (Decker & Ries, 1993; Beebe & Walley, 1991).

Crisis Intervention and Case Management

The information presented in this chapter should create an appreciation of the fact that not all crisis situations pertaining to alcohol or drugs are the same. For example, a person may present in crisis while are under the influence *(substance intoxication)* or while in a state of alcohol or drug withdrawal *(substance withdrawal)*. It is also possible that an individual may present in crisis because he or she is unable to stop using or ends up getting into trouble when using *(substance dependence)*. Other individuals may experience intermittent problems related to drug or alcohol use *(substance abuse)*. This is why it is of utmost importance to make an accurate assessment of the individual who presents with an alcohol or drug crisis. What complicates this assessment, however, is that the counselor may not be able to rely on the patient's self-report of how much of a particular substance has been ingested and over what time period. In addition, given the lack of "quality control" among drug producers/dealers, it is often impossible to determine the potency of a particular drug, such as heroin, marijuana, or cocaine. It is also not unusual for alcoholics or addicts to blame their problems on anything other than their substance use or to outright deny that they have been using at all. This should not discourage beginning counselors, as it is very much a part of the disease process. How a counselor deals with an alcoholic or addict in crisis will very much depend on the extent of the person's use at the time of intervention. For example, it would be impossible to conduct a thorough crisis interview with someone who is totally intoxicated or incoherent due to the influence of drugs. Other general recommendations for crisis counselors are listed in Box 5.1.

Let's return to the crisis case presented at the beginning of the chapter to illustrate how a crisis counselor might approach Jennifer, make an assessment, and come up with a viable plan.

BOX 5.1

General Recommendations for Crisis Counselors Working With Substance Use Disorder Patients

- It is common for alcoholic and drug addicted patients to minimize, rationalize, or outright deny the seriousness of their chemical use. Don't be put off by this.

- Don't be judgmental or blame alcoholics or addicts for their predicament. This will only add to their resistance to treatment.

- Do express concern. Studies have proven that a concerned, genuine tone of voice was more likely to result in successful treatment referrals.

- Don't get frustrated by "revolving door" patients. Addiction is a disease in which relapse is common; therefore it is not unusual to see the same patient in crisis over and over again. You never know when this crisis intervention may be the one that helps get the patient into long-term recovery.

- Do gather as much information from family members as possible. Alcoholics and addicts are not good at providing background information for a number of reasons (blackouts, repression of humiliating experiences, denial), so it always a good idea to talk with family members or significant others to gather background information and prior treatment history.

- Try to find out what has worked in the past. If an alcoholic or addict has put together any appreciable amount of sober/clean time in the past, try to find out what factors helped the patient do this. What strengths does this person have that helped him or her put together this clean time.

- Don't get roped into the "treatment won't work for me" game. Just because the alcoholic or addict has been in detox or rehab before doesn't mean that it won't work for him or her this time around.

- When in doubt about drug or alcohol use, make sure you get a toxicology screen. Alcoholics and addicts may falsify what they have taken and how much they have taken, or they may not know what substances they have taken. So when in doubt, and when possible, it is best to have a "tox screen" done.

- Don't leave intoxicated persons unattended or let them get out of your sight. A medical center and crisis screener were sued when an intoxicated patient wandered out of the emergency room and was hit and killed by a car.

Substance Intoxication: Crisis Intervention Case Example 1

> Recall that Jennifer is a 19-year-old college sophomore. She currently is on academic probation because her freshman grades were horrendous, in part due to having pledged a sorority. Jen explains that she has been smoking marijuana since high school and indicates that she currently smokes "about twice a month." When Jennifer was brought to the emergency room of the local hospital last night, she was unconscious, having passed out on the couch in her dorm room. Fortunately, when Jennifer's roommate came back to the dorm and found Jen passed out with vomit all over herself, she had the sense to call the residence assistant, who in turn called an ambulance. At the emergency room, Jen's stomach was pumped and she was given a blood test that revealed an extremely high blood alcohol level, and the presence of marijuana and Percocet in her bloodstream. The crisis counselor was called in to see Jen the next day when she regained consciousness.

Jennifer's crisis starts off as a *medical crisis.* If Jennifer's roommate had let her "sleep it off" or had tried to wake her and "talk her down," the consequences could have been disastrous. Individuals who aspirate (regurgitate) or vomit while in an intoxicated stupor can die of asphyxiation (suffocation). Therefore, most instances of *substance intoxication,* especially when a person is intoxicated to the point of being incoherent or out of touch with reality, should be handled as medical crises and the person should be brought to an emergency room or to a walk-in health center where he or she can be observed and properly treated. The worst thing one can do is to leave the person alone. People may assume that rolling intoxicated individuals onto their sides will prevent regurgitation and asphyxiation, but that is definitely not the case. In Jennifer's situation, once her medical crisis was stabilized, she would need to be evaluated by a crisis counselor familiar with substance use disorders.

In such an evaluation, once Jennifer felt comfortable enough to talk, the crisis counselor would begin by obtaining background information from Jennifer and at the same time try to determine if the incident may have represented a suicide attempt, given that Jennifer had ingested a potentially lethal combination of alcohol and drugs. People may overdose accidentally, or they may use alcohol and drugs with suicidal intentions.

How does a counselor approach the alcoholic or addict in a professional, competent manner that will be effective and will assist the individual in resolving the crisis? As in any counseling situation, it is important to first establish rapport. The person in crisis needs to know that the counselor is there to help, not to criticize or judge. Alcoholics and addicts are very attuned to judgmental attitudes. It is also important that the counselor *Listen* to the person's concerns and to the account of what he or she was able to recall. This is clearly important in Jennifer's case. Refer to the LAPC worksheet, which shows the counselor's comments about the initial intervention with Jennifer.

LISTEN	ASSESS	PLAN	COMMIT

Name: *Jennifer*   Age *19*

LISTEN

What is the client saying about the crisis? *Jennifer admits to excessive drinking, and marijuana and Percocet use.*

What happened? *Jennifer states that she went out for a "couple of beers" but ended up drinking more than intended.*

When did it happen? *Last night.*

What type of crisis was it (traumatic event, developmental, psychiatric, existential)? *At the time of admission, this was clearly a medical crisis; however, once medically stabilized this appears to be more of a developmental crisis, given the age of onset of problems.*

Did the client mention anything that indicates danger? *From a medical perspective, Jennifer was in danger of overdosing given the mixture of alcohol and Percocet.*

Other relevant information about the crisis: *Jennifer reports having had problems with alcohol in the past, especially within the past 2 years.*

ASSESS

Feeling: Is the client's predominant emotional state one of:

Anger *No*	Sadness *No*	Hopelessness *No*
Anxiety *Yes*	Panic *No*	Numbness *No*

Suicidal? If yes, complete lethality assessment/suicide. *No*

Homicidal? If yes, complete lethality assessment/violence. *No*

Acting: Is the client's behavior:

Active/restless *Yes*	Consistent with mood *Yes*
Passive/withdrawn *No*	Good eye contact *Yes*

Thinking: Is the client:

Logical/making sense *Yes*	Coherent/expressing self well *Yes*
Insightful *Somewhat*	Focused on topic *Yes*
Evasive/changing subject *No*	

Other: Any medical problems? *No*

Physical limitations? *No*

Hospitalizations? *No prior hospitalization.*

Need for hospitalization? *Will be discharged from hospital once medically cleared.*

(Continues)

PLAN

What needs to be done now? *Given lack of response to prior nonintensive counseling at university counseling center, intensive outpatient treatment is recommended.*

What alternative plans have been discussed? *None at this time, counselor will discuss plan with Jennifer and her parents.*

Are these plans reasonable? *Yes*

Can they be carried out? *Jennifer is physically able and appears motivated to carry out this plan; however, her university advisor or counselor needs to monitor her to make certain she is following through.*

COMMIT

Which plan of action has the client chosen? *Jennifer and her parents agree that she will participate in an intensive outpatient program at the medical center.*

Are there resources/support to implement the plan? *Yes, Jennifer's dorm is in walking distance to the medical center, and she can obtain a ride from other students who participate in the group. Medical insurance will cover the cost of treatment.*

Is the client motivated to implement the plan? *Yes, Jennifer is agreeable to this plan as a condition of her remaining in school. She also agrees to abstain from alcohol and all mood-altering chemicals.*

What other resources/support may be needed?

Friend *Yes*   Family members *Yes*

Neighbor *No*   Mental health provider *No*

Public agency (law enforcement, child protective services, social services)

Medical (hospitalization, medication) *Jennifer would also benefit from involvement in A.A. and/or NA.*

The next step for the counselor working with Jennifer is to *Assess* the extent and nature of her alcohol and drug use. Some say, "Why bother, most alcoholics or addicts lie anyway." Others suggest that whatever alcoholics or addicts say they are using, counselors should double the amount to get a more accurate picture of their substance use patterns. That is why, whenever possible, it is helpful to get information from significant others (e.g., roommates, friends, family, co-workers). However, it is important to note that with the exception of a life-threatening medical emergency, federal confidentiality laws pertaining to alcohol and drug cases dictate that counselors must obtain signed written releases from patients before contacting anyone, whether it be to give or gather information. In addition to getting a sense of Jennifer's alcohol and drug use leading up to her hospitalization, the counselor should also find out about Jennifer's substance use in the recent past, and whether she has had prior treatment for alcohol or drug problems, psychiatric problems, or other emotional issues. Also, the counselor should try to determine if Jennifer is considered to be at high risk for an alcohol or drug problem (see Table 5.1 for a list of risk factors).

Prior to Jennifer's being released from the hospital, it is of utmost importance that some definite *Plan* be established for continued assessment and counseling. The tendency of most individuals in situations such as Jennifer's is to deny the need for counseling once the crisis has passed. This is why it is important that definite appointment times be set before she is medically cleared to leave and that Jennifer *Commits* to following through with the plan.

Substance Withdrawal: Crisis Intervention Case Example 2

Sarah is a 28-year-old single retail manager who has been living with her boyfriend, Jon, for the past three years. Although they met while in college, Sarah and Jon did not begin dating until they met up again two years later at a birthday celebration for one of their mutual friends. Sarah had begun drinking while in high school, mostly with friends on weekends. During the summer, she would rent a house at the beach with these friends and there would be constant parties. Sarah was arrested for DWI last year, but she chalked it up to "being in the wrong place at the wrong time." Jon was really upset with her. Although he drinks, he feels that he

TABLE 5.1
Risk Factors and Protective Factors for Alcoholism and Substance Dependence

Risk Factors	Protective Factors
Family history of alcohol or drug problems	Absence of any family history of alcohol or drug problems
Family history of psychiatric problems (e.g., Bipolar Disorder, depression, antisocial personality, or neurochemical model)	Absence of any family history of psychiatric problems
History of diabetes	Absence of family history of diabetes
Prior history of trauma (e.g., childhood sexual or physical abuse)	Absence of any trauma
Friends drink and/or use drugs	Friends do not drink or use drugs and are supportive of abstinence
Family members drink and/or use drugs, encourage use, or are afraid to confront use	Family does not drink or use drugs and is supportive of abstinence

never lets his drinking get out of hand. He feels that Sarah becomes like "Jekyll and Hyde" after a few drinks. One evening at a dinner party, after Sarah consumed about a pint of tequila, Jon caught her passionately kissing one of his best friends. Sarah has sought crisis counseling today because Jon has moved out. Sarah was out drinking with her friends last night and did not come home until 4:00 a.m., only to find that Jon had left her. Sarah is upset, is crying, and doesn't know how she can live without Jon. She did not want to ruin their relationship. She feels that her life is out of control. As the crisis counselor begins to gather more information, Sarah reveals that in addition to drinking upward of a pint of hard liquor each day, she also has a "few glasses of wine" in the evening and then takes a few Valium to calm her nerves in the morning. About 30 minutes into the session, Sarah's hands are noticeably trembling.

Sarah has sought crisis counseling with the presenting complaint that her boyfriend, Jon has left her. (It is not unusual for alcoholics or addicts to present for help with many problems other than their drug or alcohol abuse.) However, as the crisis counselor gathers more information, it is obvious that Sarah has a drinking and drug problem. What is significant, although not unique about her pattern of use, is that she is a functional alcoholic who is also dependent on Valium (another depressant drug). It is likely that her use of Valium is a means of preventing the withdrawal symptoms (such as hand tremors and shakiness) that she experiences in the morning because of her drinking. Similar to the crisis of substance intoxication, substance withdrawal is also a medical emergency. The worst thing a crisis counselor could do is to let Sarah leave the office unattended. Ideally, Sarah should be medically evaluated in an emergency room. The crisis counselor's approach should be to first establish rapport with Sarah and to gather information about her recent use of alcohol and drugs in order to relay this information to the physician who will be assessing her in the emergency room. It will be important to *Listen* to her distress about Jon and to offer support (e.g., "I can see how upset you are about Jon's leaving" or "This separation must be really difficult for you right now"). It is best to stay away from statements like, "Don't worry, you'll get him back," or "I know how you feel, it's tough to go through a break up."

The most difficult scenario that arises with a case involving substance withdrawal is when the person refuses medical attention. Some states have laws that make it permissible to detain a person in an emergency room for 48 to 72 hours. The supposition of these laws is that people who are intoxicated or in substance withdrawal cannot reasonably make informed decisions regarding their treatment; however, others would argue that keeping people in emergency rooms against their will is a violation of their civil liberties. Naturally, there are horror stories of intoxicated people leaving emergency rooms against medical advice and getting killed as they crossed the street. There are no simple solutions to be found. The diagnosis of substance intoxication and substance withdrawal refer to a patient's current status at the time of the crisis intervention; however, once that crisis passes (the person is no longer under the influence of the drug or has been detoxified from the substance) the patient would still need to be evaluated to determine if he or she meets the criteria for substance abuse or dependence.

Sarah's counselor may try to find a family member or friend who can help persuade Sarah to remain in the hospital and get proper medical attention. It is important that the crisis counselor not lose patience or try to force Sarah into making a decision too hastily, as this will usually produce resistance or treatment refusal. It is better that the crisis counselor try to help diminish Sarah's fears of the detoxification process and assure her that many people are present to help see her through this difficult period with as a little distress or pain as possible.

Substance Abuse: Crisis Intervention Case Example 3

Joe is a 72-year-old retired heavy equipment operator. He was referred for an alcoholism assessment following an incident in which he had fallen stepping off of a curb after leaving a restaurant and sprained his ankle. After being examined in the emergency room, Joe was told to see his primary care physician the next day. Joe's wife, Eileen, accompanied him to the doctor's office. She explained to the doctor that Joe had fallen because he had too much to drink. Joe denied that was the reason and instead blamed the fall on losing his balance stepping off a curb. Eileen went on to explain that since his retirement, Joe had begun drinking more in the evening; instead of having his usual one or two beers, he was now consuming seven to ten beers several times a week. She also reported that Joe would drink more often on weekends, especially if they went out with other couples for dinner or if Joe went to play cards at a friend's house. Eileen mentioned that she had also been concerned because Joe would become so drunk that he was not able to get up at night to urinate and would end up wetting the bed. Joe was embarrassed and outraged when Eileen told the doctor about his "accidents," but he admitted to the doctor that what Eileen had told him was true. Joe also admitted that since retiring, he has been feeling worthless, and although he likes seeing his grandchildren, he feels he has nothing else to look forward to. Joe was agreeable to seeing a counselor.

From the information presented, Joe most likely qualifies for a diagnosis of *alcohol abuse*, given that he appears to continue using despite his use having social or interpersonal consequences (e.g., arguments with his wife over his drinking). There have been more regular instances of Joe driving after drinking. It is important to be aware that alcohol and drug abuse are growing problems among the elderly population. Joe is an excellent example of someone who, in retirement, feels stripped of his identity and purpose in life. Many older Americans find themselves confronting other issues in their "golden years," such as failing health, loss of friends, loss of status due to financial worries associated with living on a fixed income, social isolation due to lack of mobility, and loss of self-esteem associated with living an independent lifestyle (McCrady & Epstein, 1999). Although alcohol is most often the drug of choice among older Americans, drug abuse is also a growing concern. In many instances *iatrogenic addictions* occur when primary care physicians or medical specialists prescribe medications (usually for pain or anxiety) that are addictive. (An iatrogenic addiction is an addiction that comes about by treatment.) This is not to say that all older Americans will become addicted to medications that are prescribed to help them with anxiety or pain; however, there is a sizable percentage of the elderly that will become addicted to these medications and will therefore be unable to stop safely on their own.

Once various *plans* have been explored with Joe, one is chosen, and agreed upon. Research indicates that older individuals tend to remain in treatment longer when they are involved in groups with people of similar ages (McCrady & Epstein, 1999). So it is important to try to offer both Joe and Eileen some options that are appropriate and agreeable to both of them. In the event that a group does not exist for Eileen, it may be helpful to refer her to a local Al-Anon group and/or to continue to see both she and Joe for intermittent joint follow-up sessions in order to ensure that they are making progress.

Substance Dependence: Crisis Intervention Case Example 4

Frank is a 45-year-old stockbroker who owns a thriving brokerage firm. Last night he was arrested after getting into an argument with his wife. The argument got very heated and Frank ended up shoving his wife, Claire, down on the floor, which resulted in her hitting her head. She called the police and Frank was arrested for domestic violence. When asked what they were arguing about, Frank stated that about six years ago, he began using cocaine. He described his use as being occasional at first, usually with some of his golf buddies; however, over the past two years, he had begun using more consistently. He stated that on some weekends, he would rent a hotel room and would continue to snort lines of cocaine until Monday. He admitted that he would often get paranoid and would be afraid to come out of the hotel room. He would then take Valium just to calm down enough to go into his office on Monday. Frank explained that Claire doesn't do drugs and never had any interest in them whatsoever. She resented Frank's use because of the time it took him away from her and their son. Frank felt that Claire was overreacting and was being very prudish. He stated that if Claire would just get off his back, he could work this problem out on his own. He had sought crisis counseling because of the domestic violence complaint. Frank presently feels he can cut back on using cocaine, especially if he just sticks to intranasal (snorting) use and refrains from freebasing, as he has been doing the past two years. He does not feel however, that he can stop using all together, nor does he feel that he needs to. At the time of the crisis session, Frank reports feeling depressed, lethargic, and apathetic, which he attributes to his arrest.

In this case, Frank's crisis is illustrative of substance dependence. In his bravado (many cocaine dependent individuals often exhibit a sense of invulnerability), Frank declares, "I can cut back," but later admits that he probably can't stop using all together. Frank is cocaine dependent. As was pointed out previously, although an individual does not have to use on a daily basis or experience tolerance or withdrawal in order to be considered substance dependent, it appears that Frank does exhibit all of the symptoms of substance dependence to some extent. For example, he reports a progression in his cocaine use, having started with occasional use then progressing to daily use punctuated with weekend binges. His report of feeling "depressed, lethargic, and apathetic" is probably evidence of cocaine withdrawal (remember, "what goes up, must come down"). One could also make the argument that Frank is experiencing guilt and is feeling depressed over the domestic violence arrest, yet he plans to continue using despite his knowledge that his cocaine use is causing major disruptions in his marriage. It also appears that, in order to fend off his guilt, Frank blames Claire for his problems and has difficulty admitting that his cocaine addiction is the root cause of his difficulties. This is a common defense among many alcoholics and addicts.

The crisis intervention counselor working with Frank will need to establish rapport with him by *listening* to his explanation of what happened and the events leading up to the arrest. As with other crisis models (e.g., Roberts, 2000a), it would then be useful to help Frank realistically define the problem. For example, even though he would like to view Claire as "the problem," it will be necessary to provide feedback regarding the events he is describing. It will probably take some time to get Frank to focus on his cocaine use, as he is too invested in blaming Claire. The main goal of crisis sessions with individuals who are substance dependent is to get them to question their own faulty addictive logic and accept treatment. As Vernon Johnson states, the approach used in interventions is to "present reality in a receivable way." The reality of Frank's situation is that his cocaine use is out of control and is causing major problems in life functioning. The task of the crisis intervention counselor is to present this "reality in a receivable way," with the hope that Frank will commit to treatment, probably in a residential or inpatient setting in the beginning. Other modalities and sequences of treatment will be discussed in the last section of this chapter.

Family Intervention: Crisis Intervention Case Example 5

Jack Roberts is a 59-year-old attorney who has just been transported to the ER by ambulance after getting into a car accident on his way home from the country club, where he had been drinking heavily after playing golf with some friends. Jack had apparently fallen asleep at the wheel and crashed into a telephone poll. His blood alcohol level was measured at .28, which is more than twice the legal limit for most states. He is semi-conscious when his wife, Marie, and two adult daughters arrive in the ER. After Marie and the daughters are briefed on Jack's medical condition by the ER physician, a consult is requested with the medical center's crisis counselor.

Before concluding this section on intervention techniques, it is important to say a few words about family crises. In many crisis intervention settings, it is not unusual for the family to request help rather than the substance abuser. Family members who have lived with an active alcoholic or addict for years often feel powerless and frustrated in not being able to change their loved one's drinking or drug use. Most families begin to live their lives "around" their alcoholic or addict loved ones. This will sometimes work to a point, but sooner or later a crisis will occur. Family members often live in constant dread of these crises, yet they can also be pivotal points for intervention. In these instances it is important to encourage the family to "strike while the iron is hot," to take advantage of the crisis as an opportunity to intervene with the alcoholic or addict and see to it that treatment begins. The other rule of thumb in working with families in crisis is to be aware of denial in various family members. The dynamics of the chemically dependent family are often unique, not only in the various roles family members play (see the previous discussion), but also in terms of the various forms of *triangulation* and *collusion* that may occur. (Family therapists use these terms to describe family dynamics.) In triangulation, an unstable couple, for instance Jack and Marie, will often drag a third party, usually a son or daughter, into their conflicts as a means of creating a dysfunctional balance. In collusion, a parent may collude with or confide in a son or daughter who then takes sides against the other parent. Therefore, in dealing with a chemically dependent family in crisis, it is common to find a son or daughter who may defend the alcoholic parent or deny the addiction.

In Jack's situation, the counselor would begin by making certain that the Roberts have been apprised of Jack's health condition and that they are reassured that he will be okay. The counselor would then ask Marie and her daughters about their reactions when they received the call from the police. This question can be very revealing. For example, if Marie or one of her daughters were to express anger or frustration upon hearing of the accident, this may be an indication that she has dealt with the issue of drinking (or drinking and driving) in the past. It is also possible that the family may not be willing to reveal much of anything, as it is common for alcoholic families to experience what is called, "a conspiracy of silence," which is an implicit family "rule" that no one is to talk about Jack's drinking to anyone. It is also possible that one daughter may be in denial about her father's drinking problem and may have been in collusion with her father, not only to deny or ignore his behavior but also to enable him by making excuses for his behavior. Once the immediate crisis has passed, it is often helpful to explore these dynamics further; however, in the initial crisis phase of treatment, it is usually best to focus in on the more important issues at hand, for instance getting Jack to accept the need for treatment. Although one could easily infer from Jack's extreme blood alcohol level that he most likely is an alcoholic, the crisis counselor will have a better sense of the extent and duration of his drinking problem from information the family provides. If Jack is *Assessed* as being an alcoholic, then the immediate *Plan* would be to refer him to an inpatient alcoholism treatment program. In the crisis counselor's meeting with Jack, it will be important to find out his perception of the drinking and driving crash. Does he see this crisis as evidence of a drinking problem? If he is in denial of the problem, then the crisis counselor should elicit the aide of the ER physician, Jack's personal physician, and his family in insisting that he seek treatment. Even if Jack were to accept such a plan at the encouragement of his physician, his family, and the crisis counselor, it is important to mention that referrals to inpatient alcoholism programs do not always go smoothly. Since the advent of managed care, several inpatient treatment programs have closed and treatment options are limited. Also, it is often the case that if an individual is insured through a managed care plan, he or she may have limited coverage or the managed care case manager may only certify that individual to stay a few days in treatment.

Treatment Options

There are many different treatment modalities that are available to treat those with substance use disorders. It may be helpful to think of these modalities as existing on a continuum from most to least intensive. With regards to the alcoholic or drug addict, it is also necessary to think of these treatments as being sequential rather than as discrete entities (see Figure 5.1). For example, as in the case of Sarah described previously, once the initial substance withdrawal is managed effectively in a medical setting, she would then most likely be immediately transferred to an inpatient substance treatment facility for a period of about 21 to 28 days. Once she has completed the inpatient phase of treatment, she might be transferred to a halfway house, where she would work or go to school during the day while participating in group counseling and A.A. meetings in the evening at the halfway house. Or she may return home and then would immediately begin an intensive outpatient program. In an intensive outpatient program (or IOP) she would attend groups three to four nights a week while going to A.A. meetings on the weekends, as a means of reinforcing her sobriety/recovery. Usually an IOP will last three or four weeks, at which point Sarah would then most likely begin an outpatient group on a weekly basis or she may be seen for individual counseling about once a week, while she actively attends A.A. meetings in between those sessions.

Although many recovering people will often continue to attend counseling for years into their sobriety. This is not always necessary, although, it is highly recommended that the person continue to actively participate in either A.A., Narcotics Anonymous (NA), or some other 12-step program. Note that the preferred term is *recovering*, not *recovered*, as addictions are chronic lifelong diseases from which a person is never fully "cured." Twelve-step programs are the mainstay of most substance disorder treatment modalities. So, while a person may be in an inpatient program, he or she will be introduced to a 12-step philosophy on how to stay clean and sober.

Individuals without medical insurance coverage or those with managed care insurance plans may not be as fortunate as Sarah to have such a comprehensive array of treatment options at their disposal. For these individuals, their

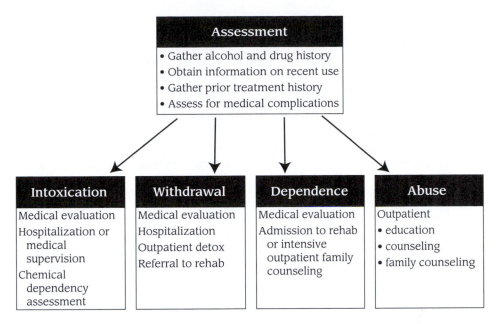

Figure 5.1 Alcohol and Drug Crisis Management

options may be limited to often overcrowded federally funded or state funded programs. These programs often have lengthy waiting lists, however, which adds to the difficulty in treating individuals effectively. From the case vignettes provided, one can see how crucial timing is when getting an alcoholic or addict to agree to treatment. Usually, this does come about in the wake of a major crisis. Unfortunately, to finally have someone agree to go into treatment and then to have them placed a lengthy waiting list is inhumane.

Most treatment programs also include some type of family counseling. Family counseling programs usually vary in terms of their length and intensity. For example, some inpatient programs offer an intensive residential family program which usually lasts for about a week. While in the program, family members often participate in both educational and counseling groups, sometimes with their addicted loved ones, other times without them. The purpose of these family programs is to assist family members in identifying how their loved one's addiction has impacted them and the role they may have played in perpetuating the addiction (e.g., the enabler, the waiverer). Naturally, the goal of such programs is to assist family members in breaking free of pathological family roles. Just as the alcoholic or addict is introduced to A.A. or NA philosophy during the inpatient treatment process, so too are the family members introduced to Al-anon and Nar-anon. (For a complete listing of 12-step programs, see Table 5.2.)

Similar to the alcoholic or addict, family members' treatment does not end once their loved one is out of crisis. Family members should ideally continue to participate in their own counseling beyond the inpatient program stay, and

TABLE 5.2
12-Step Programs

To learn more about specific 12-step programs for various types of addictions or programs for family members, call the phone numbers listed or visit the Web sites for information about meetings and services. There may also be local listings for these 12-step groups listed in the white pages of your phone book. Remember, 12-step programs are *FREE* and are very effective in helping many addicts, alcoholics, and their families.

Alcoholics Anonymous (A.A.)
World Services
Box 459
Grand Central Station
New York, NY 10163
212-870-3400
www.aa.org

Adult Children of Alcoholics
World Service Organization
PO Box 3216
Torrance, CA 90510
310-534-1815
www.adultchildren.org

Al-Anon/Alateen
For adult and teenage family members of alcoholics and other friends or relatives
Al-Anon Family Group Headquarters
1600 Corporate Landing Parkway
Virginia Beach, VA 23454-5617
888-4AL-ANON
www.al-anon.org

Co-Dependents Anonymous
For people whose lives are impacted by alcoholics or addicted individuals and who cannot seem to break free from problematic roles in which they may enable the addict or alcoholic to continue the substance abuse
PO Box 33577
Phoenix, AZ 85067-3577
602-277-7991
www.codependents.org

Debtors Anonymous
General Services Office
PO Box 920888
Needham, MA 02492-0009
Phone: 781-453-2743
Fax: 781-453-2745
www.debtorsanonymous.org

Gam-Anon
For family, friends, and significant others of people with gambling addictions
International Service Office
PO Box 157
Whitestone, NY 11357
Phone: 718-352-1671
Fax: 718-746-2571
www.gam-anon.org

Gamblers Anonymous
International Service Office
PO Box 17173
Los Angeles, CA 90017
Phone: 213-386-8789
Fax: 213-386-0030
www.gamblersanonymous.org

Narcotics Anonymous
World Service Office
PO Box 9999
Van Nuys, CA 91409
Phone: 818-773-9999
Fax: 818-700-0700
www.na.org

Overeaters Anonymous
World Service Office
PO Box 44020
Rio Rancho, NM 87174-4020
Phone: 505-891-4320
Fax: 505-891-4320
www.overeatersanonymous.org

Sexaholics Anonymous (S.A.)
PO Box 111910
Nashville, TN 37222
Phone: 615-331-6230
Fax: 615-331-6901
www.sa.org

Sex Addicts Anonymous (S.A.A.)
International Service Office
PO Box 70949
Houston, TX 77270
800-477-8191
www.saa-recovery.org

(Continues)

TABLE 5.2
12-Step Programs *(Continued)*

Sexual Compulsives Anonymous (S.C.A.)
International Service Office
PO Box 1585
Old Chelsea Station
New York, NY 10011
800-977-HEAL
www.sca-recovery.org

Sex and Love Addicts Anonymous (S.L.A.A.)
The Augustine Fellowship
PO Box 338
Norwood, MA 02062-0338
781-255-8825
www.slaafws.org

S-Anon International Family Groups
For family members and significant others of sex addicts
PO Box 111242
Nashville, TN 37222-1242
615-833-3152
www.sanon.org

Solvency
Ideas and support for those in debt and compulsive spenders, and listings for Debtors Anonymous meetings
www.solvency.org

Sober Space
Information on A.A. meetings across the United States by state; also lists phone numbers for local A.A. Intergroups and e-mail addresses by state
www.soberspace.com

Living Cyber
A.A. interaction on the internet; get a list of online A.A. meetings by typing in "meetings" in the search box; A.A. related Web chats and message boards
www.livingcyber.org

New Beginnings
An e-mail Narcotics Anonymous group; members from all over the world e-mail and share via the Internet twice a week; this site can be viewed in English, Spanish, Portuguese, and Italian
www.netmegs.com/na-nbg

Original Group
Download a copy of the A.A. Big Book in Windows 95 Format
www.originalgroup.com/on-the-net/bb_index.html

continue to attend Al-anon and Nar-anon meetings regularly. A question arises in terms of when is the best time to begin couples counseling or family counseling with the alcoholic or addict present. This is not always a black or white issue. Obviously, the alcoholic or addict must be stable enough in recovery to be capable of hearing sometimes not-too-flattering feedback from family members. Sometimes, family members see the initial counseling sessions as a safe means to vent all their anger and resentment towards the alcoholic or addict. In some instances, if this is handled similarly to an intervention, it can certainly help to break down any remnants of denial. However, the caveat, is that the alcoholic or addict must be stabilized enough to withstand the anger. This is why some addiction treatment providers prefer to hold off on any heavy duty family or couples counseling until the alcoholic or addict is well into recovery (perhaps at least 6 to 12 months sober). The problem with this approach is that many more couples break up during recovery than they do during active addiction, so the question remains whether it is truly better to hold off on couples/family counseling. Research studies seem to suggest however, that there is a better prognosis for those families who do participate in treatment when compared to those who don't.

SOURCES OF CHAPTER ENRICHMENT

Print Sources

Goodwin, D. W. (1984). Studies of familial alcoholism: A review. *Archives of general psychiatry, 45*, 14–17.

McCrady, B. S., & Epstein, E. E. (Eds.). (1999). *Addictions: A comprehensive guidebook.* Oxford, UK: Oxford University Press.

Johnson, V. (1980). *I'll quit tomorrow: A practical guide to alcoholism treatment.* San Francisco, CA: Harper Collins.

Stanton, M. D., & Todd, T. C. (1982). *The family therapy of drug abuse and addiction.* New York: Guilford Press.

Vaillant, G. E. (1995). *The natural history of alcoholism revisited.* Cambridge, MA: Harvard University Press.

Internet Sources

National Institute of Alcohol Abuse & Alcoholism (NIAAA) (http://www.niaaa .nih.gov) NIAAA is located in Washington, DC. This site contains a plethora of useful information, including incidence and prevalence statistics; factual information about alcohol, alcohol abuse, and alcoholism; mortality statistics; treatment resources; and "Frequently Asked Questions." This is an excellent Web site for gaining some good basic knowledge about alcohol.

National Institute of Drug Abuse (NIDA) (http://www.nida.nih.gov) The NIDA is located in Washington, DC. This Web site is similar to the NIAAA site cited above, but it deals specifically with drugs of abuse. It also contains a great deal of factual information about incidence and prevalence rates, up-to-date information about a variety of drugs, treatment resources, and other worthwhile statistics.

Substance Abuse & Mental Health Services Administration (http://www.samhsa.gov) SAMHSA is an agency of the U.S. Department of Health & Human Services. This site contains up-to-date information on incidence and prevalence rates, treatment resources, and information on drugs and alcohol.

National Clearinghouse of Alcohol and Drug Information (http://ncadi.samsha.gov) The National Clearinghouse of Alcohol and Drug Information is a service of the Substance Abuse & Mental Health Services Administration (SAMHSA), which is an agency of the U.S. Department of Health & Human Services. This site provides excellent up-to-date information on topics pertaining to drugs and alcohol. Each drug of choice has a separate page that contains vital information about the effects of the drug, as well as the dangers and consequences associated with it. There is also information about treatment resources. This page is quite useful for those providing education and/or prevention services to a variety of individuals from different backgrounds, as the site contains specific pages for various groups (e.g., teens, elderly, gay and lesbians, as well as a variety of racial and ethnic minorities).

National Council on Alcoholism and Drug Dependence (http://www.ncadd.org) This site contains useful, up-to-date information on alcohol and drugs, as well as treatment services.

Alcohol & Drug Abuse Commission (http://www.aadac.com) This Web site contains a lot of information pertaining to drugs and alcohol, negative effects, and treatment options.

The Web of Addictions (http://www.webofaddictions.com) This is an excellent Web site that provides a great deal of information for those with addictive illnesses. The page contains links to many other resources and mailing lists. A review of the Web site can be found on Dr. Grohol's Web site at http://www.grohol.com/reviews.htm.

CHAPTER 6

Threats of Suicide, Homicide, and Other Violent Acts

Susan is a 24-year-old divorced mother of a 10-month-old daughter. She called the hotline of the local mental health clinic today because she felt so upset she could not get out of bed. Susan explained to the hotline crisis worker that she has felt this way for the past three months. Susan described feeling "lifeless and hopeless" that she has no energy to do anything. She also said that nothing is really enjoyable to her anymore, and as a result, she has become more and more reclusive and prefers to be left alone. Since her husband left her for one of her best friends, she feels she doesn't "have anything to live for." When questioned directly, she denied feeling suicidal, but then stated that she tried to cut her wrists about four weeks ago when she received the final divorce papers, but "lost the nerve" and could not go through with it. "Besides," she said, "I could not leave my baby all alone, with no one to look out for her."

Of all the different types of crises that are covered in this text, crises that have the potential for severe injury or loss of life are often the most upsetting, anxiety provoking, and complex for counselors. Yet when these crises are successfully resolved, crisis counselors may take some comfort in knowing that their efforts may have saved lives. The types of crises presented in this chapter are those involving suicidal and homicidal threats, as well as other threats of violence that may result in severe injury or death. Suicidal crises are extremely problematic to manage in terms of ascertaining that the suicidal individual will be safe. In some instances this is easier than in others. In Susan's case, ensuring her safety is made difficult by the fact that her initial contact is made through a crisis hotline. Homicidal crises are also difficult, and often frightening, to manage. Crisis counselors are frequently called upon to assess the lethality of direct threats—as well as veiled threats—of violence, which may have homicidal implications. Lethality is a measure of the degree of danger in a crisis situation. The goal in managing crises involving homicidal and violent threats is naturally to prevent harm from coming to others. Therefore, the assessment of lethality often determines what steps will be taken in an intervention.

Suicidal Crises

One of the driving forces behind most suicides is unendurable psychological pain (Schneidman, 1985). William Styron (1990), the well-known novelist who suffered from depression, referred to this pain as "a howling tempest in the brain." Indeed, the three most painful emotions often associated with suicide are self-hate, aloneness, and murderous hatred (Maltsberger, 1992).

Scope and Definition of the Problem

The statistics regarding suicide are rather alarming. Suicide ranks among the leading causes of death, not only in the United States, but in many industrialized countries (Malley, Kush & Bogo, 1994). In the United States, there were 30,903 suicide deaths in 1996 and 28,332 in 2000. In 2001, there were more than 30,000 deaths related to suicide, roughly equivalent to more than 80 suicides per day, or one suicide every 20 minutes. Suicides outnumbered homicides three to two, and were twice as common as deaths related to HIV and AIDS (National Institute of Mental Health, 2002). Young people between the ages of 15 and 24 are considered to be a high-risk group because suicide ranks among the leading causes of death in this age group. In fact, between 1950 and 1996, suicide rates within this age group tripled (Peters, Kochanek, & Murphy, 1998; Anderson, 2001). During 2000, suicide was the fifth leading cause of death in the 5- to 14-year-old age group, the third leading cause of death in the 15- to 24-year-old age group (accidents and homicides are the other leading causes of death in this age group); and the fourth leading cause of death for the 25- to 44-year-old age group. Firearms were used in the majority of the suicide deaths in the 15- to 24-year-old age group. However, it should be noted that injuries from firearms were the leading cause of death for both adult men and women (Peters, Kochanek, & Murphy, 1998). Therefore, according to Maris (1992), the issues of suicide prevention and gun control are very much intertwined.

According to demographic statistics, suicide is more prevalent in European American males, however, the rates of suicide among African American males between 15 and 24 years old have been increasing dramatically (Kachur, Potter, James, & Powell, 1995). Table 6.1 indicates that suicide is among the leading causes of death in African Americans, Native Americans, and Asian/Pacific Islander Americans.

Adolescents and young adults are not the only group at risk for suicidal behavior. Males 45 years and older constitute the other high-risk group. Research literature suggests that the risk of suicide in men increases with age. This risk is compounded if there is a chronic medical condition present,

TABLE 6.1
Ranking of Suicide Among Leading Causes of Death in the
United States for Selected Age Groups by Race and Sex, 1999

	Male				
	Age Group				
	10–14	15–19	20–24	25–34	35–44
Caucasian	3rd	2nd	2nd	2nd	4th
African American	7th	3rd	3rd	5th	7th
American Indian	4th	2nd	2nd	2nd	4th
Asian/Island Pacific	3rd	3rd	2nd	2nd	4th

	Female				
	Age Group				
	10–14	15–19	20–24	25–34	35–44
Caucasian	6th	a	4th	3rd	4th
African American	7th	5th	6th	10th	a
American Indian	a	2nd	3rd	3rd	7th
Asian/Island Pacific	5th	2nd	2nd	3rd	5th

a These combined factors fell outside of the top ten leading causes.

Note. Derived from "Deaths: Leading Causes for 1999," by R. N. Anderson,
2001, *National Vital Statistics Report, 49*(11), Hyattsville, MD: National Center
for Health Statistics. Available at http://www.cdc.gov/nchs/data/nvsr
/nvsr49/nvsr49_11.pdf.

especially if that condition involves chronic pain. Risk can also be compounded by several other factors including particular psychiatric illnesses, alcohol and drug abuse, and living alone. The psychiatric disorders most often associated with suicide include Schizophrenia, Depression (both Major Depression and Bipolar Depression), and Substance Use Disorders (alcohol and drug dependencies). Research indicates that approximately 10% of Schizophrenics end up committing suicide. Risk factors for suicidality in this population include being male, younger than 30 years old, and unemployed; having a high level of education, chronic relapses, prior depression in the last episode of active schizophrenic symptoms, and a recent hospital discharge. Schizophrenics who commit suicide are often painfully aware of their condition, which often results in feelings of inadequacy and hopelessness. They rarely communicate their suicide intentions to others. In addition, alcohol and drug abuse will exacerbate suicidal risk (Tsuang, Fleming, & Simpson, 1999). The risk of suicide is also increased when people have endured severe psychological trauma. According to Chu (1999), individuals who have been subject to severe childhood physical or sexual abuse often manifest two traits that place them at substantial risk for suicide—profound mistrust and self-hate.

Substance Use Disorders also increase the risk for suicide in the general population. Intuitively, drinking or drug use will often intensify an already existing depression and will add to feelings of hopelessness and helplessness. Alcohol and drug intoxication will often disinhibit people, which makes the likelihood of suicidal action much greater. Mood-altering chemicals can also increase the chances of indirect suicidality, as when someone "accidentally" overdoses or "accidentally" is killed in a car accident (Weiss & Hufford, 1999).

Lifetime data indicates that men outnumber women 4.6 to 1 in their suicide completion rates (Shaffer, Gould, & Hicks, 1994; Centers for Disease Control and Prevention, 1998). However, adolescent and adult women outnumber men in nonfatal suicide attempt rates and in overall rates of depressive illness (Andrews & Lewinsohn, 1992; Garrison, McKeown, & Valois, 1993). The lifetime data on suicide attempts, however, suggests there is no difference between men and women (Andrews & Lewinsohn, 1992; Beautrais, Joyce, & Mulder, 1996; Petronis, Samuels, & Moscicki, 1990).

Table 6.2 presents a list of risk factors associated with suicide. Naturally, this is just a partial list. Several predictors must be taken into account when assessing someone who may be suicidal. For example, suicidal risk is considered to be greater when the individual is male; is 45 years old or older; is separated, widowed, or divorced; lives alone; is unemployed or retired; is in poor physical health; has a mental disorder; is an alcoholic; has had medical care within the past six months; has a suicidal plan involving firearms, hanging, jumping, or drowning; has made a prior attempt in the warmer months; made the prior attempt at home and was discovered immediately; does not report suicidal intent to others; and leaves a suicide note. The difficulty in assessing a patient based upon risk factors is that a person may exhibit three or four risk factors and actually be at lower risk for suicide than somebody who only exhibits one (e.g., a depressed African American teenaged male with undefined suicidal ideas might be at lower suicidal risk than a European American female of the same age who has a prior history of suicide attempts). Therefore, assessment of risk needs to be done on a case-by-case basis.

In spite of efforts to improve our ability to assess, predict, and prevent suicide based upon lists of risk factors, there are limitations to this approach. Motto (1999) pointed to the fact that some risk factors may have no significance at all. Motto provides an example of a man who was hospitalized two years earlier for a serious suicide attempt presently reports not having any suicidal thoughts because his divorce finally came through. The research literature indicates that individuals who are divorced are at higher risk for suicide, yet for this individual, being able to extricate himself from a miserable marriage was apparently the key to ridding himself of hopeless feelings. In another example, Linehan (1999) described a rather high functioning professional individual who had an extensive support system. But he committed suicide because of his guilt over being a burden to those to whom he felt closest and who had taken care of him.

Assessing Suicidal Risk

When people are assessed for suicidal risk in crisis situations, usually their entire histories and family histories are taken into account, as well as their current mental status (see Box 6.1). A mental status exam usually includes an

TABLE 6.2
Risk Factors Associated with Suicide

General Risk Factors

- A past history of suicide gestures or attempts (it is a myth that those who talk about suicide rarely act on those threats; all suicidal threats, statements, or comments should be taken seriously)
- A family history of suicide or depressive psychiatric illness
- Active drug or alcohol use/abuse/dependence (alcohol and drugs may have a disinhibiting effect, making the person more likely to act on suicidal feelings or ideas)
- A history of psychiatric disorder; the following disorders often have the highest rates of suicide: Bipolar Disorder, Schizophrenia, Major Depression, alcohol or drug dependence
- A history of severe trauma, such as sexual molestation, incest, sexual abuse
- Isolation from others (i.e., either lives alone or is recently separated, divorced, or widowed)
- Radical shifts in behavior or mood, such as giving away prized possessions, saying goodbye to loved ones, or taking care of unfinished business; there may also be changes in sleep or eating habits and work or school behavior, as well as anxiety and irritability
- Expression of a profound sense of hopelessness or helplessness ("no matter what I do or say, nothing will ever change or be different. I will never be able to change," or "I just can't go on living without him/her")
- Chronic medical condition or a medical condition that causes chronic pain
- Suicidal ideation or a plan and means to carry out that plan
- Living alone or divorced, separated, or widowed

Risk Factors for Adolescents and Young Adults

- Family history of suicide
- Male (higher suicide rate than females)
- History of previous attempts
- Native American
- Psychiatric diagnosis: mood disorders and substance abuse
- White (higher suicide rate than Blacks)
- Mini-epidemic in community
- History of delinquent or semi-delinquent behavior, even without depression in current mental state
- Access to firearms (when other factors are present)

(Continues)

TABLE 6.2
Risk Factors Associated with Suicide *(Continued)*

Risk Factors for Adults Older Than 30

- Family history of suicide
- Male (higher suicide rate than females)
- History of previous attempts
- Native American
- Psychiatric diagnosis: mood disorder, schizophrenia, alcoholism
- Single, especially separated, divorced, or widowed
- Lack of social supports
- Concurrent medical illness or illnesses
- Unemployed
- Decline in socioeconomic status
- Psychological turmoil
- History of violence
- Access to a weapon or firearm

Note. Adapted from various chapters in *The Harvard Medical School Guide to Suicide Assessment and Intervention,* by D. G. Jacobs (Ed.), 1999, San Francisco: Jossey-Bass.

assessment of a person's present physical appearance, behavior, speech, emotional expression, thought processes, perception, attention and concentration abilities, memory, judgment, intellectual functioning, and ability to form insight (Maxmen & Ward, 1995). If a counselor is using a mental status exam to determine if a person is suicidal, he or she might expect to see depressive type affect or sometimes an agitated depression. In agitated depression, the person expresses primarily depressive thoughts. However, the person is in so much emotional pain that it is difficult for him or her to slow down or even to sit still. An individual in an agitated depression might pace around the room restlessly, wring his or her hands, or talk rapidly. This is a very different presentation from a person who is suffering from a more typical depression, which usually manifests as slowed speech and movements, lethargy, hopelessness, helplessness, and a sense of despair. In making a suicide assessment, there are also some commercially available suicide assessment measures—the Beck Scale for Suicide Ideation (Beck, 1991), Suicide Probability Scale (Cull & Gill, 1989), Beck Hopelessness Scale (Beck, 1993), Adult Suicidal Ideation Questionnaire (Reynolds, 1991), Suicidal Ideation Questionnaire (for adolescents) (Reynolds, 1992), Suicidal Behavior History Form (Reynolds & Mazza, 1993), and the Children's Depression Inventory (Kessler et al., 1996).

Although cognitively and/or intellectually, there may be no overtly unusual thoughts, it is common for suicidal individuals to either keep their thoughts hidden or to have rather elaborate justifications for why the world would be a better place without them. This lapse of reasoning or judgment may be evident only in relation to their suicidal thoughts. Their memory, problem

---

BOX 6.1

SAD PERSONS: A Mnemonic for Assessing Suicide Risk

Sex (male)
Age (adolescent or elderly)
Depression

Previous suicide attempts
Ethanol (alcohol) use
Rational thinking loss (psychosis)
Social supports lacking
Organized plan to commit suicide
No spouse (divorced, widowed, or single)
Sickness (physical illness)

Note. From "Evaluation of Suicidal Patients: The SAD PERSONS Scale," by W. M. Patterson, H. H. Dohn, J. M. Bird, and G. A Patterson, 1983, *Psychosomatics, 24,* 343–349. Reprinted with permission.

---

solving skills, attention, and concentration abilities may be otherwise intact. It is even more disconcerting when a person presents in a crisis state, but purposely refrains from divulging any suicidal ideation. Motto (1999), for example, described individuals who suffer from "emotional exhaustion" who will consistently deny any active suicidal thoughts and who appear to function well on a daily basis. These individuals are often "too tired to go on any longer" (p. 228) and at that point will take their lives without any rhyme or reason. Even attempts to find a triggering event are often futile, although a minor issue sometimes surfaces as being "the last straw." In such cases, where suicidal ideas may not be directly or overtly communicated, it is important to listen for subtle clues, such as vague statements similar to the following:

- "She'd be better off without me."
- "What difference does it make anyway if I live or die."
- "I just can't stand the pain anymore."
- "I have a way to solve everything."
- "Life has lost its meaning for me."
- "Nobody needs me anymore."
- "If (such and such) happens, I just don't think I can go on."
- "You won't have to worry about me much longer."
- "I'm going to take care of it."

These statements may indirectly allude to suicidal intent.

One of the rules of assessment often taught to mental health graduate students and psychiatric residents is, "When in doubt about suicidal intent, ask directly about it." One of the myths regarding suicide is that talking about it will cause the person to think about suicide and/or to carry out suicidal actions. This is not true. If anything, many individuals will be quite open about their suicidal thoughts or feelings when asked directly. (See Box 6.2 for more examples of myths about suicide.) In such instances, the counselor may raise a question such as, "I've been listening to what you've said about not finding life worthwhile anymore, and I was wondering if you're feeling so down, so helpless, that you may be having suicidal thoughts?" If the client were to respond affirmatively that he or she had considered suicide, then the most important information to gather would be how recently those thoughts had occurred, had the client formulated a plan or method for committing suicide, had the client made any type of suicidal gesture or attempt in the past and if so, what happened. It would also be important to ask if this person has access to a means of committing suicide (e.g., access to firearms, pills, weapons). If so, does the client also have a plan to act on these thoughts? Does he or she know of anyone who has tried or succeeded in committing suicide, especially family members? In some instances there may be behavioral clues. Molin (1986) described a phenomenon called "covert suicide," which is a series of progressively more serious suicidal gestures or "accidents" that a person may engage in prior to making a suicide attempt. This type of suicidal behavior is common in adolescents who abuse alcohol and drugs (Cavaiola & Lavender, 1999).

Unfortunately, there are instances of individuals with suicidal intent who give absolutely no clues regarding their self-destructive intentions. This is naturally the most frightening situation. However, because many suicidal individuals are ambivalent and confused (Schneidman, 1985), they may provide some indirect clues or indications. Example of behavioral clues include giving away prized possessions or telling friends and loved ones how much they have meant, as if saying goodbye. Research indicates that individuals who commit suicide will often give clues to those around them (Capuzzi, 1994; Capuzzi & Golden, 1988) that may reflect their ambivalence toward life.

Another startling factor in suicide counters the myth that once a person's depression has lifted, the suicidal crisis is over. Frequently, as a depressed individual begins to "feel better," the suicidal risk *increases*. This may seem paradoxical; however, in the throes of deep depression, many individuals simply lack the energy to carry through with suicidal behavior. But once the depression begins to lift, the person feels sufficient energy to carry through with suicidal intentions. This type of situation is always difficult to assess, which is why any counselor working with someone who has a history of suicidal behavior or intent will usually monitor how the person is feeling and his or her progress on a regular basis. Also, antidepressants can take several weeks before they become effective, so another crisis can occur after the onset of treatment when the person may feel a sense of failure for not feeling any better.

BOX 6.2

Myths of Suicide

1. *Myth:* Individuals who are suicidal will usually convey their feelings to others, even if subtly.

   Fact: Not all individuals will convey their suicidal ideas or intent to others.

2. *Myth:* Once the person's mood has lifted, the danger of suicide has passed.

   Fact: In many instances, the lifting of a person's mood may be a sign that they he or she has made the decision to commit suicide and therefore is feeling some relief, just by having made the decision. In many instances, people who are in deep depression lack the energy to carry through with suicidal intentions and will only act once their mood has lifted and they are feeling more energetic.

3. *Myth:* Talking about suicide with someone will cause him or her to become even more suicidal or to carry through with suicidal acts.

   Fact: If a counselor is in doubt or is suspecting that someone is harboring suicidal thoughts, it is better to bring these concerns up directly in a nonjudgmental manner. It is also better to ask specific questions rather than to merely ask, "Are you suicidal?" to which the person could simply reply, "No, I'm not."

4. Myth: Suicidal people are insane.

   Fact: Although many individuals who attempt suicide may be in the throes of depression, alcoholism, or schizophrenia, they are usually not insane. Even with schizophrenia, people may be more likely to act on suicidal feelings when they are in remission.

5. *Myth:* All suicides are impulsive.

   Fact: Although some people commit suicide suddenly or in the midst of an emotional crisis, the majority of suicides are well-planned and well thought out.

6. *Myth:* All suicides are about revenge.

   Fact: There are some who feel that "behind every suicide, there's a homicide"; however, this is not the only motive for suicide. Most individuals who attempt suicide are attempting to seek relief from emotional and/or physical pain.

It is important for crisis counselors to keep in mind as they assess someone who may be at potential risk for suicide that hopelessness is one of the most important predictors of suicide (Reinecke, 2000). Hopelessness refers to a cognitive set of negative expectations that people hold about themselves and the future, including an inability to change themselves and situations in the future (Beck, 1967 and 1986; Dyer & Kreitman, 1984; Weishaar & Beck, 1990). Hopelessness is a common symptom of depression, but has been found to differentiate between suicidal and non-suicidal individuals with equal levels of depression (Ellis & Ratliff, 1986). Also, hopelessness is a good long-term predictor of those who eventually do commit suicide (Beck, Brown, & Steer, 1989; Beck & Steer, 1989; Fawcett, et al., 1990).

Crisis Intervention With Suicidal Individuals

Crisis intervention that involves some type of suicidal threat usually will begin with a risk assessment. As described in the last section, there are several risk factors that may help to ascertain whether a person is at high risk of committing suicide. What should be clear, though, is that some risk factors or correlates will weigh more heavily than others. Linehan (1999), for example, outlined a number of factors that are associated with immediate risk for suicide attempts. See Table 6.3 for a list of the indicators and circumstances of an immediate or imminent suicidal danger or risk. It should be noted that some of the items listed are also listed in Table 6.2. What distinguishes this list in Table 6.3, however, is that these items are associated with imminent or immediate risk, which is of tremendous importance to crisis counselors who are assessing individuals in the immediate throes of a suicidal crisis. The direct indicators include obvious expression of any suicidal threats, plans, prior attempts, and suicidal ideas. The indirect indicators, however, include the more subtle but serious indicators, such as recent disruptions in interpersonal relationships, indifference or dissatisfaction with one's therapy, current hopelessness or anger or both, recent medical care, and indirect references to one's own death or arrangements pertaining to one's death (e.g., giving away prized possessions, referring to a will, funeral arrangements). Current circumstances include major depression (either agitated depression or significant depressive affect), alcohol consumption, isolation, precautions to conceal suicidal plan, recent incarceration in jail or prison, and recent media publicity about a suicide.

Linehan (1999) provided a useful model for counseling individuals who are in the throes of a suicidal crisis; the model provides a series of steps (see Table 6.4) that crisis counselors can take in order to effectively manage suicidal behaviors. This series of steps helps guide the crisis counselor through a specific action plan to make certain the patient will be safe. Most often, the plan will require that a psychiatric evaluation be performed in an emergency room, so that if inpatient hospitalization is recommended, it can be expedited. Once patient safety is ensured, the crisis counselor can begin to address the suicidal ideations, motivations, and reasons why the patient views suicide as a solution to his or her current situation or problem.

TABLE 6.3
Indicators and Circumstances of Imminent Risk for Attempted Suicide or Suicide

Direct Indicators of Imminent Risk for Suicide or Attempted Suicide

1. Suicide threats
2. Suicide planning or preparation
3. Suicide attempt in the last year, especially if suicide intent was expressed at the time
4. Suicidal ideation

Indirect Indicators of Imminent Risk for Suicide or Attempted Suicide

1. Patient's shift into suicide or attempted suicide risk population
2. Recent disruption or loss of interpersonal relationship; negative environmental changes in past month
3. Indifference to or dissatisfaction with therapy; elopements and early pass return by hospitalized patients
4. Current hopelessness or anger or both; increased psychological perturbation
5. Recent medical care
6. Indirect references to own death; arrangements for death

Circumstances Associated With Suicide or Attempted Suicide in the Next Several Hours or Days

1. Major depression with
   a. severe agitation, psychic anxiety, panic attacks; severe obsessional rumination or compulsive behaviors
   b. global insomnia
   c. severe anhedonia (inability to experience pleasure in anything)
   d. diminished concentration, indecision
2. Alcohol consumption
3. Suicide note written or in progress
4. Methods available or easily obtained
5. Isolation
6. Precautions against discovery or intervention; deception or concealment about timing, place, and so forth
7. First twenty-four hours of jail incarceration
8. Recent media publicity about suicide

Note. From "Standard protocol for assessing and treating suicidal behaviors for patients in treatment" (p. 158), by M. M. Linehan, in *The Harvard Medical School Guide to Suicide Assessment and Intervention,* by D. G. Jacobs (Ed.), 1999, San Francisco: Jossey-Bass. Copyright © 1999 by the President and Fellows of Harvard College. Reprinted with permission.

The following case example was presented briefly at the beginning of this chapter. What makes this case especially difficult is that Susan has called a crisis hotline. Therefore, it is more difficult to ensure her safety. More case detail is also provided.

TABLE 6.4
Management of Acute Suicidal Behaviors and Crisis Intervention

- Assess risk of immediate suicide or parasuicide
- Explore the problem now
  - Identify key events that have set off current emotional response
  - Formulate and summarize the problem situation with the patient
- Address high-risk environment factors
  - Remove or convince the patient to remove lethal items
  - Maintain contact when suicide risk is imminent and high
  - Communicate with patient's network
  - Intervene to stop ongoing traumatic events
  - Recommend or consider hospitalization
  - Remove or counteract modeling of suicide behaviors
- Address behavioral high-risk factors
  - Pay attention to affect rather than content
  - Focus on affect tolerance
  - Consider short-term somatic treatment
  - Generate hope and reasons for living
- Focus on problem solving
  - Emphatically instruct patient not to commit suicide
  - Persist with statements that suicide is not a good solution, that a better one can be found
  - Predict future consequences of various plans of action
  - Confront the patient's ideas or behavior directly
  - Give advice and make direct suggestions
  - Offer solutions from the perspective of the other skills the patient is learning in therapy
  - Clarify and reinforce adaptive responses on the part of the patient, especially adaptive problem-solving ideas or prior adaptive responses in similar situations
  - Identify factors interfering with productive plans of action
- Commit to a plan of action
  - Reassess suicidal potential
  - Anticipate a recurrence of the crisis response

Note. From "Standard protocol for assessing and treating suicidal behaviors for patients in treatment" (p. 187) by M. M. Linehan, in *The Harvard Medical School Guide to Suicide Assessment and Intervention,* by D. G. Jacobs (Ed.), 1999, San Francisco: Jossey-Bass. Copyright © 1999 by the President and Fellows of Harvard College. Reprinted with permission.

THE HIGH RISK INDIVIDUAL: CRISIS INTERVENTION CASE EXAMPLE 1

Susan is a 24-year-old divorced mother of a 10-month-old daughter. She called the hotline of the local mental health clinic today because she felt so upset she could not get out of bed. Susan explained to the hotline crisis worker that she has felt this way for the past three months. Susan described feeling "lifeless and hopeless" that she has no energy to do anything. She also said that nothing is really enjoyable to her anymore, and as a result, she has become more and more reclusive and prefers to be left alone. Since her husband left her for one of her best friends, she feels she doesn't "have anything to live for." When questioned directly, she denied feeling suicidal, but then stated that she tried to cut her wrists about four weeks ago when she received the final divorce papers, but "lost the nerve" and could not go through with it. "Besides," she said, "I could not leave my baby all alone, with no one to look out for her." Susan mentioned that she has no family living in the area, and her closest relatives live about 200 miles away and they have not been very supportive of her.

In Susan's case, we see an individual who is considered to be at high risk for suicide. Even though she claims that she tried to cut her wrists four weeks ago and was unable to go through with it, there is still a real danger of a future, potentially fatal suicide attempt. Susan is young. She and her baby live alone without any support. She has experienced the trauma of a marital separation in which her husband left her for her best friend. Susan's recent suicide attempt occurred when she was served with divorce papers. What makes this case difficult to assess is that the initial contact occurred when Susan called a psychiatric hotline. If she had presented at a clinic or emergency room, this assessment could have been conducted face-to-face, which offers many advantages. However, crisis counselors are usually quite limited in how much information they will be able to obtain over the phone. Obviously, the crisis counselor working with Susan would first need to establish rapport or try to connect with her. Asking Susan about her baby or some other aspects of her life that would be less threatening might help accomplish this. Also, the crisis counselor will need to convey a willingness to listen to Susan's problems nonjudgmentally and convey to Susan that he or she is there to help her work out some solutions to these problems. The counselor needs to be very definite in convincing Susan that treatment works, that he or she will help Susan explore effective solutions to her problems, and that he or she will she see Susan through her current emotional crisis. It is of utmost importance to provide hope (Bohen, 2002). This is sometimes difficult, as many suicidal individuals will often feel that there are no solutions, so suicide is perceived as their only viable alternative. However, Susan did call the crisis hotline, which can be viewed as a positive step and perhaps as a cry for help. The crisis counselor basically needs to create an ally in that part of Susan that wants to live, that part of her personality that wants to continue to be a good parent to her daughter, or that part of her personality that gave her the courage to call the hotline.

Susan goes on to explain to the crisis counselor that she had sought counseling after her mother died and it really helped. She also had contacted her aunt to stay with her. These factors may be seen as positive signs. At this point, the counselor is able to persuade Susan to come down to the mental health clinic, where she can speak with her in person. Susan agrees because she feels some trust in the crisis counselor and is willing to get help. Susan makes an agreement with the counselor that she will come to the center and she will bring her aunt with her. They set up a specific meeting time. Susan allows the counselor to speak to her aunt over the phone, in order to make certain that Susan will make the appointment. If the crisis counselor had assessed Susan as being in danger at that particular moment and she was alone, then it would have been necessary for the counselor to trace the call through the telephone operator and to have the police or a mobile mental health outreach team sent to Susan's home. If that were the case, Susan would then have been brought to the local emergency room or mental health clinic for assessment and probably would be admitted to a hospital for observation.

Once Susan is assessed at the mental health clinic, it is determined that she is not actively suicidal and can be treated on an outpatient basis with a combination of psychotherapy and antidepressant medication. With the support of her therapist and her aunt, Susan agrees to a "No Suicide Contract." According to Motto (1999), contracts may be a useful therapeutic tool; however, this will depend on whether there is a strong, mutually trusting relationship with the therapist. Contracts can be formal written documents that the therapist, the patient, and a significant other would sign (in this instance, Susan's aunt would be involved in the contract), or they can be simple verbal agreements (e.g., "Would you agree to call me or come in for a session if you're feeling overwhelmed or feeling like you might hurt yourself?"). Contracts are still a subject of research study and debate (Davidson, Wagner, & Range, 1995; Egan, 1997; Miller, 1999). However, when lethality is judged to be low, they do have a place in crisis management.

INTERVENTION PRACTICES   In any situation involving a suicidal person, the most important step is to make certain that individual will be *safe*. It is always better to err on the side of caution. There may be instances when a person who intends to commit suicide tells a counselor, friends, or family what he or she thinks they want to hear to convince them that the crisis has passed. In Susan's case, for example, the crisis counselor might have been lead to think that the crisis had passed and that Susan was feeling better. Therefore, it is always preferable to have a potentially suicidal client evaluated by a psychiatrist or psychologist immediately. Given the inherent danger of a suicidal crisis, it is always best that crisis counselors inform their supervisors immediately. The question arises, "What if the patient refuses to be evaluated?" This is not uncommon, as suicidal individuals will often retract their suicidal statements once they know that people are paying attention to them and or are taking steps to make certain they will be safe. Here again, it is best to err on the side of caution. If the person refuses to be evaluated, the person may need to be transported by ambulance or the police to the nearest emergency room, where a complete psychiatric evaluation can be completed. If inpatient hospitalization is recommended and the person refuses, then most states provide some procedure for an involuntary hospitalization or commitment. According to Frierson, Melikian, and Wadman (2002), there are essentially three categories of potentially suicidal individuals: (1) patients with suicidal ideation, plan, and intent; (2) patients with ideation and plan but without intent; and (3) patients with ideation but no plan or intent. Patients that fall within the first group (especially when they have accompanying psychosocial stressors and access to a lethal means of suicide), should be psychiatrically hospitalized (either voluntarily or involuntarily if necessary). Patients that fall within the second group (suicidal ideation and plan but without intent) may be treated on an outpatient basis provided they have a good social support network and no access to lethal means of suicide. Some patients within this group, however, may require hospitalization if their environments cannot be assured as being safe or they are not adequately supervised. For patients in the third group, outpatient treatment is recommended, again though, only if the environment is safe (e.g., all weapons are removed from the dwelling) and there is adequate social support and supervision. For patients in the second and third groups, their willingness and motivation to seek treatment and follow through with therapy naturally will play a role in determining their suitability for outpatient treatment.

There is also the question of whether parents or a guardian should be notified in the event that their son or daughter has expressed suicidal intent. In an instance involving a child or adolescent, there is no question that parents need to be informed immediately and be involved in every step of the treatment planning process. Although it is always preferable to have the child or adolescent's consent to notify his or her parent or guardian, this is where ethical dictates regarding confidentiality are superseded by the safety of the patient. When the parent or parents works along with the counselor to help resolve the crisis, this collaborative effort helps to provide support to the child or teenager and sends the message that both counselor and family are working together to keep the patient alive and to make sure that he or she receives help in managing the problems (or depression) that precipitated the crisis. This collaborative approach represents the best-case scenario; however, what happens when the family refuses to have their child or adolescent evaluated. This may occur in instances when parents deny the seriousness of the suicidal threat, making such statements as, "Oh, she's threatened to kill herself a million times. A day doesn't go by where she doesn't threaten to kill herself." Another scenario might involve parents who are part of the reason behind a child's suicidal threats, as in instances of family members physically or sexually abusing children. These families often are very secretive and want no part of any outside intervention, to keep the abuse from coming to light. If a parent is refusing to have his or her child or teenage properly evaluated, the crisis counselor may report the case to the state child protective services agency (even when the case does not involve known physical or sexual abuse). A parent's refusal to have his or her suicidal child or teen evaluated could constitute neglect, which is also a form of child endangerment. In such a situation, the child protective agency worker would make an initial assessment and would then make certain a psychiatrist or psychologist properly evaluates the child or adolescent.

What would happen though if the son or daughter is not a child or adolescent, but a young adult, for example a college student. Confidentiality regulations and professional ethical guidelines are clear in specifying that information discussed in counseling sessions remains strictly confidential, *except* in instances involving danger to self or others. Many counselors, psychologists, and treatment agencies use an informed consent to treatment form, which is signed by patients at the onset of treatment, that specifies that confidentiality can be broken in instances of suicidal or homicidal threat or in instances of child abuse. In a recent lawsuit filed against the Massachusetts Institute of Technology, it is alleged that MIT administrators had not acted responsibly in preventing the death of an MIT student who purposely set herself on fire in her dorm room (Sontag, 2002). The suit alleges that the MIT staff did not inform the parents of their daughter's suicidal threats. The next case illustrates problems that arise when suicidal threats are vague or retracted.

THE VAGUE THREAT: CRISIS INTERVENTION CASE EXAMPLE 2

> Cheri is 18 years old and is a junior at Essex University. Her roommate and friends have noticed that Cheri has become more and more isolated over the past two months. She hardly leaves her dorm room and has not been going to the dining hall to eat with them as she had been doing. When they try to include her, Cheri tells them that she has a lot on her mind and that she wants to be left alone to "think things out." Her roommate knows that Cheri has been worried about her parents who are having marital difficulties because her mother found out that her father was having an affair. She is also aware that Cheri has not been happy with majoring in education; however, her parents had pushed her into a career in which she could earn a living after receiving her bachelor's degree. One day, when Cheri is at class, her roommate comes across what appears to be a suicide note on Cheri's computer.

If Cheri were to openly agree that she had written the suicide note and agree to be seen voluntarily at the nearest mental health clinic, college counseling center, or local medical center, this would be a pretty simple case in which to intervene. As mentioned earlier, one of the myths regarding suicide is that talking about it will somehow bring on the desire to carry through with the act. This is not the case. It is much better to speak openly, nonjudgmentally, and frankly about suicidal feelings than to dance around the subject. After a thorough suicide assessment is conducted, the counselor can then begin to develop a plan to ensure that Cheri will be safe, whether it involves a brief hospitalization or some intensive outpatient contact with her. If Cheri were actively suicidal and were she to express a plan of suicide, then hospitalization would be the safest recommendation.

The Aftermath of Suicide: Helping the Family and Significant Others

In spite of crisis counselors' and therapists' best efforts, all suicides cannot be prevented. Even the most intensive efforts to provide treatment (both inpatient hospitalization or outpatient treatment), the best efforts of family members, and the most compulsive treatment protocols will not prevent suicides (Steffens & Blazer, 1999). As Toynbee (1969) stated in his book *Man's Concern with Death,* "There are always two parties to a death; the person who dies and the survivors who are bereaved ... and in the proportion of suffering, the survivor takes the brunt." In instances of suicide, the "brunt" of the bereavement can be much more intense. Family members, significant others, and therapists are often racked with guilt and doubt. Survivors will often obsess over what they "would've, could've, or should've" done in order to prevent their loved ones from taking their own lives. Unfortunately, because these feelings of grief and guilt are so intense, there is often a tendency to project the blame onto someone else, such as the health care provider, the counselor, the doctor, or the teacher. This was well portrayed in the film *Dead Poets Society* (Haft, Witt & Thomas, 1989), in which the grieving, overbearing father blames his son's suicide on the teacher who encouraged the son's dreams of becoming an actor. The teacher becomes a perfect target for the father's anger and a perfect way to avoid examining his role in his son's death. Fortunately, in addition to individual and group counseling for suicide survivors, there are also many self-help groups, some of which have professionals available for counseling. For example, Survivors of Suicide is a self-help group that offers support for family members and friends of people who have died by suicide. Information about these groups can be found in the "Sources of Chapter Enrichment" section at the end of the chapter.

Homicidal and Violent Crises

This section of the chapter will address those individuals who may be likely to act out violently, either in terms of a homicidal threat or some other threat to harm others.

Scope of the Problem

When viewing the national statistics pertaining to homicide and assault, there is both good news and bad. The good news is that the overall rates of homicide and assault appear to be on the decline from ten years ago. The bad news is that for some groups, homicide still ranks among the ten leading causes of death. For example, for Hispanics and African Americans, homicide ranks as the sixth leading cause of death (Anderson, 2001). Similarly, crimes of violence have declined precipitously; however, there were still 5.3 million violent crimes committed in 2002 (Bureau of Justice Statistics, 2003).

Assessing Homicidal and Violence Risk

The prediction of homicidal and violent behavior is a daunting task, although not one that is totally impossible. Predictors of violence include a prior history of violent behavior, age, social stressors, substance abuse, personality traits, and psychopathology. The best predictor of future violence is a past history of violent behavior. Then, there are particular personality traits that are often associated with violent individuals, such as low frustration tolerance, impulsivity, immaturity, poor problem solving, and viewing violence as glamorous or a viable solution to life's problems. Three types of mental disorders (psychopathology) are often associated with violence and homicidal behavior: Intermittent Explosive Disorder, Paranoid Schizophrenia, and Antisocial Personality Disorder. While not all individuals with Antisocial Personality Disorders are violent, many will resort to violence in order to achieve certain goals, for example a violent assault in a robbery or rape or an abuser who uses violence as a means of control and intimidation. Some psychopaths' violent behavior is impulsive and spontaneous, while other psychopaths can be very calculating in their violent behavior (Hare, 1993).

Given that one of the best predictors of violent behavior is a past history of such behavior (Litwack, Kirschner, & Wack, 1993; McNeil & Binder, 1991; Meloy, 1987; Monahan, 1995; Mulvey & Lidz, 1995; Slovic & Monahan, 1995; Truscott, Evens, & Mansell, 1995), it is often necessary to thoroughly explore past history and to gather prior legal and treatment records as quickly as possible. Individuals with criminal histories, including assault and battery offenses, arson, sexual assault, weapons possession, aggravated felonies, domestic violence, drunk and disorderly, property damage, reckless and/or drunk driving, assaultive behavior while hospitalized, and homicide, could be considered at high risk for future violent behavior (Blumenreich & Lewis, 1993; Klassen & O'Connor, 1988). This risk is further increased when the individual is male and has a history of prior victimization (Cavaiola & Schiff, 1988). Although women can also become violent and assaultive, it should be noted that the majority of women imprisoned for murder committed the acts as "crimes of passion," for example the murder of a spouse, boyfriend, or lover in the heat of a jealous rage or an act of self-defense against a physically abusive partner.

Violent behavior can also be situational, for example "road rage" may cause a person to act out violently, as could becoming outraged by a boss or coworker. Violent behavior can also be exacerbated when individuals are under the influence of alcohol or drugs. Because alcohol intake can have a disinhibiting effect, it is not unexpected that there are correlations between criminally violent behavior and alcohol use (Bradford, Greenberg, & Motayne, 1992). Other mood-altering chemicals also associated with a propensity towards violence include stimulant drugs such as amphetamines and cocaine. It is noted that violent behavior (e.g., accidents, suicide, and homicide) are the leading causes of death among stimulant users (Warner, 1993). Violent behavior has also been associated with certain types of hallucinogens, particularly PCP (phencyclidine); however, some research suggests that PCP does not induce violence in individuals unless they are prone to violence (Brecher, Wang, Wong, & Morgan, 1988). Steroids have also been known to increase violent behavior, sometimes called "roid rage" (Pope & Katz, 1990, 1994). Similarly, some types of inhalant abuse have also been linked to violent behavior and delinquency in adolescents (Reed & May, 1984) and in adults who inhale solvents (Dinwiddie, 1994).

Crisis Intervention With Homicidal or Violent Individuals

The ability to effectively manage individuals who become aggressive or violent is an essential skill for any crisis counselor, police officer, teacher, nurse, or anyone who is involved in a human service industry, including customer service representatives, consumer complaint representatives, human resource personnel, and flight attendants. All of the aforementioned individuals may have to deal with people who become aggressive or violent. At one time, it was thought that only corrections and police officers who worked with violent criminal types or psychiatric aides working with potentially violent psychiatric patients needed to be trained to manage violent or aggressive behavior. Today, we know that this is simply not the case. The ability to manage violent behavior is essential for anyone working in any of the human services fields. This would include teachers (especially special education teachers who work with children or adolescents who have problems with self-esteem, impulse control difficulties, and low frustration tolerance), counselors, social workers, psychologists, and medical personnel.

The goal of crisis intervention with violent or aggressive individuals is to provide safe, nonharmful behavior management (Crisis Prevention Institute, 1999). Given that individuals may act out either verbally or physically, it is important to match the intervention to the type of aggressive behavior being displayed. For example, with someone who is acting out verbally, it would be inappropriate and over-reactive to respond by using physical force. Similarly, verbal interventions are usually not effective with someone who is physically violent.

According to the Crisis Prevention Institute (1999), there are four crisis development levels and specific ways in which a human service worker can intervene appropriately at each level, in order to prevent the crisis from escalating. Level I is the Anxiety Level. At this level, a behavioral change in the individual may be observed, usually an increase in agitation or restlessness. In such a scenario, a supportive approach is called for. This may consist of an empathic remark or actively listening to what is bothering the person. In order to be supportive, it is important not to be judgmental or dismissive of the person's feelings. At Level I, crises are often kept from escalating simply by hearing the person out and validating his or her frustration. A counselor simply remarking, "I hear you," can often help to diffuse the crisis.

In Level II, the Defensive Level, the client loses rationality, and may begin to lose control. A patient at this level is considered to be highly volatile because he or she may attempt to gain power by trying to "push the counselor's buttons." The individual may do this by making personal verbal attacks, such as abusive comments about age, weight, race, sex or family members. This behavior is often meant to test the limits, to see how far he or she can push the counselor or if he or she can elicit a reaction, which then gives the agitated individual control over the situation. This type of irrationality tends to yield irrationality in the counselor, instead of a professional response. At this point, if a shouting match develops security personnel would probably be called to intervene. However, it is preferable for the counselor to set limits in a firm, yet calm and rational, manner. This can be accomplished by giving the agitated person a choice and knowledge of the consequences if the behavior continues. For example, a counselor might say, "Jeff, I can see that you're angry about the situation, but yelling and screaming is only upsetting others and making the situation worse for yourself. Would you rather get a cup of coffee and talk about the situation or would you rather go and lay down for a bit to calm down?" If a person is backed into a corner, he or she usually has no choice but to come out swinging. If given an option or a choice, the individual can save face and hopefully will not chose to escalate the situation. The key at this level is not to get into a no-win power struggle (e.g., "Sit down and shut up, or I'll sit you down myself"). This will naturally only make things worse. It is also best not to give ultimatums or to threaten the person into compliance (e.g., "If you don't sit down, I'm having you taken out of here in handcuffs" or "If you don't shut your mouth, we're filing charges"). Being able to set limits is a practiced skill that requires a calm, professional manner and approach. If the client is acting like a belligerent child, don't fight fire with fire; it is important to maintain control.

Level III, The Acting Out Person, occurs when all verbal means of managing the crisis have been exhausted and the agitated person has lost control over his or her behavior. Physical intervention and restraint of the person is a last resort to managing such a situation because of the potential for harm to both the patient and the counselor. There are also legal implications of physically restraining someone. A hands-on approach would never be used unless it was quite certain that all means of verbal intervention had been exhausted. In these instances, safe, noninjurious restraint techniques (such as the "basket hold") are often used to help keep both the patient and others present safe. This type of physical intervention is naturally never done as a punitive measure, nor with the intention of inflicting pain.

In Level IV, the Tension Reduction Level, the patient begins to "come down" from the peak level of expended energy in Level III. The person who was angry, aggressive, and hostile becomes emotionally spent and begins to appear withdrawn. The patient may also express some remorse, as he or she begins to regain some control and sense of rationality. The person may be aware that he or she lost control and this may bring about feelings of fear or guilt. This is one of the most opportune times to talk with the person. It is best to present a contract to refrain from further violence (e.g., "Jeffrey, if you remain calm, I can sit over here and we can talk about what happened"). It is also important to let the agitated person know what you're doing and why (e.g., "Jeffrey, we're going to move into the office so we can talk some more").

According to the CPI training guide, the sooner you establish therapeutic communication, the sooner the agitated person will regain control and become more rational. Box 6.3 provides some guidelines for crisis counselors working with potentially violent or agitated individuals.

THE LAPC MODEL: CRISIS INTERVENTION CASE EXAMPLE 3

Richard is a 43-year-old separated father of two. He is seeking counseling at the recommendation of a coworker who is concerned about Richard's "threatening remarks" and depressive statements. This coworker is also worried about Richard's increased use of alcohol and explosive temper outbursts at work. Richard explains that he recently separated from his wife, Carol, after 20 years of marriage and that he doesn't know if he can go on without her. He is restless and angry as he describes how his wife "kicked him out of his home" because she wanted to "find herself." Richard is convinced she is seeing a guy she works with at her part-time job. Richard states that the thought of them together drives him crazy and

---

BOX 6.3

Guidelines for Working with Potentially Violent Individuals

- Don't "stare the person down." Making too much direct eye contact can be perceived as threatening (just as it is with dogs, cats, and primates who "square off" against one another).

- Use a calm tone of voice. Speak slowly and clearly the more agitated you become, the more agitated the other person will become.

- Move slowly and/or telegraph your movements. Don't make sudden moves that may be mistaken for threatening movements. By telegraphing your movements, your telling the person what you are doing and why (e.g., "I'm going to stand up and move over here, so I can hear you better").

- Be aware of any throwable objects in the room.

- Don't let yourself be cornered; be aware of your exit possibilities in case you need to get out quickly.

- Keep assistance nearby, but let one counselor do the talking. Too many counselors talking to the agitated person will often just increase the level of agitation or confusion.

- Don't use threats or ultimatums; remember that your goal is to defuse the situation, not to punish the individual.

apparently, this is where his threats are focused. Richard has made some vague threats about killing his wife and boyfriend if he ever caught them together and has also threatened to wait for the boyfriend after work and beat him up. Richard denies any domestic abuse history in his relationship with his wife. Richard is currently living alone in a rented room and has few friends other than his coworker, whom he seems to trust and confide in. Richard also confided in his coworker that he owns both a handgun and a rifle.

Richard's situation represents a crisis that has the potential for violent behavior, with both homicidal and suicidal outcomes. This type of crisis would be one of the most frightening because of it's many inherent dangers; yet one should also note that Richard does not appear to fit into any one of the diagnostic groups that are most likely to act out aggressively. Instead, the catalyst of his crisis was the recent marital separation and Richard's suspicions and fears that his wife is now involved in another relationship. His sexual jealousy fuels his anger and fear and his alcohol abuse makes the likelihood of violent behavior even greater. The fact that Richard has a means of carrying out his plans for vengeance (because he owns firearms), also lends more urgency to this crisis. The research literature on murder-suicide also suggests that this is a high risk situation. Marzuk, Tardiff, and Hirsch (1992) found the average age of murder-suicide perpetrators to be 39.6 years old. Approximately, 93% to 97% are Caucasian (Copeland, 1985; Currens et al., 1991), while 85% of the victims are female (Hanzlick & Koponen, 1994). The principal method is firearms, which are used in 80% to 94% of the cases (Copeland, 1985; Currens et al., 1991). The central theme of most murder-suicides is that the perpetrator is overly attached to a relationship that is threatened with dissolution, which leads to the destruction of the relationship and self (Nock & Marzuck, 1999). Murder-suicide between spouses and lovers accounts for 50% to 75% of all murder-suicides in the United States (Dorpat, 1966; Palmer & Humphrey, 1980; Allen, 1983; Currens et al., 1991). These relationships are often characterized by emotional abusiveness and sexual jealousy.

The crisis counselor working with Richard must therefore make an assessment of the potential for both violence/homicide and suicide, and come up with a strategy that will ensure the safety of all those involved. The counselor would begin by *Listening* to Richard's feelings of anger and betrayal and providing him with emotional support. The counselor would then begin to *Assess* the seriousness of Richard's intentions to harm his wife and her boyfriend. It would be helpful to review the Lethality Assessment Form (see Table 6.5), which provides a brief outline for assessing the risk of violence. In the *Planning* phase, it is hoped that Richard would be agreeable to an immediate psychiatric evaluation. Brief hospitalization may be needed to help stabilize him emotionally. However, what if Richard refused? What if he were intent on his plan to carry out violence towards Carol and her lover? What if Richard were to storm

TABLE 6.5
Lethality Assessment Form—Homicide/Violent Threat

1.	Is there a past history of any of the following:			
	■ violent behavior	☐ yes	☐ no
	■ property destruction	☐ yes	☐ no
	■ attempted homicide	☐ yes	☐ no
	■ other criminal behaviors	☐ yes	☐ no
	■ intimate partner violence	☐ yes	☐ no
	■ other family violence	☐ yes	☐ no
	■ bullying of others	☐ yes	☐ no
	■ child abuse (client)	☐ yes	☐ no
	■ incarceration	☐ yes	☐ no
	■ job loss due to threats	☐ yes	☐ no
	■ school expulsion	☐ yes	☐ no
	■ animal cruelty	☐ yes	☐ no
	■ psychiatric treatment	☐ yes	☐ no
	■ alcohol/drug abuse	☐ yes	☐ no
	If yes, specify substances abused _____		
2.	Present threats of violence?	☐ yes	☐ no
3.	Violent or homicidal plan?	☐ yes	☐ no
4.	Recent homicidal plan or behavior?	☐ yes	☐ no
5.	Violent ideation or obsessions?	☐ yes	☐ no
6.	Means or methods to carry out plan?	☐ yes	☐ no
7.	Recent disruptions in interpersonal relationships (e.g., separation)	☐ yes	☐ no

out in the middle of the session? What would the crisis counselor do? In an instance of either homicidal or suicidal threat, in order to ensure safety, the counselor would need to report these threats to the police. In keeping with the *Tarasoff v. Board of Regents of the University of California* (1976) ruling (explained later in this chapter), the counselor would also need to consider whether to report the threats to both Carol and her boyfriend. Even if Richard agrees to be admitted to a hospital, there would still need to be a consideration of whether to notify Carol and her boyfriend of the threats. It is likely, given the homicidal and suicidal threats, that if Richard were to try to sign himself out of the hospital, he would be involuntarily committed; however, under the *Tarasoff* ruling, potential victims need to be notified of such threats.

When people in crisis become agitated to the point of threatening violence (either verbally or through physical actions, for example slamming a fist on the table), then crisis counselors need to employ *defusing* techniques. The following are some defusing strategies that might be used with a potentially violent individual:

- *Understand the mindset of the hostile or potentially violent person.* Potentially violent individuals often have a compelling need to communicate their grievances to someone now! Even if their perceptions of certain situations are skewed, they believe they are in the right. In an overwhelming number of cases, the client just wants to be heard and to be treated with fairness.

- *Practice "active listening".* Stop what you are doing and give the person your full attention. Listen to what is really being said. Use silence and paraphrasing. Ask clarifying, open-ended questions.

- *Build trust, provide help, and avoid confrontation.* Be calm, courteous, respectful, and patient. It is important to be open and honest, but don't make promises you can't keep. Never belittle, embarrass, or verbally attack a potentially violent person (or any patient).

- *Allow a total airing of the grievance without comment or judgment.* While the person is airing the grievance, make eye contact, but don't stare (that can be perceived as a challenge). Let the person have his or her say while ignoring challenges or insults. Don't take venting personally; redirect attention to the real issues.

- *Allow the aggrieved party to suggest a solution.* A person will more readily agree to a resolution that he or she has helped to formulate.

- *Move towards a win-win solution.* Preserve the individual's dignity. Switch focus from what can't be done to what can be done (Bohen, 2002, p. 27).

There may be times, however, when you will need to call in additional resources (a supervisor, security, another counselor), even if the person does not consent, or call the police if you feel you are in danger.

Issues of Confidentiality and Duty to Warn

All counselors are taught the importance of maintaining confidentiality. The ability for the counselor and client to form a therapeutic relationship often is based on trust in the fact that the counselor will not divulge any information revealed by the client unless the client specifically authorizes the release of such information. Confidentiality is protected by legal, ethical, and moral principles. Legally, for example, the communications of certain professionals (i.e., attorneys, medical doctors, clergy, and depending on the state in which they practice, some psychologists, nurse practitioners, social workers, and counselors) are protected under the legal concept of "privileged communication." This means that information revealed to them in the context of their professional relationships cannot be revealed. Ethical standards are those guidelines developed by each profession for establishing codes of conduct. Ethical standards are not laws, but are developed to guide professionals in appropriate conduct.

Confidentiality is an ethical standard that is addressed by most professional associations, such as the American Counseling Association, the American Psychological Association, and the National Association of Social Workers. For example, Standard of Practice Nine (SP-9) in Section B: Confidentiality of the *Code of Ethics and Standards of Practice* of the American Counseling Association states, "Counselors must keep information related to counseling services confidential unless disclosure is in the best interest of clients, is required for the welfare of others, or is required by law. When disclosure is required, only information that is essential is revealed and the client is informed of such disclosure" (American Counseling Association, 1995). While violation of ethical standards will not necessarily result in legal consequences, it may result in censure or suspension by the professional boards that oversee that profession. There is also a moral obligation that helping professionals have to do no harm to their clients. Confidentiality, therefore, also can be viewed as a moral obligation of any counselor or helping professional.

In instances involving lethality, there will often be situations in which confidentiality and client safety (or the safety of others) are at odds. This dilemma has been illustrated in some of the case vignettes presented in this chapter. When clients reveal that they are going to harm themselves or someone else, helping professionals are faced with the dilemma of whether to inform the authorities, potential victims of the threats, and significant others, such as family members. The *Code of Ethics and Standards of Practice* of the American Counseling Association (1995) makes note of these exceptions in Section B: Confidentiality, part c: Exceptions: "The general requirement that counselors keep information confidential does not apply when disclosure is required to prevent clear and imminent danger to the client or others or when legal requirements demand that confidential information be revealed. Counselors should consult with other professionals when in doubt as to the validity of an exception." For example, if a client were to reveal suicidal intentions to a counselor and that counselor did not take responsible action to prevent the suicide from occurring, it is likely that the counselor could be sued for negligence. However, given that same scenario, if the counselor notified the authorities in order to have the client evaluated and admitted to a psychiatric unit for observation, the counselor could be sued by the client for breaching confidentiality. What many treatment agencies and helping professionals do is use a written informed consent form. This form usually spells out several aspects of the counseling process (e.g., risks/benefits of treatment, fees, missed appointments, estimated length of treatment) and also explains the nature of confidentiality and the limits thereof. So the form may include a statement to the effect that "everything you say will be held in strictest confidence and can only be released with your written consent; however confidential information can be disclosed in the event of a threat to self or others in order to prevent harm." While using an informed consent form is a sound practice and helps reduce the liability of the helping professional, the caveat is that it may signal to a potentially suicidal or homicidal client not to divulge information of this type.

The duty to warn potential victims of violent acts came about as the result of a landmark court case in California, which is often referred to as the Tarasoff ruling (*Tarasoff v. Board of Regents of the University of California,* 1976). The Tarasoff case involved the murder of a University of California student, Tatiana Tarasoff, by a male graduate student, Prosenjit Poddar. In the course of a therapy session with the university counseling center psychologist, Dr. Lawrence Moore, Poddar had confided his intent to murder his girlfriend whom he had been stalking. Poddar had allegedly not identified this female student, however, the therapist figured out who it was. Taking these threats seriously, Dr. Moore had initiated proceedings to have Poddar committed for psychiatric evaluation. Moore also had orally notified two campus police officers and also had notified the university police chief in a written letter. Subsequently, Poddar was taken into custody for observation but was later released with the agreement that he would stay away from Tatiana. Neither Moore nor the campus police notified Tatiana Tarasoff of the threats to her life. The therapist's supervisor at the university health center requested that the letter the therapist had written be returned and directed that the letter and all notes pertaining to the case be destroyed. Two months after being released, Poddar stabbed and killed Tatiana Tarasoff on the front porch of her parents' home. Tatiana's parents sued the university and the court ruled that when a therapist determines that a patient presents a serious danger of violence to another, then there is an obligation for that therapist to use reasonable care to protect the intended victim against that danger (*Tarasoff v. Regents of University of California,* 1976). Presently, several states have adopted similar statutes that limit the privilege of confidentiality when there is a danger to others. This is similar to restrictions for attorneys, who are sworn to keep clients' communications confidential except when the information pertains to the execution of a future crime (Stern, 2001). There are certain conditions that must be present, however, before a therapist could be considered liable for a failure to warn: (a) a therapist-patient relationship existed, (b) the therapist knew or should have known of the violent tendencies of the patient, (c) the victim was a "foreseeable" victim of the patient, (d) the therapist did not take the necessary steps to discharge his or her duty to protect, and (e) the failure to warn was the proximate cause of the victim's injuries. Since the original Tarasoff ruling, many courts have limited the duty to warn to only those situations in which a victim is readily identifiable (Remley & Herlihy, 2001); however, other courts have extended the duty to warn to include unknown victims. For example, a Washington State court ruled that a psychiatrist could be held liable for injuries sustained by a traffic accident victim who was injured by a drug-abusing patient released from inpatient care by the psychiatrist, subsequently running a red light while under the influence of drugs (*Petersen v. State of Washington,* 1983).

For crisis counselors, as well as mental health and school counselors, these rulings raise many difficult and often ambiguous issues. As Remley and Herlihy (2001) pointed out, the ACA *Code of Ethics and Standards of Practice* guidelines pertaining to the exception to confidentiality (quoted above) presume that counselors be able to predict dangerousness. However, even when the most thorough risk assessment is performed, it is obvious that not all human behavior can be predicted. What if the client was only venting feelings of anger? What if the threat is vague or brought up in the heat of the moment, and the counselor does not have evidence that it will be carried out? What if the potential victim is unknown to the therapist (as is often the case), or what if the therapist has no way to contact this person? For example, as Stern (2001) pointed out, a warning from an unknown therapist may invoke fear that the therapist has no way to allay, or the therapist may have no way to enhance protection of that potential victim.

Once a determination is made that a client is a danger to others, the question then arises, what constitutes "necessary steps to prevent harm"? Once potential victims have been warned, there are other steps that can be taken to prevent harm. According to Remley and Herlihy (2001), the choices can range from the least intrusive action (e.g., obtaining a written commitment from the client not to harm anyone) to involuntary commitment to a psychiatric facility, with many options in between. Whatever is decided to be the responsible course of action, it is always recommended that one consult with other mental health professionals, especially those who specialize in working with potentially dangerous clients.

In the instance of suicidal intent, confidentiality can also be breached in order to ensure the safety of the client. The counselor would begin with a thorough suicide risk assessment and then, depending on the level of suicidality, the counselor might begin to work with the client's family or significant others to arrange for a voluntary hospitalization. If this does not work, then involuntary commitment procedures should be initiated. In order to prevent being held liable (either for a failure to act responsibly or for breaching confidentiality), it is important that the crisis counselor do a thorough suicide risk assessment and document the findings as a means of justifying the recommendations that will be made to prevent harm. It has been noted, "The law does not require that counselors always be correct in making their assessments of suicide risk, but the law does require that counselors make those assessments from an informed position and that they fulfill their professional obligations" (Remley & Herlihy, 2001, p. 100).

SOURCES OF CHAPTER ENRICHMENT

Print Sources

Jacobs, D. G. (Ed.) (1999). *The Harvard Medical School guide to suicide assessment and intervention.* San Francisco: Jossey-Bass.

Litwack, T., Kirschner, S., & Wack, R. (1993). The assessment of dangerousness and prediction of violence: Recent research and future prospects. *Psychiatric Quarterly, 64,* 245–273.

Maris, R. W. (1992). The relationship of nonfatal suicide attempts to completed suicides. In Maris, R. W., Berman, A. L., Maltsberger, J. T., & Yufit, R. I. (Eds.), *Assessment and prediction of suicide* (pp. 362–380). New York: Guilford Press.

McNeil, D., & Binder, R. (1991). Clinical assessment of risk of violence among psychiatric inpatients. *American Journal of Psychiatry, 148,* 1317–1321.

Internet Sources

American Association of Suicidology (http://www.suicidology.org) This association provides a tremendous amount of information pertaining to suicide. The AAS sponsors conferences and provides trainings throughout the United States. This is an excellent Web site for information.

American Foundation for Suicide Prevention (http://www.afsp.org) AFSP is a national organization founded in 1987 that provides information about suicide prevention programs, up-to-date research on suicide prevention, and directories of survivor support groups for family and friends who have lost loved ones by suicide. The foundation also provides information on suicide statistics, prevention, and how to survive a loss by suicide. This is an excellent Web site. The American Foundation for Suicide Prevention's International Headquarters are located at 120 Wall Street, 22nd Floor, New York, New York 10005, or they can be reached by phone at 888-333-AFSP or at 212-363-3500. Some of the survivor support groups that are listed in the AFSP directories include Heartbeat and Ray of Hope/Survivors of Suicide. Heartbeat is an organization that provides mutual support for those who have lost a loved one through suicide. It provides information and referrals, phone support, speakers on bereavement, and chapter development guidelines to establish local meetings. Write to Heartbeat, 2015 Devon St., Colorado Springs, CO 80909 or call 719-596-2575. Ray of Hope/Survivors of Suicide was founded in 1977. It provides mutual support for after-suicide bereavement. Educational materials on suicide postvention are also available, as well as books on grief and bereavement following suicide. Telephone consulting is also available.

Centre for Suicide Prevention (http://www.suicideinfo.ca) The SIEC is a computer-assisted resource library containing print and audiovisual materials on suicide, suicidal behaviors, and suicide bereavement. This Web site also provides a "Suicide Helpcard" which can be downloaded and distributed for free. The Helpcard provides useful information on how to help someone who is expressing suicidal ideas or intent.

CHAPTER 7

Rape and Sexual Assault

Mary is a 19-year-old college sophomore. One night after studying late at the library, she was attacked and sexually assaulted by a group of young, intoxicated fraternity members. They laughed as they assaulted her, stating that she deserved it; when finished, they left her as if nothing had happened. Immediately following the assault, Mary utilized the campus emergency phone. The campus police found her lying on the ground crying hysterically, and they escorted her to the local hospital. There they gathered a report while she was being examined. Mary was offered counseling services at the hospital but refused them. The campus counseling services contacted her the following day and urged her to come in for counseling, stating that the campus police were required to report all incidents to the center. Mary reluctantly scheduled an appointment.

*R*ape, once considered to be an unfortunate fate suffered by an unfortunate few at the hands of some mentally disturbed men, has grown significantly in the past three decades as a subject of inquiry for scholarly research (Odem & Clay-Warner, 1998). The prototype of the antisocial rapist depicted in movies bears a resemblance to only a very small percentage of men who rape (Strong & DeVault, 1994).

The issue of rape reached research-worthy proportions due, in large part, to the feminist movement of the 1960s and 1970s, which served not only to focus attention on violence against women but also to alter forever society's way of thinking about the sexual victimization of women (Odem & Clay-Warner, 1998; Scully, 1990). Prior to the acceptance of the topic as a professional and scientific research endeavor, rape had a long history of being minimized and overlooked as a societal problem (Russell & Bolen, 2000). When Rhett Butler ignored all of Scarlett O'Hara's clearly stated refusals of a physical/sexual encounter in the 1939 classic movie, *Gone With the Wind,* and carried her up the grand staircase to the bedroom anyway, the movie made quite a statement about where it stood regarding one of the more prevalent of the rape myths (see next section): when a woman says "no," she really means "yes." Her blissful appearance the following morning reinforced this myth.

Similarly, with the advent of women's liberation and the legitimization of female sexuality, many people were skeptical that a woman who really did not consent could be raped (Odem & Clay-Warner, 1998). Perhaps it was based on Lerner's (1980) "belief in a just world" theory that people, in order to protect themselves from thoughts of tragedy and misfortune, have a need to believe that individuals "get what they deserve." That is, it is reassuring for an individual to believe that a woman had been raped because of her scanty attire or her alluring appearance. All women had to do was avoid such attire or such an appearance to avoid being raped; if they didn't deserve it, it wouldn't happen to them.

It was not unusual for rape victims to be faulted for playing a role in their own rapes, even by the criminal justice system. Margolin (1972) documented the case of a well-known attorney who began a rape trial by placing a soda bottle on a table in the courtroom, spinning it, and demonstrating to the jury how difficult it was to insert a pencil into its opening while in motion. The implication to the jury was clear: if she really wanted to fend off her attacker, she would have been able to do so.

In this chapter we will examine definitional issues of rape and sexual assault and look at rape statistics and how they are affected by unreported rapes. We will then consider reasons why men rape and how women are affected by rape. Finally, we will look at crisis intervention and treatment of rape victims.

Definitional Issues

Although the terms *sexual assault* and *rape* are used interchangeably in everyday language, this is usually not the case in research studies (Russell & Bolen, 2000). Individual states vary in their definitions of these terms, and the lack of definitional uniformity among national surveys tracking the occurrence of rape and sexual assault can cause inconsistencies in their results. There is less consensus among researchers on how to define rape than sexual assault, thus contributing to differences in incidence figures (Russell & Bolen, 2000). For a detailed description of the different methodologies used to collect incidence data, and for an analysis of the surveys themselves, the reader is referred to Russell and Bolen's work (2000); these authors reviewed the data from eight different surveys and asserted the fact that, despite some differences in the data, each survey revealed that rape was a serious epidemic in the United States.

In this chapter we examine three of these surveys, which track the prevalence of rape and sexual assault and which provide comprehensive sources of data on these problems. The surveys include the National Crime Victimization Survey (Bureau of Justice Statistics, 2001), the National Violence Against Women Survey (National Institute of Justice & the Centers for Disease Control and Prevention, 2000), and the Uniform Crime Reports (Federal Bureau of Investigation, 2000).

The U.S. Department of Justice's bi-annual *National Crime Victimization Survey* (NCVS) utilizes a definition of rape that includes forced sexual intercourse involving psychological coercion and physical force. The definition also considers vaginal, oral, or anal penetration by the perpetrator or by a foreign object. The survey's definition for sexual assault includes a wide range of victimizations distinct from rape or attempted rape, such as unwanted sexual contact with or without the use of force, fondling, and verbal threats.

This twice-yearly survey includes data from approximately 45,000 households and 100,000 people and reports individual data for both rape and sexual assault, as well as composite data for both crimes in combination. Data are collected for individual victims, both male and female, beginning with the age of 12 years. However, the inclusion of the far less serious crime of sexual assault and the extension of respondents to the age of 12 years (unlike the 18-year minimum age of most surveys) generally results in greater numbers of victims than those found in other surveys.

The *National Violence Against Women Survey* (NVAW) is sponsored by both the National Institute of Justice and the Centers for Disease Control and Prevention. Data are collected on multiple offenses against women from the age of 18 years. Conducted annually via telephone interviews with a representative sample of 8,000 women and 8,000 men throughout the country, the NVAW gathers rape statistics for both lifetime occurrence and those committed within the previous year. Its definition of rape is, "An event that occurs without the victim's consent and involves the use of threat or force to penetrate the victim's vagina or anus by penis, tongue, fingers, or object or the victim's mouth by penis."

The *Uniform Crime Report* (UCR) is the annual statistical report published by the Federal Bureau of Investigation (FBI); it tracks eight offenses known to the police, including rape. It defines rape as the carnal knowledge of a female forcibly and against her will. Assaults or attempts to commit rape by force or threat of force are also included; however, statutory rape (without force) and other sex offenses are excluded.

This definition of rape is narrower than other definitions, and the term *carnal knowledge* is not defined. It also excludes the acts of oral and anal penetration, and it does not account for the condition of a woman unable to consent due to a state of incapacity brought on by drugs, unconsciousness, or the like. Another limitation of the UCR statistics has to do with its source of data: crimes of rape originally reported to local police jurisdictions. Since studies suggest that only 16% to 39% of victims report their rapes to the authorities, the UCR data collection may be confounded not only by the narrowness of its definition but also by the lack of consistent reporting of rapes. Its findings, therefore, are somewhat limited.

Wife or *spouse rape and acquaintance rape* (aka *date rape*) are not listed as separate offenses in any of these surveys, but are instead subsumed under the more general category of rape. Wife or spouse rape is the term used to describe sexual acts perpetrated against a woman without her consent and/or against her will by her husband or ex-husband. It is currently considered a crime in all fifty states (Bergen, 1996; Mahoney &Williams, 1998). Acquaintance/date rape is considered the most frequent form of rape reported and may account for the majority of all rapes (Sue, Sue, & Sue, 2003). A crime committed within the context of a friendship or dating relationship, acquaintance rape is considered a significant problem on college campuses, where most of them occur (Meadows, 1998; Sue et al., 2003). Acquaintance rape often involves the use of alcohol (Martin & Hummer, 1989) or of one of the date rape drugs, such as the sedatives rohypnol or GHB (gamma-hydroxybutyrate), which are surreptitiously administered to the victim and are used to incapacitate her and make her susceptible to a sexual assault (Meadows, 1998).

Despite the state-by-state differences in the definition of rape, the Federal Criminal Code (Title 18, Chapter 109A, Sections 2241-2242) does not use the term *rape*, but defines instead two different types of sexual abuse, *aggravated sexual abuse* and *sexual abuse*, a typology based upon the degree of force or the threat of force used. These terms are defined as follows in the Code:

Section 2241. Aggravated sexual abuse
   a. By Force or Threat.—Whoever ... knowingly causes another person to engage in a sexual act—
      1. by using force against that other person; or
      2. by threatening or placing the other person in fear that any person will be subjected to death, serious bodily injury, or kidnapping; ...
   b. By Other Means.—Whoever ... knowingly—
      1. renders another person unconscious and thereby engages in a sexual act with that other person; or
      2. administers to another person by force or threat of force, or without the knowledge or permission of that person, a drug, intoxicant, or other similar substance and thereby—
         a. substantially impairs the ability of that other person to appraise or control conduct; and
         b. engages in a sexual act with that other person; or attempts to do so. ...

Section 2242. Sexual abuse
   Whoever ... knowingly—
      1. causes another person to engage in a sexual act by threatening or placing that other person in fear (other than by threatening or placing that other person in fear that any person will be subjected to death, serious bodily injury, or kidnapping); or
      2. engages in a sexual act with another person if that other person is
         a. incapable of appraising the nature of the condition; or
         b. physically incapable of declining participation in, or communicating unwillingness to engage in, that sexual act; or attempts to do so. ...

The Federal Criminal Code also addresses *abusive sexual contact*, a term congruent with other definitions of sexual assault. It refers to acts of intentional sexual touching without penetration which are designed to humiliate the victim or to arouse or gratify the perpetrator's sexual desire. *Sexual abuse of a minor or ward* (a sex act with a person between the ages of 12 and 15) and *sexual abuse resulting in death* (any of the above acts leading to the death of the victim) also are included in the code.

Incidence of Rape And Sexual Assault

The aforementioned definitional issues notwithstanding, researchers and surveys that track the crime of rape offer staggering numbers. The NVAW survey (1998; 2000) approximated that a total of 17.7 million American women have been raped during their lifetimes. In the 12 months prior to the survey, the total number of rape victims was determined to be 302,091 women. The NCVS (Bureau of Justice Statistics, 2001) estimated that more than 260,000 rapes or sexual assaults occurred in 2000. Although the Rape, Abuse, and Incest National Network (2001) documented an overall decline in the number of sexual assaults between 1993 and 2001, it still placed the total number at 248,000 in 2001. RAINN estimated that in 2001, an American was sexually assaulted every two minutes.

The stereotype of the stranger lurking in the bushes looking for a victim is no longer a useful or even an appropriate image of the typical perpetrator; 66% of all victims know their assailants. Friends or acquaintances account for 48% of the assailants known to victims, and another 18% are intimates or other relatives. Only 34% of reported rapes are committed by perpetrators who are considered strangers to the victims. Similarly, approximately 4 out of 10 sexual assaults take place in the victim's own home, with another 2 out of 10 occurring in the home of a friend.

Unreported Rapes: The Confounding of the Statistics

Any survey reporting the incidence of rape or sexual assault must contend with a confounding variable that clouds the results and leads to only a minimal estimate of the number of rape cases: the alarming number of cases that are never reported to the police. Estimates run as low as only 16% of rapes being reported, while the NCVS (2000) placed the number at 39%. The NVAW estimated that approximately 20% of all rapes are reported to the police, with the number being somewhat smaller (17.2%) for those reporting instances of intimate partner rapes. Wright (1991) claimed that the three primary reasons for failure to report cases of rape to the police are

- considering the rape a private matter;
- fearing reprisals from the rapist or his family and friends; and
- believing that the police would be inefficient, ineffective, or insensitive.

Still others (Kilpatrick, Edmunds, & Seymour, 1992) found that the main reasons were related to victims' concerns over their families and friends learning of the rape, media publicity about the crime, and people blaming them for the attack. NVAW found a similar pattern in reasons for not reporting intimate partner rape. In the order of expressed importance by the respondents, NVAW found the following reasons:

1. fear of perpetrator;
2. belief that the rape was a minor, one-time incident;
3. feelings of shame; wish to keep it a private matter;
4. belief that police would be unable to do anything about it;
5. wish to protect the attacker, the relationship, or the children;
6. wish to handle it themselves; and
7. sense that the police wouldn't believe them.

Researchers have estimated that self-blaming attributions are found in as many as 74% of rape victims presenting for treatment (Frazier, 1990). They have found that victims of acquaintance rape have more blame attributed to them than do stranger rape victims (Bridges & McGrail, 1989; Pollard, 1992; Quackenbush, 1989; Tetreault & Barnett, 1987). When accusations of sexual assault are made, unbalanced attention is given to the pre-existing relationship between the victim and the perpetrator and to the behavior of the victim rather than to the perpetrator's intentions and the nature of the act (Batemen, 1991). Quackenbush (1989) also found that people tend to assign more blame to the victim of an acquaintance rape compared to the victim of stranger rape. Weller (1992) noted that this phenomenon makes it difficult to prosecute acquaintance rape cases.

Factoring in large numbers of unreported cases of rape, and considering the low probability of convicting prosecuted perpetrators, the National Center for Policy Analysis, using U.S. Department of Justice (2000) statistics, estimated that only about 6% of rapists, 1 out of 16, ever spends a day in jail.

Why Men Rape

No single theory holds the key to the question of why men rape; rather a combination of societal, relational, and individual factors is needed to explain the perpetuation of rape (Malamuth, 1998). Research suggests that there are simply too many different kinds of rape for a single theory to provide a sufficient explanation for all of them (Kendall & Hammen, 1998). An exploration of each of these factors is beyond the scope of this chapter, but several explanations will be posited in this section.

Social-Cultural Explanations

Although culture is a factor in rape, the exact nature of the relationship between the two remains a topic of incomplete discussion (Odem & Clay-Warner, 1998). The feminist perspective views rape as an act of men's social control over women in a patriarchal society that values males over females (Brownmiller,

1975; Mooney, 2000). It asserts that the traditional socialization process encourages males to associate power and superiority with masculinity and submissiveness and passivity with femininity (Odem & Clay-Warner, 1998).

This perspective contradicts the popular belief that rape is a sexually motivated offense committed by only a few disordered, abnormal men. It proposes that the act of rape is not the impulsive or irrational act of the few, but rather a common act of control committed by the many (Brownmiller, 1975). It is not an act of sexual deviance, but rather an act of violence and aggression against women, with power being the principal motive (Strong & DeVault, 1994). Contemporary research also contradicts the image of the deviant sex fiend as the typical rapist. Kendall found that no more than approximately 10% of all rapes are committed for purposes of sexual pleasure (Kendall & Hammen, 1998). According to Mosher and Tomkins (1987), society's emphasis on male power and aggression, in combination with traditional sex roles, has helped to develop rape-permissive attitudes in both men and women.

Cognitive-Behavioral Explanations

Over the years, cognitive-behavioral research has contributed to the emerging profile of men who rape. Below are some of the explanations offered by different cognitive-behavioral researchers of sexual violence toward women:

- *Response control deficit:* The inability of sexually aggressive men to suppress (or control) their sexual arousal leads to a propensity to commit sexual crimes (Hall, 1989).

- *Response compatibility:* In men who have learned to respond to the stimulus of sexual arousal with aggressive behavior, sexual stimuli become paired with aggression responses (Blader & Marshall, 1989).

- *Deviant stimulus control:* Responses to sexual stimuli are acquired through classical conditioning or through instrumental learning. Non-rapists' sexual stimuli include descriptions of normal sexual acts or of attractive women. Rapists, however, become conditioned to stimuli that include descriptions of violence, pain, humiliation, and fear (Barbaree, 1990).

- *Disinhibition of arousal to rape stimuli:* Certain emotional or cognitive states may increase the possibility of performing rape. If a man's inhibitions have been lowered by alcohol or drug intoxication, and if he harbors previous anger directed at the victim, he is more probable to commit sexual assault or rape. Barbaree and Marshall (1991) demonstrated that when given permissive instructions about arousal and rape, more men demonstrated a reduced discrimination between consensual and non-consensual sex.

- *Belief in rape myths:* Rape myths are stereotypical beliefs about rape that can serve to place women in a disempowered position (Bohner, 1998). They can be defined as "descriptive or prescriptive beliefs about rape (i.e., about its causes, context, consequences, perpetrators, victims, and their interaction) that serve to deny, trivialize or justify sexual violence exerted by men against women" (Bohner, 1998, p. 14). The myths that only certain women are likely to be raped (those who behave indecently or show other moral deficits) and that women are not susceptible to rape if they carry themselves in a certain manner function to obscure and deny the personal vulnerability of all women (Lonsway & Fitzgerald, 1994). In addition, rape myth acceptance in men is associated with a greater rape proclivity (Malamuth, 1981; Malamuth & Check, 1983), and research suggests that the belief in rape stereotypes is the most powerful predictor of men's sexual aggression (Scully, 1990). Men who express acceptance of the myths tend to use more coercive and aggressive approaches to sexual influence, and their attitudes are associated with greater hostility toward women (Malamuth, 1996; Brehm, Kassin, & Fein, 2002).

These rape myths allow men to justify sexual aggression, and they fall into four major categories (Scully, 1990):

1. Victim precipitation: The belief that certain characteristics or behaviors of women actually cause men to rape ("She asked for it by the way she acted/dressed.")

2. Victim responsibility: The belief that women could avoid rape if they really tried ("She couldn't have fought very hard at all, otherwise she would have scared him off.")

3. Victim participation: The belief that women ask for and secretly enjoy rape ("I could tell by the way she looked at me that she really wanted it.")

4. False accusation: The belief that women charge men with rape just to punish them ("She's just saying that I raped her, just to get back at me for going out with her friend.")

Interpersonal Explanations

The tendency to respond to threats to self-esteem contributes to overall elevated levels of interpersonal difficulties (Rhodewalt, Madrian, & Cheney, 1998). Other research (Baumeister, Catanese, & Wallace, 2002) also supported this as a motivating factor for rapists. For example, when rejected as a potential suitor, the narcissistic rapist does not manage this insult to his self-esteem well (i.e., rejection leads to rape).

Social Learning Theory Explanations

The social learning model suggests that rape and violence towards women is learned through social modeling or through media representation. Rape and aggression are learned through imitation, observation, modeling, and desensitization to violence against women (Weiche & Richards, 1995). These early learning experiences can occur through the media or within a family milieu that promotes violence as a means of attaining one's goals.

Psychopathology Explanations

The most common diagnosis in sexual offenders is Antisocial Personality Disorder (APD) (Brown & Forth, 1997). Mental health professionals have identified typologies describing various antisocial behavior that include criminal activity; aggression; impulsivity; and lack of empathy, guilt, or remorse. Rape is a common antisocial behavior among men with APD, especially given their lack of conscience and incapacity for empathy (Hare, 1993). This pathology is notable early in childhood and adolescence and tends to progress throughout the lifespan.

In general, researchers (Hall & Hirschman, 1991) have proposed four main characteristics that discriminate rapists from other men. First, rapists are more likely to have engaged in sexually aggressive or other antisocial conduct on prior occasions. Second, men who rape are more likely to endorse callous attitudes toward women, including sexual aggression—endorsing rape myths (Malamuth, 1996). Third, men who rape experience high levels of sexual arousal to rape stimuli; engaging in rape fantasies occupies much of their time. Finally, periodic episodes of depression or hostility lead to loss of control and aggressive behavior toward women; these acts generally are accompanied by alcohol or substance abuse.

The Aftermath of Rape

Although data derived from the National Women's Study (1991) indicated that more than two thirds of rape victim respondents (70%) reported no physical injuries suffered as a result of the rape, the psychological injuries of a sexual attack are far more devastating and debilitating than the physical ones (Sue et al., 2003). Rape is a crisis event that causes significant upheaval in the victim's psychological functioning for a considerable period of time (Tobolowsky, 2000).

Studies that have examined the long-term effects of rape have found significant problems with fear, social adjustment, depression, and sexual disorders in women who had been raped six years earlier (Kilpatrick et al., 1985). Other researchers (Burnam et al., 1988) have found that sexual assault resulted in substance use disorders (both alcohol and drug dependence) and anxiety disorders, such as phobia, Panic Disorder, and Obsessive-Compulsive Disorder.

The trauma of rape produces aftereffects that are reminiscent of the diagnostic condition of Posttraumatic Stress Disorder (PTSD) from the American Psychiatric Association's *Diagnostic and Statistical Manual of Mental Disorders, Fourth Edition, Text Revision* (*DSM-IV-TR*) (2000). This diagnosis involves experiencing a traumatic event followed by feelings of fear, horror, or helplessness, along with multiple other symptoms. These other debilitating psychological effects may include repetitive nightmares, intrusive thoughts of the event, flashbacks, mental distress, and various physiological reactions. Hyperarousal (insomnia, irritability, poor concentration) and a numbing of general responsiveness (avoidance of familiar people or activities, feelings of detachment or isolation) also are part of this clinical syndrome.

Indeed, the vast majority of rape victims appear to experience PTSD, sometimes months after the event (Koss, 1993). Studies demonstrate that the diagnosis of PTSD is appropriate for anywhere from 83% to 94% of rape survivors (Kubany, Leisen, Kaplan, & Kelley, 2000; Foa, Rothbaum, Riggs, & Murdock, 1991). Even 3 months after the assault, PTSD symptoms persisted for 47% of the victims, and 16.5% of victims still had evidence of PTSD 17 years later (Foa et al., 1991). Ensink and Van Berlo (2000) also reported sexual problems (fear of and/or avoidance of sexual contact with their partners) to be as common as PTSD in rape victims. Foa and Rothbaum (1998) addressed the possible magnitude of the problem of rape-related aftereffects; using data from other research sources, they approximated that there were about 1.5 million adult female rape victims with chronic cases of PTSD. Despite the prevalence of PTSD among rape survivors, PTSD was studied directly only in the most recent studies, since many of them were carried out prior to the general acceptance of PTSD as a diagnostic category, and because these studies described symptoms only and not diagnoses (Tobolowsky, 2000).

Prior to the introduction of the diagnosis of PTSD in 1980 in the Third Edition of the *Diagnostic and Statistical Manual of Mental Disorders* (DSM-III), another syndrome, Rape Trauma Syndrome (RTS), which included several PTSD-like symptoms specific to the experience of rape, was proposed (Burgess & Holmstrom, 1974). RTS is a two-phase syndrome.

1. *Acute phase: Disorganization*—Lasting from a few days to several weeks, during the acute phase the rape victim will experience a complete disruption of her life, along with depression, fear, and self-blame. During this phase, she may adopt either of two styles of responding to the rape:
   - *expressed reaction*, which is a very expressive emotional reaction involving anger, fear, rage, anxiety, depression, restlessness, or even laughing and joking; or
   - *controlled reaction*, which is an absence of a reaction of any kind. In a controlled reaction, the victim shows little response to the rape and appears quite calm. Beneath this facade, however, lie feelings of tension, depression, and irritability.

2. *Long-term phase: Reorganization*—This phase may last for several years. It begins when the victim begins to deal directly with her feelings and to reorganize different parts of her life. Anxieties may linger, however, as may fears of sex or a lack of sexual desire. Recovery in this phase depends on several factors, including the victim's age, general personality style, and her support system.

Treatment and Intervention

Many experts in the field of trauma study have stressed the critical need for immediate intervention after a trauma in order to prevent chronic problems resulting from the event (Bell, 1995). However, as noted earlier in this chapter, the very low probability that a rape victim will report or disclose the assault to anyone, including family or close friends, crisis centers, police, or mental health professionals, essentially either delays or avoids the intervention entirely. As a result, the victim is denied access to resources that may be potentially helpful, including treatment for medical and psychological issues and for related health problems, such as sexually transmitted diseases (Koss, Woodruff, & Koss, 1991). Furthermore, many victims who seek treatment years after their assaults still receive psychiatric diagnoses of Anxiety Disorder, Depressive Disorder, or substance dependence (Kilpatrick, Saunders, Veronen, Best, & Von, 1987).

Crisis intervention and therapy groups for trauma victims are the most common approaches used in rape crisis centers (Koss & Harvey, 1991; Foa & Rothbaum, 1998). Therapy can be a long-term process that typically takes place in the reorganization phase of RTS. The next section will examine some of the most widely used long-term therapeutic approaches; a discussion of the crisis intervention work of the acute phase will follow.

Long-Term Therapeutic Options

Therapeutic methods used with rape victims have included systematic desensitization, cognitive therapy, stress inoculation training, eye movement desensitization and reprocessing (EMDR), cognitive processing therapy, and traditional psychoanalytic therapy (Foa et al., 1991). In addition, group therapy has been effective with rape victims by decreasing shame through a supportive environment, by challenging self-blaming cognitions, by providing social support, and by reducing victims' experiences of isolation and aloneness (Koss & Harvey, 1991).

Tomasulo (1998) proposed the following therapeutic benefits of group therapy:

- *Hope:* seeing other rape survivors able to cope with everyday situations
- *Universality:* realizing that they were not alone, and their reactions not unusual
- *Information:* learning about other resources for survivors
- *Altruism:* providing the opportunity to help other victims in the group
- *Corrective recapitulation of the primary family group:* replicating a positive or accepting family experience (the rape survivor may be lacking this support in her family)
- *Development of socializing techniques:* providing opportunities to develop new social skills
- *Imitative behavior:* providing effective coping models for the other rape survivors in the group

- *Interpersonal learning:* learning what other survivors have been through and how they have coped
- *Catharsis:* providing an opportunity to express the entire gamut of emotions that rape victims experience
- *Existential factors:* offering the realization that horrible things do happen to good people without rhyme or reason and that trauma is part of the human condition

Researchers have also examined the efficacy of more traditional psychodynamic psychotherapy methods in the treatment of PTSD (Foa & Rothbaum, 1998). Due to the difficulties in defining both the therapy methods and the measurement standards themselves, the information from these studies has been quite limited and open to various interpretations. The largest number of controlled studies of PTSD treatment involve cognitive-behavioral approaches (Foa & Rothbaum, 1998). These approaches for rape also overlap considerably with the treatment of PTSD (Davison, Neale, & Kring, 2004).

In *exposure treatment*, a method used also in the treatment of phobias, clients are exposed, either in real life (in vivo) or in imagination only, to those things that they fear. For example, height-phobic (acrophobia) therapy clients are exposed to their fear of heights by spending sessions with their therapists on the top floor of tall buildings or by imagining themselves, under the therapists' guidance, scaling great heights in the absence of a negative outcome. Once habituation takes place (becoming accustomed to the formerly feared object), the fears subside.

Similarly, exposing PTSD sufferers (i.e., rape victims) to those thoughts, images, and feelings associated with the attack in the presence of a trained therapist also serves to reduce rape-related fears and anxieties. That is, by having victims relive and describe the attacks in vivid detail, the fears associated with the rape/trauma are extinguished (eliminated) over several sessions (Rothbaum & Foa, 1992). As with phobia treatment, repeated exposure to the feared stimulus (the rape) without negative consequences accompanying it allows for release of the fear and for newer, more rational information about the event to emerge (Nietzel, Speltz, McCauley, & Bernstein, 1998). Outcome studies attest to its effectiveness as a treatment modality for PTSD (Foa & Rothbaum, 1998).

Cognitive processing therapy, a variant of direct exposure treatment, involves the element of exposure in addition to cognitive restructuring techniques (Resick, 1992; Nietzel et al., 1998). The addition of the cognitive therapy component allows for the identification of and treatment of the self-defeating and self-blaming cognitions (thoughts) resulting from the rape. That is, the victim who blames herself for the assault can learn to attribute the event to other more salient aspects of the attack that were beyond her control.

PTSD treatment also has included components of systematic desensitization, stress inoculation training, and anxiety management training. These approaches involve the elements of relaxation training, thought-stopping, and some cognitive restructuring techniques. Although they each add to the efficacy of the exposure approach, they have not proven to be as effective as exposure alone due to the latter's simplicity to administer and to its often ver-ified efficacy via empirical study (Foa & Rothbaum, 1998).

Crisis Intervention: The LAPC Model in the Immediate Aftermath of the Assault

Before exploring the following case examples of rape victims vis-à-vis the Listen-Assess-Plan-Commit (LAPC) model of crisis intervention, it is important to stress at this point a critical component in responding to a report of rape: the need for medical attention. Of paramount importance is tending to the possible injuries to the victim, but the medical ministrations of a trained professional also are vital in order to test for sexually transmitted diseases and AIDS, and for the proper gathering of medical evidence, should the victim decide to press charges against the perpetrator (Meadows, 1998).

States and local communities vary in the protocol followed in responding to the report of rape. Members of sexual assault response teams (SART) are spe-cially trained individuals who can be summoned when a report of rape is made by a victim. They consist of a member of law enforcement, a medical profes-sional (sexual assault nurse examiner) trained to provide care and collect evi-dence, and a rape victim advocate who provides support and access to appropriate community resources. The specific training that members of SART receive serves to avoid the secondary victimization of rape victims (Campbell & Raja, 1999). *Secondary victimization* is a term for insensitive behaviors and atti-tudes exhibited by social service providers that imply blame toward the victims for their attacks and consequently victimize them yet again.

STRANGER RAPE: CRISIS INTERVENTION CASE EXAMPLE 1

Maura is a 50-year-old single professional woman who prides herself on her appearance and her physical condition. Midway through one of her early morning runs through the local park, she was suddenly pulled into the bushes. A stranger threw her to the ground, held a knife to her throat, and began to remove her clothes. He became agitated and started shak-ing her. She tried to remember something she once had read about sur-viving a rape or sexual assault, but she was unable to recall what she was supposed to do to protect herself. Her attacker proceeded to rape her. When he was finished, he kicked her a few times before disappearing into the morning fog. Maura lay there in the bushes for what seemed like an eternity before she pulled up her jogging shorts and made her way home. She didn't tell anyone about the rape.

Eight months later, Maura was in a counselor's office at the insis-tence of a friend who could not understand the sudden and dramatic changes in her behavior. She had gained one hundred pounds in eight months. She struggled with sleeping and had recurring nightmares about the assault. When she was not at work, she was at home in front of the

television, eating. The slightest noise startled her; she had difficulty concentrating, and at times, she felt as if she were "leaving herself." Most bother-
some to her was the numbing that she experienced any time a man came
near her. She even felt uncomfortable around, as if threatened by, her close
male friends. The thought of sexual intimacy was abhorrent to her.

Although no case of rape can be considered "typical" because of the individual-
ity of the victim's personality, coping style, history of previous traumas, and
strength of family/support system, there are some elements of Maura's case that
are common in incidents of rape. Elements of PTSD, a common aftereffect of
rape, were present in Maura's post-rape behavior; she exhibited those behaviors
and affect that are typical for a PTSD diagnosis. Her nightmares and flashbacks,
her level of agitation, her edginess, her avoidance of familiar settings and activities, and her discomfort with men and with sexual relations were indicative of
PTSD. Other factors that are common among victims of rape were Maura's failure to report the attack to the authorities and her excessive weight gain.

Since she had not reported the rape to the proper authorities, Maura was not
able to access the medical attention she may have needed at the time. She also
was not able to benefit from a referral system which would have connected her
with a support system consisting of an array of social, community, and advocacy
groups. Additionally, she decided to cope with the aftermath of the rape on her
own, preferring to forego the supportive network of family and friends that may
have assisted her in recovery, although her friend did provide the impetus for
her to seek out the services of a counselor. However, as noted earlier, not reporting a rape experience is far more common than reporting one.

The LAPC model of crisis intervention provides clear steps for intervening
with Maura, and the LAPC worksheet shows the comments the counselor
working with Maura recorded. In the *Listen* phase, as Maura told her story for
the first time, the counselor listened intently. During this step, the goal of the
counselor was to use active listening in an attempt to understand what meaning the rape had for Maura. The counselor avoided attributing personal
assumptions about the rape experience and began to understand instead
Maura's unique perspective on the attack. In other words, besides the trauma
of the assault, what were the salient factors unique to Maura? Her middle-age
independence on which she had prided herself, now shattered? Her typical
ability to problem-solve in the face of personal and professional challenges,
now ruined? Her health-conscious sense of invincibility, now a thing of the
past? Her explanations for not reporting or reaching out to family? To friends?

The counselor's role is to listen, to offer support, to be nonjudgmental, and
to assure Maura that the assault was not her fault. "Why" questions should be
avoided (see chapter 2). Questions concerning "why" she was jogging by herself at that time or in that location imply blame and undoubtedly would reinforce the self-blaming tendencies Maura, like many rape victims, may be
experiencing. In fact, the counselor should be prepared to dispute any self-
defeating, self-blaming statements that arise.

In the *Plan* phase, other supportive social or community resources should
be explained and explored for Maura, if she decides to access them. These

LISTEN	ASSESS	PLAN	COMMIT

Name: *Maura*   Age *50*

LISTEN

What is the client saying about the crisis? *Maura had little to say about her assault, keeping it a secret from her friends and family. The intervention of a concerned friend who was worried about the sudden changes in Maura's behavior and appearance resulted in Maura's agreeing to see a counselor, albeit 8 months after the attack.*

What happened? *A forcible rape by a stranger.*

When did it happen? *Eight months before Maura sought treatment.*

What type of crisis was it (traumatic event, developmental, psychiatric, existential)? *Traumatic event.*

Did the client mention anything that indicated danger? *There was no suicidal ideation or intent assessed. However, her feelings of safety have been shattered. She feared a repeat attack by the assailant, so she purchased a firearm for protection.*

Other relevant information about the crisis: *She has gained a hundred pounds, and she has curtailed the many professional and social activities she had enjoyed for years.*

ASSESS

Feelings: Is the client's predominant emotional state one of:

Anger *Yes*   Sadness *Yes*   Hopelessness *Yes*

Anxiety *Yes*   Panic *Yes*   Numbness *Yes*

Suicidal? If yes, complete lethality assessment/suicide. *No*

Homicidal? If yes, complete lethality assessment/violence. *No*

Acting: Is the client's behavior:

Active/restless *No*   Consistent with mood *Yes*

Passive/withdrawn *Yes*   Good eye contact *No*

Thinking: Is the client:

Logical/making sense *No*   Coherent/expressing self well *No*

Insightful *No*   Focused on topic *No*

Evasive/changing subject *Yes*

Other: Any medical problems? *Medical needs were not assessed at the time of the rape due to non-reporting. Psychological needs more paramount now over physical ones.*

Physical limitations? *Only those that are self-imposed*

Need for hospitalization? *None rape-related*   *(Continues)*

PLAN

What needs to be done now? *Continuation of treatment and development of a detailed plan for recovery.*

What alternative plans have been discussed? *Disclosing the rape to her family. Making a police report of the rape. Returning to some of her exercise and social routines she enjoyed previously.*

Are these plans reasonable? *Yes*

Can they be carried out? *Yes, although motivation for treatment is still not high; she was brought to treatment by a friend.*

COMMIT

Which plan of action has the client chosen? *Maura is considering returning to therapy for weekly sessions. She agreed to work out a plan for telling her family what happened.*

Are there resources/support to implement the plan? *Yes*

Is the client motivated to implement the plan? *Yes*

What other resources/supports may be needed?

Friend *Yes*   Family member *Yes*

Neighbor *Yes*   Mental health provider *Yes*

Public agency (law enforcement, child protective services, social services) *Yes*

Medical (hospitalization, medication) *Yes*

---

resources could assist her in reestablishing her pre-crisis level of functioning, and help her disclose the rape to other friends or family members. (Note: The counselor also must respect Maura's decisions regarding recovery throughout treatment; other needs should be addressed by Maura.)

ACQUAINTANCE RAPE: CRISIS INTERVENTION CASE EXAMPLE 2

Marcie is a 23-year-old female in her senior year at a large urban university. Marcie invited classmates to her place so they could complete an assignment. Everyone except Marcie was enjoying a few beers while they worked. As the night wore on, her classmates left one by one. Kevin stayed behind to help clear the dishes. When he came out of the kitchen, he had beers for himself and Marcie. She thanked him and began to enjoy a cold one at the end of a long, hard day. Soon, Marcie noticed that she could hardly hold her eyes open. She began to have some difficulty breathing, her body would not move, and as she tried to push herself out of the chair, nothing happened. Through the confusion and disorientation, she realized that she had been drugged.

Kevin had put something in her beer. She was aware of his disrobing and raping her, but she was powerless to stop him. She simply could not lift her arms. Marcie's friend, Lynne, arrived at the apartment several days later. She was worried because Marcie had not been to work or class; she also was not answering the telephone or her cell phone. Since this was not like Marcie, Lynne went to her house, pushed the door open, and found her in a fetal position on the bed. She had not eaten nor slept in 48 hours. Lynne started to call 911, but Marcie became hysterical. So she simply helped Marcie get dressed, gathered her friend's clothes off the floor, placed them in a bag, and drove her friend to the college counselor's office.

As with the case of Maura, the counselor utilized the LAPC model of crisis intervention with Marcie. In the *Listening* phase of the intervention, the counselor allowed Marcie to talk and acknowledged, via active listening and supportive feedback, what Marcie had experienced. She gave space in the interview for Marcie to discharge emotion. Rapport was established. The counselor was aware that returning control of her life to Marcie was an important step in the treatment process. She attended to Marcie's nonverbal cues as much as to her verbal communication. Allowing Marcie to exercise her choice over where to sit in the counselor's office was an attempt to empower Marcie.

The *Listening* phase of the intervention allowed the counselor to acknowledge Marcie's feelings related to the rape. If a counselor is able to listen and to validate the thoughts and feelings of the victim, the likelihood that the client will be revictimized in the helping process is minimized significantly. Once the establishment of rapport enabled Marcie to feel safe, she was able to tell the counselor all that she was able to recollect.

The *Assessment* phase of the intervention with Marcie then began. Her feelings included fear of another attack, since the perpetrator remained on campus as a student; anxiety and agitation; and depression, as she tended to blame herself for arranging the initial gathering. Her thoughts also took on a life of their own: If people found out, what would they think of her? What would this mean for future romantic relationships? Would she ever feel safe again?

The *Planning* stage then began, as the counselor was able to gather information about the rape in order to determine what possible plans should be discussed with Marcie. The counselor determined that there was an immediate need for medical treatment, that her client had been drugged, and that there was a rapist on campus who might also endanger other unsuspecting female students. The counselor empowered Marcie to make decisions regarding her medical care. She also explored what social support was available to Marcie by finding out if any of her friends were willing to accompany her and the counselor to the medical center. The counselor then explored whether there was anyone else Marcie wanted to tell. The counselor discussed each of these plans with Marcie; they seemed reasonable and able to be implemented without undue delay. *Commitment* to the plans chosen was the next step in the intervention process. Marcie agreed to access medical attention, to report the rape to the campus police, and to utilize the social support provided by two of her close friends in implementing these plans.

In general, the crisis intervention counselor confronted several challenges. In the space of an hour or less, the tasks were to build a rapport with a new client, identify the problem and assess the situation, prioritize issues, develop and implement a plan of action, bring about closure, and arrange for follow-up. In Marcie's case, the counselor moved through each recommended phase while tending to the emotional needs of a client who still showed symptoms of shock as the result of trauma. It was evident from the information that Marcie provided to the counselor that she typically made wise decisions. The counselor incorporated this information and used an identified strength to bring about the desired outcome. If the counselor instead had focused solely on symptomotology, Marcie may not have become willing to take care of her medical needs.

SEXUAL ASSAULT: CRISIS INTERVENTION CASE EXAMPLE 3

Large crowds gathered to watch the parade. The August heat was particularly unbearable, so Amy, a 26-year-old newlywed, decided to wear a pair of shorts and a halter top. Believing she was appropriately attired, a very important issue for Amy, she left her apartment to meet her friends. Many of them were dressed similarly. Amy is very modest and was just beginning to establish her new life with her husband. She and her friends were enjoying the parade when they noticed some commotion, a group of men pulling the strings on several women's string bikinis and then splashing them with water. The men were behaving aggressively, and the women appeared frightened. Before Amy could react, the crowd of men moved toward her and her friends. She tried desperately to get away, but the men proceeded to hold her and to take off her top, laughing and shooting water guns at her and her friends. As the men moved to another group of women, Amy frantically searched for her halter top. Other men began to approach her, touching her breasts while she screamed and cried for them to stop. The police then arrived, and the men scattered. Thanks to the videotapes of several people filming the parade, Amy had the opportunity to press charges against the assailants. However, she chose not to, feeling ashamed and wishing to keep her husband from finding out what had happened to her. She felt as though it was her fault because of the way she was dressed; she also feared that her husband would be angry with her. The police officers took her and several other women to the police station as material witnesses. There they met a crisis counselor. Amy spoke briefly with her but did not make a decision on what to do.

Amy's case includes several issues that were not pertinent to the cases of Maura and Marcie. Amy, a newlywed, harbored considerable fears over the repercussions she would experience if her husband learned of the incident. She also had started to blame herself for the assault, faulting herself for the attire she wore on that hot day. Her encounter with the crisis counselor at the police station was not one that she initiated, thus her reluctance to seek services and to draw more attention to the attack than she considered necessary. Even her refusal to follow up with the counselor had to be respected. The

---

| LISTEN | ASSESS | PLAN | COMMIT |

Name: *Amy*   Age *26*

LISTEN

What is the client saying about the crisis? *Amy feels ashamed and believes it to be her fault; she does not want her husband to know.*

What happened? *Amy was sexually assaulted by a group of men.*

When did it happen? *This occurred while at a parade earlier in the day.*

What type of crisis was it (traumatic event, developmental, psychiatric, existential)? *Traumatic event.*

Did the client mention anything that indicated danger? *No*

Other relevant information about the crisis: *Amy is a very modest person, recently married, and fears her husband will be angry with her.*

ASSESS

Feelings: Is the client's predominant emotional state one of:

Anger *No*	Sadness *No*	Hopelessness *No*
Anxiety *Yes*	Panic *No*	Numbness *No*

Suicidal? If yes, complete lethality assessment/suicide. *No*

Homicidal? If yes, complete lethality assessment/violence. *No*

Acting: Is the client's behavior:

Active/restless *No*	Consistent with mood *Yes*
Passive/withdrawn *Yes*	Good eye contact *Yes*

Thinking: Is the client:

Logical/making sense *Yes*	Coherent/expressing self well *Yes*
Insightful *No*	Focused on topic *No*
Evasive/changing subject *No*	

Other: Any medical problems? *No*

Physical limitations? *No*

Hospitalizations *No*

Need for hospitalization? *No*

(Continues)

PLAN

What needs to be done now? *Ongoing support and reassurance, reduction of her anxiety, and assistance for her to recognize that it is not her fault.*

What alternative plans have been discussed? *Developing with her a plan to inform her husband of the attack.*

Are these plans reasonable? *Yes*

Can they be carried out? *Yes*

COMMIT

Which plan of action has the client chosen? *Amy will attend one session and make a decision from there.*

Are there resources/support to implement the plan? *Yes*

Is the client motivated to implement the plan? *Yes*

What other resources/supports may be needed?

Friend *No*   Family member *Husband*

Neighbor *No*   Mental health provider *Crisis counselor*

Public agency (law enforcement, child protective services, social services) *No*

Medical (hospitalization, medication) *No*

---

police also did not notify her husband against her wishes. The counselor provided her with some pamphlets that offered information regarding other resources. There are times when the only role that a crisis intervention mental health worker can play in helping a sexual assault victim is to provide support and information. Amy's case is examined in the Listen Assess Plan Commit (LAPC) worksheet.

SOURCES OF CHAPTER ENRICHMENT

Print Sources

Bryden, D., & Lengnick, S. (1996). Criminal law: Rape in the criminal justice system. *Journal of Criminal Law & Criminology, 87,* 1194–1395.

Burgess, A. W. (1983). Rape trauma syndrome. *Behavioral Sciences & the Law, 1,* 97–113.

Coppin, C. B. (2000). *Everything you need to know about healing from rape trauma.* New York: Rosen Publishing Group Inc.

Foa, E. B., & Rothbaum, B. O. (1998). *Treating the trauma of rape: Cognitive behavioral therapy for PTSD*. New York: Guilford Press.

Foa, E. B., & Rothbaum, B. O. (1991). Treatment of posttraumatic stress disorder in rape victims: A comparison between cognitive-behavioral procedure in counseling. *Journal of Consulting & Clinical Psychology, 59,* 715–723.

Frankfurt, H. G. (1971). Freedom of the will and the concept of a person. *Journal of Philosophy, 1,* 5–20.

Kaminker, L. (1998). *Everything you need to know about sexual assault*. New York: Rosen Publishing Group Inc.

La Valle, J. (1996). *Everything you need to know when you are the male survivor of rape or sexual assault*. New York: Rosen Publishing Group Inc.

McEvoy, A. W., & Brookings, J. B. (1984). *If she's raped: A book for husbands, fathers, and male friends*. Holmes Beach, FL: Learning Publications.

Norris, F. H. (1992). Epidemiology of trauma: Frequency and impact of different potentially traumatic events on different demographic groups. *Journal of Consulting and Clinical Psychology, 60,* 409–418.

Pineau, L. (1989). Date rape: A feminist analysis. *Law & Philosophy, 8,* 217–243.

Russell, D. E. H. (1977). *The politics of rape: The victim's perspective*. New York: Stein and Day.

Schulhofer, S. J. (1998). *Unwanted sex: The culture of intimidation and the failure of law*. Cambridge, MA: Harvard University Press.

Taslitz, A. E. (1999). *Rape and the culture of the courtroom*. New York: New York University Press.

Wertheimer, A. (1987). Coercion. Princeton, NJ: Princeton University Press.

Internet Sources

Rape, Abuse, and Incest National Network (http://www.rainn.org) The nation's largest anti-sexual assault organization, RAINN operates the National Sexual Assault Hotline (1-800-656-HOPE) and carries out programs for the prevention of sexual assault and for assistance to victims.

Bureau of Justice Statistics (http://www.ojp.gov/bjs/) This site offers various statistics. It is helpful for those survivors who may need to know that they are not alone. This is also a great resource for people doing research.

Men Against Sexual Assault (University of Rochester) (http://sa.rochester.edu/masa/) This site is designed for men against rape, but can be useful for anyone. It includes statistical information, as well as quizzes to test your knowledge of the prevalence of rape and the myths that surround sexual assault.

CHAPTER 8

Loss and Bereavement

Robert was 55 years old and had been married to Betty for 28 years. They had two daughters, ages 24 and 22. About 8 months ago, Robert began to experience stomach pains and also began losing weight. His primary care physician did several blood tests and suspected cancer. It was later confirmed by an oncologist that Robert had an advanced case of pancreatic cancer. Within 4 months of the confirmed diagnosis, Robert died at home, where hospice workers had been caring for him. All of Robert's family was devastated by his death, especially his wife, Betty. Betty was referred for crisis counseling by an emergency room physician who examined her for chest pains and having difficulty catching her breath.

*T*his chapter deals with the types of crises that come about as a result of loss, such as the death of a spouse or partner, divorce, loss of one's job, the death of a pet, major health changes, and financial losses. Whether these losses come about suddenly or are expected, for example if death occurs after a long period of chronic illness or divorce follows years of marital problems, the reactions to the losses are intense and difficult to work through. However, not all losses will result in a person experiencing a bereavement crisis. For example, a wife whose husband has died after a long battle with prostate cancer most certainly experiences grief reactions, yet there may also be a sense of relief that he is no longer suffering. Also, the time period from when the initial diagnosis was made to the time of death allowed the wife to prepare for this loss emotionally. If a crisis period were to occur, it may have been more likely at the time of the initial diagnosis. Yet even with time to prepare, many surviving family members and significant others are thrown into crisis. This chapter will explore the types of crisis situations that may occur as a result of loss and how crisis counselors help people to manage these types of crises.

Defining Grief and Crises of Bereavement

In her seminal work on grief, Rando (1984) makes important distinctions between three terms that will be used throughout this chapter: grief, mourning, and bereavement. She defines *grief* as "the process of psychological, social, and somatic reactions to the perception of loss. This implies that grief is (a) manifested in each of the psychological, social, and somatic realms; (b) a continuing development involving many changes; (c) a natural, expectable reaction (in fact, the absence of it is abnormal in most cases); (d) the reaction to the experience of many kinds of loss, not necessarily death alone; and (e) based upon the unique, individualistic perception of loss by the griever, that is, it is not necessary to have the loss recognized or validated by others for the person to experience grief" (p. 15). Rando defines *mourning* as having two historical meanings. The first involves a wide range of intrapsychic processes, both conscious and unconscious, brought on by the experience of loss; the second involves the cultural response to grief. Implied here is that there is no one acceptable style of mourning. Rando defines *bereavement* as "The state of having suffered a loss" (p. 16). Losses can take many forms, including the death of a spouse or partner, divorce, the death of pet, moving, graduation, the end of an addiction, major health changes, financial changes brought about by retirement, the aftermath of holidays, legal problems, and empty nest. Yet not all of the losses included in this list are necessarily associated with grieving. Rando (1984) suggests that losses can be either physical or tangible, such as losing a desired possession or the death of friend, or they can be symbolic, such as a divorce or losing job status because of a demotion.

Types of Grief Reactions

Grief is normal in the face of loss, however there are many factors that influence how one experiences feelings of grief. In spite of the similarities that are often found in bereavement processes, there are many variations in how each individual grieves. This is seen within families in which siblings grieve the loss of a parent very differently and parents grieve the loss of a child in their own unique ways. What is important however is to refrain from making judgments about what constitutes the "right or proper" way to grieve. The reasoning behind this will become more evident throughout this chapter.

Normal grief can be experienced on several levels and in several different ways, which accounts for why there tends to be quite a bit of variation in how people grieve. For example, on an *affective* or emotional level, feelings of sadness, despair, guilt, loneliness, anxiety, helplessness, hopelessness, disinterest or apathy with regards to work or school, or feelings of emancipation and relief are all common reactions. On a *cognitive* or thinking level, one may experience shock, disbelief, preoccupation, or self-deprecation, which may manifest in the form of "would've, could've or should've" (e.g., "I should have told my son how much I loved him while he was still alive"). On a *behavioral and somatic* level, one may experience disturbed sleep, a loss of appetite, crying, a tendency to sigh, fatigue, or a loss of desire to interact with others. Some may experience physical symptoms, such as panic attacks, feelings of emptiness, heart palpitations, loss of sexual desire or increased sexual drive, hollowness or aching in their stomachs, headaches, muscle pain or muscle weakness, and other physical manifestations of their grief. It is not unusual for grief to be expressed more through physical problems than emotionally or cognitively. Such is the case with Betty, described in the opening vignette.

Pathological Reactions to Grief

A question that often arises is, "When does normal grief cross over into problematic or pathological grief?" Similarly, "How does bereavement differ from depression?" Although it is common that most crisis intervention and grief counselors refrain from diagnosing or pathologizing reactions that are considered normal, sometimes normal grief can cross over into pathological condition. The following case example illustrates such a situation:

> Sara is a 20-year-old college student who had been dating Jason for the past 2 years. They talked about the possibility of getting married after college, depending on whether or not Jason got into law school. Their plans ended however when Jason was killed in a fire in his apartment complex off campus. Sara presented at the student counseling center on campus distraught and crying. She felt she just could not go on living without Jason and explained that she had not only thought about suicide but also had a means of carrying out her plan, by taking pills she had stored.

This case example demonstrates not only a pathological reaction to grief, but also illustrates how intense sudden, unexpected grief can be. Sara was serious about suicide as evidenced not only by suicidal ideation, but also by having a plan and a means to carry out that plan. Some studies conclude that approximately 12% to 15% of bereaved individuals will experience intense and prolonged reactions to their losses (Clayton, Desmarais, & Winokur, 1968; Zisook, Shuchter, & Lyons, 1987; Parkes & Weiss, 1983).

There are some key distinctions between normal grieving and depression and ways to distinguish the symptoms. Schneider (1984) provided a useful way to distinguish these symptoms, which are shown in Table 8.1. As can be seen in the table, although the symptoms of normal grieving and depression may overlap in several areas, they are qualitatively quite different. Worden (1982) suggested that distinctions be made between normal, difficult, and pathological grief. Determinants of normal grief reactions will be discussed in the next section. Difficult reactions are often exhibited when the conditions of the person's death are exceptionally arduous, such as the death of a young child in an accidental shooting, the death of an infant or a new spouse, or deaths that occur as the result of tragedy, such as the terrorist bombings of September 11, 2001.

TABLE 8.1
Key Differences Between Grieving and Depression

	Grieving	Depression
Loss	Recognizable loss by bereaved	May be no recognizable loss by the depressed, or it is seen as punishment
Mood states	Quick shifts from sadness to more normal states in same day; variability in mood; psychomotor activity level, verbal communication, appetite, and sexual interest within same day/week	Sadness mixed with anger; tension or absence of energy; consistent sense of depletion, psychomotor retardation, anorexia with weight loss, sexual interest is down; or there is agitation, compulsive eating, sexuality or verbal output
Expression of sadness	Weeping	Difficulty in weeping or in controlling weeping
Expression of anger	Open anger and hostility	Absence of externally directed anger & hostility
Dreams, fantasies, & imagery	Vivid, clear dreams, fantasy and capacity for imagery, particularly involving the loss	Relatively little access to dreams; high capacity for fantasy or imagery of a self-destructive nature; severe insomnia, early morning awakening
Sleep disturbance	Disturbing dreams, episodic difficulties in getting to sleep	Severe insomnia, early morning awakening
Pleasure	Variable restriction of pleasure	Persistent restrictions of pleasure
Self concept	Sees self as to blame for not providing adequately for lost object; tendency to experience the world as empty, preoccupation with lost object or person	Sees self as bad because of being depressed; tendency to experience self as worthless; preoccupation with self; suicidal ideas and feelings
Responsiveness	Responds to warmth and reassurance	Responds to repeated promises, pressure and urging, and unresponsive to most stimuli
Reactions of others	Tendency for others to feel sympathy for griever, to want to touch or hold the person who is grieving	Tendency to feel irritation toward the depressed; others rarely feel like touching or reaching out to the depressed

Note. From *Stress, Loss and Grief,* by J. Schneider, 1984, New York: Aspen Publishers, Inc. Reprinted with permission.

Pathological grief reactions are often characterized by major psychiatric symptoms, such as severe depression, suicidal ideation, extreme agitation, or restlessness. Although there is no time frame in which grief feelings should be resolved, pathological reactions are often as intense several years after the loved one died as they were at the time of death. Another way to think about pathological grief reactions is that when a person suffers a loss and experiences a crisis as a result of that loss, it is natural that he or she will be immobilized for a period of time by the loss. Even once the person does resume everyday activities, he or she may just be "going through the motions." In a pathological grief reaction, the mourner continues to remain immobilized even after months or years have passed. The person may be unable to work, to attend religious services, or to engage in any meaningful social contact.

Finally, another distinction needs to be made, regarding crisis intervention counseling and ongoing bereavement counseling. Naturally, not everyone who experiences a loss will access formal counseling services. A great deal of grief counseling is done informally with the help of family, friends, clergy, and sometimes coworkers. For those who do access formal counseling, crisis bereavement counseling would usually constitute the initial contact the bereaved person makes to seek formal counseling. This might occur in the immediate aftermath of the loss or tragedy, however many individuals will access formal counseling in crisis sometimes several months (or possibly even years) after their loss (this is explored in the case vignettes throughout the chapter). Why is this? Just as trauma reactions can have a delayed onset, so too can grief reactions.

Much of how a person reacts to loss will be determined by several factors, which are presented in the next section.

Determinants of Grief Reactions

Grief can take many forms from individual to individual, in part because of the many factors that can influence grief reactions. For example, in the list of affective reactions provided previously, feelings of sadness or loneliness are obvious grief reactions. But what about feelings of relief or emancipation? A death that comes about after a lengthy, chronic, and painful illness may bring about feelings of relief as well as sadness. In a highly abusive relationship with a possessive, alcoholic spouse, death may bring about feelings of emancipation in the surviving spouse and children. The loss of a part of one's body, such as a limb or a breast, can bring about grief reactions; so too can a loss of mobility due to paralysis. Rando (1984) provides a listing of many psychological factors that can influence the grief reaction. They are discussed in the following sections.

THE MEANING OF THE LOSS   The unique nature and meaning of the loss sustained or the relationship severed affects the extent and severity of the grief. As Rando pointed out, some people may grieve more intensely over the death of a pet than over the death of a sibling. This suggests that the impact of the loss is very much determined by the nature and meaning of the relationship to the individual.

THE ROLES OF THE DECEASED AND THE GRIEVER IN THE FAMILY OR SOCIAL SYSTEM   Here again, the nature and quality of the relationship will determine the intensity of the grief reaction. When one loses a spouse, it can represent the loss of a companion, a friend, a lover, an income provider, an accountant, a gardener, a babysitter, a chauffeur (Parkes, 1970). Therefore, when a loved one dies, surviving family members are often forced to assume new roles, and it may take time for the family to regain its sense of balance. In providing effective crisis intervention, it is important that the crisis counselor take into account the role of the deceased in the survivor's life.

COPING ABILITY, LEVEL OF MATURITY, AND INTELLIGENCE   Coping with grief will be determined in part by how the person has coped with crisis in the past. Has this individual coped with other crises in a positive way? According to Rando (1984), "Most will cope with grief using the responses they have become familiar with. The mourner will tend to grieve (and the dying patient will tend to die) in much the same manner in which the rest of her life has been conducted" (p. 45). Individual grief reactions can also be determined by the behaviors of the individual mourner: avoidance of painful stimuli; distraction; excessive use of drugs, alcohol, or food; obsessive rumination; impulsive behavior; prayer; rationalization or intellectualization; and whether one engages in contact with others. Level of maturity also plays an important role. For example, an over-indulged 38-year-old daughter might make a hysterical scene every time she visited the oncology ward where her dying father was being treated.

Just as individuals will grieve based upon their abilities to cope with loss in the past, so too will families cope as they have coped with crisis in the past. It is no surprise that grief will bring out the best or worst in families. Families that have a strong identity, that value trust and honesty, that value the opinions and feelings of each family member will often be supportive in their grief. Conversely, families that have had strained interactions will tend to become even more dysfunctional in the face of a bereavement crisis. For example, some families have spent years contesting a will and family members will communicate with one another only through their attorneys.

PAST EXPERIENCE WITH LOSS AND DEATH   Current reactions to loss are very much influenced by one's past experiences with grief. For example, a person who as a young child perceived the death of his grandparent as being a horrific experience because his father had a major falling out with his aunt and uncle over the grandfather's estate would rightfully perceive grieving as a dangerous enterprise that could result in even more loss. On the other hand, a person who perceives grieving as a process that helps to bond family and community members together, and in doing so allows them to work through their feelings, will naturally have different expectations of the grieving process. Although crisis intervention focuses more on the here-and-now, it is important that crisis counselors understand the client's past experiences with loss and death to effectively intervene in the present.

CULTURAL AND RELIGIOUS/PHILOSOPHICAL BACKGROUND   As has been emphasized throughout this text, it is of utmost importance in any counseling endeavor to take culture, race, ethnicity, and social milieu into account. This is especially true in crisis counseling with the bereaved. Multicultural influences can greatly affect the expression and process of grief. For example, grief reactions of individuals from highly expressive cultures, races, or religions will be much different from those individuals from less expressive cultures. A New Orleans African American funeral procession complete with a seven piece jazz band is very different from a New England Protestant funeral of sixth generation New Englanders. In order to understand these rituals, one must understand the cultural context. In the New Orleans African American and Creole community, death is viewed as a graduation, or emancipation, from the struggles of life and a promise of paradise in the life hereafter. In the Anglo-Saxon Protestant tradition, extreme forms of emotional expression are often frowned upon. Instead rationality and a stoic, "stiff upper lip" attitude is expected. It is important that crisis counselors take these cultural factors into account and not be fooled into thinking that because a client does not express grief outwardly, the grief is not as heartfelt as in someone who does.

AGE   Children, adolescents, and adults all grieve differently. Even among adults, there are tremendous variations in grief reactions, influenced by whether the griever is young, middle aged, or elderly, as well as previously mentioned factors. For example, elderly people who have experienced the death of their peers may become outwardly impervious to the death of yet another friend or loved one.

Children and adolescents also tend to express their grief differently. As with adults, a lack of outward expression of grief should not be misinterpreted as a lack of emotional distress. In the aftermath of parent's death, a child may regress developmentally by becoming more dependent on the surviving parent or by exhibiting certain behaviors, such as thumb sucking, bedwetting, or "baby talk." When one parent dies, the child often feels the pain of losing both parents, because the surviving parent is also experiencing grief and may seem unavailable to the child. In addition, the surviving parent must now take on new roles, deal with financial problems, and take on the tasks of becoming a single parent. Adolescents (and some children) may be more prone to "acting out" behaviors, such as getting into fights or having trouble in school. Some teenagers may resort to drug or alcohol use to avoid the pain of the loss, while others may throw themselves into a whirlwind of activity.

The age of the deceased is also a factor. Death of the elderly is perceived as being inevitable, whereas the death of a young adult is perceived as tragic, eliciting such comments as "They were cut down in the prime of their life" or "They had their whole lives ahead of them; what a pity to be taken at so young an age." Age is often a relative factor, though. As Rando (1984) points out, given the case of an 80-year-old man who loses his 78-year-old wife, "Age is irrelevant to him—he has lost his life's companion" (p. 49).

CHARACTERISTICS OF THE DECEASED In addition to age, the character of the deceased will also influence grief reactions. A well-known, well-loved high school student who died in an accident involving a drunk driver had mourners lined up around the block of the funeral home. As Rando (1984) pointed out there is a "... tendency for our society to approve of grief for those who are good and worthwhile but not for those who are bad. The death of a criminal in the midst of a robbery does not arouse much social concern" (p. 49–50).

PERCEPTION OF THE DECEASED'S FULFILLMENT IN LIFE Frequently, when the bereaved perceive the deceased as having lived a full life, the death can be more readily accepted and grief work can take place. When a child or a young person dies, there is always a sense that the youth was robbed or cheated out of a full life. When a young psychology graduate student died in a car accident, the pain of his death was magnified by the fact that this was an individual with so much promise and a true commitment to helping others.

CONCURRENT STRESSES OR CRISES A person who is experiencing ongoing stressors (e.g., a physical illness, job loss, financial problems, or other interpersonal stressors) will have difficulty in the grief process. For example, a couple who were considering divorce, because the wife had had an affair, were 2 months into marital counseling when the husband was struck by a hit and run driver and instantly killed. The wife's grief was naturally compounded by her guilt over having had the affair. Families who lost loved ones in the World Trade Center attack reported several concurrent crises, such as being badgered by the media, being called by the New York City Medical Examiner to identify remains, and fears about the long-term impact of the loss on their children.

THE SUDDENNESS OR EXPECTEDNESS OF THE DEATH It is generally accepted that when death is expected, as with terminal illnesses, there is time for anticipatory grieving to take place. For example, unfinished business can be taken care of and loved ones can prepare for the loss and say farewell to the dying person. A client once commented that when her father finally died after a long fight with cancer, she was struck by the fact that she did not cry or mourn as she thought she might. In exploring this unexpected reaction, it was clear that she had been mourning her father's loss throughout all the months of his illness and felt relief when he died. When a death is sudden, however, this is not the case. The shock of a sudden, unexpected loss can often be immobilizing. Such was the case with those who lost loved ones in the September 11 attacks. They had expected to see their loved ones again, and so did not get an opportunity to say goodbye. Unexpected losses and deaths resulting from violence will often overwhelm a person's coping abilities (Murphy, Johnson, & Cain, 1998; Parkes & Weiss, 1983).

The aftermath of a disastrous fire that occurred more than 60 years ago is said to have marked the inception of crisis intervention. On November 28, 1942, a fire broke out in the kitchen of the Cocoanut Grove nightclub in Boston, and

493 people were killed. (Most were trampled to death due to poorly marked exits!) Erich Lindemann, a clinician who was working at Massachusetts General Hospital at the time, offered the first "crisis intervention" services to the survivors and grieving loved ones (Lindemann, 1944). The experience led Lindemann to the conclusion that acute grief reactions are a normal response to tragic deaths. Lindemann defined five characteristics of acute grief: (a) somatic distress, (b) preoccupation with the image of the deceased, (c) guilt, (d) hostile reactions, and (e) loss of patterns of conduct (daily life disruptions).

The Grieving Process

As discussed in the previous section, the grieving process varies based on the circumstances of the death, particularly whether the death was expected or sudden. In this section we examine the grieving process, including the emotions that, in many cases, begin before death actually occurs.

Grieving and the Terminally Ill

When an individual is terminally ill, both the dying patient and the family go through a grieving process before death actually occurs. Perhaps the most well-known work on the grieving process was done by Elizabeth Kubler-Ross (1969), a Swiss psychiatrist who was working with terminally ill children and adults when she developed her stage theory. What is noteworthy is that when Kubler-Ross first wrote about death and dying, it was from the perspective of the dying individual. However, it was later concluded that members of the dying individual's family went through the same stages. More recently, Kubler-Ross's stages have been applied to describe the process by which individual's come to accept any medical illness (including mental illness and substance use disorders). The stages are described in the following list.

1. *Denial and isolation:* Denial is a natural initial reaction to the dying process. Denial is also considered to be a healthy reaction, as it may help the individual continue functioning on a daily basis. It may also help to cushion the patient from the initial shock or despair.

2. *Anger:* Once the reality of the illness begins to set in, denial begins to decrease and anger takes center stage. Patients may question, "Why me?" and their anger may be directed at doctors, health professionals, family members, or God. They may experience rage, bitterness, and envy.

3. *Bargaining:* The bargaining stage can take different forms, but usually is characterized by a secret pact made with God in which the dying patient agrees to change or do something in return for more time or a return of health. One woman who was diagnosed with uterine cancer secretly prayed that her life be spared until she could see her daughter graduate from high school.

4. *Depression:* This stage occurs when the inevitability of death is prominent and overwhelming. As with clinical depression, feelings of hopelessness, helplessness, and despair are paramount.

5. *Acceptance:* Not all individuals reach this stage. Perhaps the best way to characterize this stage is being at peace. The patient is no longer wrestling emotionally with the inevitability of death. Family members may reach a point of acceptance when they can reflect back on their loved one's life with fond memories now devoid of the sharp pain that grief often brings. The dying patient may appear to be void of feeling, and begins to disengage from life or disengage from battling the illness.

There are several important points to discuss about Kubler-Ross's stages. First, not everyone experiences these stages in sequence, even though these stages are said to be sequential. From clinical observation, we find that people often bounce between stages at various points during the course of their illness. So it is not unusual, for example, for a person to feel depressed one week and to return to anger the next or denial and isolation after that. This does not negate the importance of this stage model. Instead, it is important for counselors to roll with these changes and to be able to work with patients or family members, no matter where they are in their grief at any particular moment in time. Second, in doing crisis intervention in bereavement situations, it is possible for individuals to present in any of these stages (except for acceptance, because with acceptance, there is usually no stated crisis). So, patients in crisis may present when feeling anger, bargaining, or when depressed. Please keep in mind that prior to Kubler-Ross's work, no one really took the time to talk with dying patients, to listen to their feelings and their needs. Her work not only pioneered the field of grief counseling, but also made course work in grief counseling and communication with dying patients and their families mandatory in many medical schools.

Phases of Mourning

Whether death was sudden or protracted, family members go through a process of mourning. John Bowlby (1980), who is best known for his work on attachment theory and separation/loss as viewed from a psychodynamic perspective, and Parkes (1970), described four phases of mourning.

1. *Numbing:* Shock and disbelief prevail in this phase. Often, the bereaved experience varying degrees of denial.

2. *Yearning and searching:* The bereaved individual often demonstrates strong urges to find, recover, or reunite with the lost loved one. Feelings of anger, restlessness, and irritability are most evident in this stage. Strong preoccupations with visual memories of the deceased are also present.

3. *Disorganization and despair:* This phase is marked by the bereaved giving up the search for the deceased. Feelings of depression are most prevalent in this phase, along with an inability to look to the future or see purpose in life.

4. *Reorganization:* In this phase, the bereaved breaks the intense attachment to the deceased and begins to establish ties to others. There is a gradual return to former interests and appetites.

The Tasks of Mourning

Related to the phases of mourning are the tasks or goals of the bereavement process. These tasks are somewhat analogous to developmental tasks. For example, there is a general time frame that demarcates the developmental stage of adolescence (sometime between the ages of 13 and 19). However, in order to move beyond this stage, teens must complete particular tasks relevant to this stage, such as forming a sense of identity, making career decisions, defining interpersonal relationships, and separating from the family of origin. In mourning, various essential tasks have been described. Worden (1982) for example, has described four primary tasks.

1. *Accepting the reality of the loss:* As in Kubler-Ross's stages, denial is often encountered when dealing with a dying patient or a family member who has lost a loved one. One grieving widow continued to set a place at the dinner table for her husband for several months after he died. She demonstrated that she had reached some acceptance of his death when she stopped doing this and when she gave his clothes to a local homeless shelter.

2. *Experiencing the pain of the grief:* One of the most difficult tasks in grief work is expressing and experiencing the feelings associated with grief, whether they be feelings of rage, guilt, or depression. Anthropologists explain that feelings of anger towards loved ones who have died are normal and may have fostered important funeral rituals. For example, placing tombstones on graves became a way of "holding down" the spirits of the deceased who might come back and attack us. The twenty-one gun salute is said to have originated in primitive tribes who would throw rocks and spears into the air with the intent of driving the deceased's spirit away. These traditions exist because of our natural anger at the deceased.

3. *Adjusting to an environment in which the deceased is missing:* Coping with the loss of a loved one is difficult enough; however, coping in the environment without the loved one is even more of challenge. Whether it be a widow who is learning where to have her car repaired, a widower who is learning to cook for himself, or a child who is learning to pick out her own clothes in the morning or braid her own hair, the challenges of learning these new skills is an essential element of the grief process.

4. *Withdrawing emotional energy and reinvesting it in another relationship:* The very thought of withdrawing emotional energy from the deceased may be viewed as disloyalty or may be accompanied by a sense of betrayal or guilt. Parents who experience the death of a child often report that they find themselves pulling away from their surviving child or children. It may take years for a person who has lost a loved one, particularly a

spouse or significant other, to trust and love again, to reinvest emotions in another person. This process takes time, and there may be cause for concern if a person develops another love relationship too quickly. In one such instance, a widower quickly become involved with another woman about 3 months after his wife died, rationalizing that he just wasn't meant to live alone. After a quick marriage, he soon realized that he and his new bride were very different. Although he had thought she possessed many of the same character traits of his deceased wife, he now found he had deluded himself into fabricating these similarities. This couple grew more and more miserable with each passing month as the conflict between them took over their day-to-day interactions. It was no surprise when they announced that they had decided to divorce.

Crisis Intervention in Bereavement and Loss

Although there are no hard and fast rules when it comes to crisis intervention in bereavement situations, there are some guidelines that might be useful for counselors as they are working with people in the throes of these types of crises. Worden (1982) offers the following guidelines for crisis bereavement counseling.

- *Help the survivor to actualize the loss.* It is important for crisis counselors to allow the person to talk about the loss, including the details of what happened and how the death occurred.

- *Help the survivor to identify and express feelings.* Don't assume that clients will be able to identify their feelings readily. They may be burdened with guilt, anxiety, or anger, but may be unaware of these feelings. Therefore, it is important that counselors listen for affect as clients tell the stories of their loved ones' deaths. Body language and facial expression can also provide cues to affective state. If a client is having difficulty with guilty feelings, the counselor could approach this issue by asking, "If there was something you could have changed when Jane was alive, what would it have been?"

- *Assist the survivor to live without the deceased.* In this task, basic crisis counseling skills to help the client explore alternative approaches to problem solving are useful. It is important to remind clients that they often do not need to make major decisions right away and to allow themselves time to make decisions.

- *Facilitate emotional withdrawal from the deceased.* Counselors can encourage clients to take steps towards moving on with their lives in subtle ways, for example by reestablishing connections with friends or supportive family members.

- *Provide time to grieve.* It is important to allow clients time and space to grieve. In doing so, the counselor can help the client to anticipate difficult times and milestones. Holidays and the anniversary of the death are particularly difficult. Anniversary reactions are common, often triggered by changes in season or other cues in the immediate environment. With regards to milestones, grief groups often employ the concept of "2 weeks, 2 months, and 2 years." The first 2 weeks following the loved one's death are naturally the most difficult in terms of getting through the initial shock, including dealing with funeral preparations and visits from extended family and friends. After 2 months, much of the initial support of family and friends may have begun to recede and the bereaved begins to acknowledge the loss in a different way. At the 2 year mark, the person has been through all of the major holidays, birthdays, and anniversaries at least twice and now may find that the intensity of the grief has changed.

- *Interpret "normal" behavior.* As alluded to earlier, clients will often question whether their reactions are normal or not. One widow questioned whether it was normal to cry whenever she was in church several months after her husband had died. While he was alive, she and her husband had been actively involved in their local church and his funeral service was held in this same church. Naturally, each time she was in church, the painful memories of the funeral service came flooding back.

- *Allow for individual differences.* Grief reactions tend to be idiosyncratic. Some people will grieve openly and intensely, others will grieve quietly and privately. Some will cry everyday for weeks or months, others not at all. It is important for counselors to be sensitive to individual differences in grieving styles.

- *Provide continued support.* If the counselor will not be involved in the long-term, it is important that he or she provides for a support network. Since crisis counseling is time-limited, it is important to connect clients with bereavement support groups with which they can identify. For example, there are support groups that are specific to couples who have lost children, such as Compassionate Friends. There are other groups that support individuals who have lost a loved one to suicide. One 32-year-old widow was referred to a hospital-based bereavement group after her husband died of leukemia. When she went to the group, she began to feel angrier and angrier with each passing week. In exploring her anger, she happened to mention to her counselor that the majority of the widows in the group were more than 60 years old. She explained her anger by exclaiming, "They have had a full life with their husbands. I was only married for 5 years when Ted died. I feel cheated." Her anger was appropriate and dissipated when the counselor found a group comprised of younger widows and widowers who were feeling much of the same anguish that she was.

- *Examine defenses and coping systems.* It is important to look for how the client copes with day-to-day life and what resources exist that can assist the person in enhancing his or her coping abilities. With regards to defenses, it is important to determine to what extent psychological defense mechanisms, such as denial, rationalization, or minimization, are utilized and how effective or ineffective they might be.

BOX 8.1

Good Grief and Bad

The new grief counseling industry tries to help lessen the pain of loss. That's its first mistake.

By Lorenzo Albacete

Soon after my ordination to the Catholic priesthood, on my very first "night on duty" in the parish where I was assigned, I answered a phone call from a woman whose sister had just died in a plane crash. She wasn't sure whether she believed in God, but she just wanted to talk with someone. I thought about her recently when I heard that "grief counselors" would be sent to console the passengers of a cruise that the victims of the Air France Concorde crash had planned to board.

Grief counseling has become an industry. An Internet search reveals thousands of grief counseling Web sites, hundreds of advice-filled books, herbs, acupuncture, "therapeutic touching," help for those whose pet has died and certified "bereavement facilitators," one of whom promises to "facilitate a reunion" with the departed.

Grief is a multi-layered experience. Grief counselors are largely trained to recognize grief's psychological and physical effects, as well as various ways in which people of different cultures, ages, sexes and so on, experience them. When Msgr. Ronald Marino spent three weeks with the families of T.W.A. Flight 800's victims, he said, "I did not go as a professional grief counselor; I went as a priest." The difference? Professional counselors, as Marino put it, "leave the 'ultimate questions' to the clergy."

I'd be the last to suggest that only the clergy can deal with those questions, but I do think they are unavoidable at such a time. The roots of grief arise from a wound deeper than the psychological or cultural. It is at that level in ourselves where we decide what we can or cannot expect of life, what is just or unjust, what is the purpose and value of our existence. To the degree that grief counseling ever ignores those questions, it does not deal with grief; it leads us to suppress it.

When his closest friend died, St. Augustine said that he became a "great riddle" to himself. His wound was so profound it was a challenge to his identity. Traditional religious consolation—which points our attention beyond this life, toward a reality beyond our understanding—was no comfort. If he told his soul to hope in God, he wrote, it was useless, "because the dearest friend my soul had lost was an actual man, both truer and better than the imagined deity he was ordered to put his hope in." Tears had taken the place of his friend in his heart.

Grief is the crying of the heart, and the human heart will resist being soothed by ideas and abstractions. Not long ago, I saw an interview with the dramatist Dennis Potter conducted shortly before his death from cancer. Potter, who during the interview took a morphine-based painkiller, had only one request left to make of life: the time to finish his last play. (He got his wish.)

My friends saw his dedication to his art as a triumph of the human spirit, and everyone was deeply inspired. Everyone except me, that is. I found the interview depressing. To me, the unavoidable reality was that Dennis Potter was dead, that he would never write again. The "survival of the human spirit" didn't console me. This wasn't about the human spirit; this was about one man, Dennis Potter, and he had not survived.

In this life—even for me, a priest— "life after death" is an abstraction that can never replace the loss of a living, breathing person. I remembered the words of Ivan, stricken by injustice in "The Brothers Karamazov": "I must have retribution, or I shall destroy myself. And retribution not somewhere in the infinity of space and time, but here on earth, and so that I could see it myself. ... And if I'm dead by that time, let them resurrect me, for if it happens without me, it will be too unfair. Surely, the reason for my suffering was not that I as well as my deeds and sufferings might serve as manure for some future harmony for someone else."

I suspect that today we are not supposed to expect that much of life. We are supposed to settle for less. What, then, do we expect of grief counselors? To help us suppress these embarrassing expectations of the heart? Is consolation after all a lowering of expectations? If anything, I am consoled by the Book of Job, which derides those who tried to explain Job's suffering to him. God does not seek to console him; He just shows up and this is enough. It was not explanations Job wanted, but solidarity, compassion, love.

In Helen Whitney's program about Pope John Paul II last year on "Frontline," Germaine Greer wept, recalling the suffering children she saw in Africa. "And if God exists," she cried, "I hate him." I was asked to offer the response of faith. My faith told me that those children would live again to see the day of justice. But since she is not a believer, I could only tell her that I experience the same sense of horror, and that she was right to cry out for justice. For me, that's the counseling that respects all the human dimensions of that grief. As Monsignor Marino told me, when you are moved by the reality of a tragedy, "God instantly gives you the credentials for grief counseling." That solidarity in suffering cannot be professionalized.

That is why on that first night on duty in my parish, I told the woman who had lost her sister that I would come over to her apartment. I brought some doughnuts and coffee with me. I wasn't there to discuss theology, or propose intellectual answers to the questioning in her heart. I told her that although I believed that her sister had not died forever, I shared the demands of her grief, and we sat in her kitchen to eat doughnuts and drink coffee.

Lorenzo Albacete, a Roman Catholic priest, is a professor of theology at St. Joseph's Seminary in Yonkers.

Reprinted with permission from the *New York Times,* August 27, 2000, Section 6

Terminal Illness: Crisis Intervention Case Example 1

At the beginning of the chapter, we described a bereavement crisis situation involving the death of Robert due to pancreatic cancer. Shortly thereafter, Betty, his widow, had been seen in the emergency room complaining of chest pains and shortness of breath.

> Betty is a 56-year-old mother of two daughters, ages 24 and 22. Three months ago, her husband Robert died of pancreatic cancer. Approximately 8 months ago, he had complained of nausea, upper stomach pain, and was losing weight even though he was not dieting. His physician suspected cancer and had Robert see an oncologist, who made the diagnosis. Robert died within 4 months of being diagnosed. He and Betty had shared many happy years together, and they were both very proud of their two daughters. The oldest daughter was married right after graduating college and she and her husband were living in Paris, both working for a large international investment company. The youngest daughter lived at home while completing her bachelor's degree at a local college. She had just been accepted to graduate school when her father was diagnosed. Betty was referred for crisis counseling at the recommendation of the emergency room physician who examined her for complaints of chest pains and difficulty breathing.

In this case example, Betty has just experienced the loss of her husband and her daughter may be moving away soon to go to graduate school. The goal of the initial crisis intervention session is to move from a discussion of Betty's medical symptoms to a discussion about her grief. There are many individuals who feel that in order to be strong, they must not talk about their grief nor express their emotions to others. As recommended by Worden (1982), it is important that Betty express and identify her feelings of grief. As part of the *Listening* process, it is important that the counselor validates Betty's feeling of numbness as being a normal reaction. The counselor should also encourage Betty to talk more about what she has been going through, both before Bob died and since.

It is important to allow Betty time and space to grieve. It is important to *Assess* possible complicating factors to Betty's grief, such as her daughter's pending move. In the *Planning* process, the counselor should realize how important it will be to get Betty connected with a support group as soon as possible, since she has been quite isolated in her grief. It is hoped that after Betty talks about her grief and her life with Bob, she will be receptive to a referral to a support group.

LISTEN	ASSESS	PLAN	COMMIT

Name: *Betty*   Age *56*

LISTEN

What is the client saying about the crisis? *Betty complains of chest pains and shortness of breath, but later begins to talk about the death of her husband and her grief.*

What happened? *Death of husband*

When did it happen? *2 months ago*

What type of crisis was it (traumatic event, developmental, psychiatric, existential)? *Developmental, husband's cancer developed over the course of several months*

Did the client mention anything that indicated danger? *No*

Other relevant information about the crisis: *Betty is also grieving about her daughter leaving for graduate school.*

ASSESS

Feelings: Is the client's predominant emotional state one of:

Anger *No*   Sadness *Yes*   Hopelessness *Yes*

Anxiety *Yes*   Panic *Yes*   Numbness *No*

Suicidal? If yes, complete lethality assessment/suicide. *No*

Homicidal? If yes, complete lethality assessment/violence. *No*

Acting: Is the client's behavior:

Active/restless *Yes*   Consistent with mood *Yes*

Passive/withdrawn *No*   Good eye contact *Yes*

Thinking: Is the client:

Logical/making sense *Yes*   Coherent/expressing self well *Yes*

Insightful *Yes*   Focused on topic *Yes*

Evasive/changing subject *No*

Other: Any medical problems? *Yes*

Physical limitations? *No*

Hospitalizations? *No*

Need for hospitalization? *Possible*

(Continues)

PLAN

What needs to be done now? *Betty needs to be reassured that she will be able to get through her current panic*

What alternative plans have been discussed? *Ongoing individual counseling and/or group counseling*

Are these plans reasonable? *Yes*

Can they be carried out? *Yes*

COMMIT

Which plan of action has the client chosen? *Group counseling*

Are there resources/support to implement the plan? *Yes*

Is the client motivated to implement the plan? *Yes, well motivated*

What other resources/supports may be needed?

Friend *Yes*   Family member *Daughter*

Neighbor *No*   Mental health provider *grief counselor, bereavement support group*

Public agency (law enforcement, child protective services, social services) *No*

Medical (hospitalization, medication) *No*

Traumatic Death: Crisis Intervention Case Example 2

> Jack is a 64-year-old retired New York City police officer. He was very proud of his youngest son, Frank, who had just completed training at the New York City Police Academy and had been assigned to a precinct in lower Manhattan in the summer of 2001. Frank was one of the police officers killed in the World Trade Center attacks. For several days after September 11, Jack walked around in a state of shock. He could not believe that his son was gone. Every day for 4 months, Jack walked to Ground Zero, somehow with the hope that he would find his son or that his body would be recovered. He refused to believe that his son was dead. Jack finally sought counseling through his parish priest as a result of the prodding of his wife and some of his closest friends.

In this case example, Jack's bereavement is complicated by the tragic nature of the event that resulted in his son's death, but his grief is not pathological. His visits to Ground Zero every day are what Bowlby (1980) refers to in his stages of grief as "yearning and searching." Jack is now moving into the phase of "disorganization and despair," according to Bowlby's model. This is the point at which Jack was willing to seek assistance with the encouragement of his parish priest and his wife.

The counselor begins by *Listening* to Jack's story of where he was on September 11, what he was doing at the time of the attacks, and when he began to realize that his son was on duty that day and that he may have rushed to the scene. The main initial goal of the counselor is to create an environment in which Jack will feel comfortable expressing any of his feelings. The counselor also tries to normalize Jack's various feelings, including some of the guilt he feels for having encouraged his son to pursue a career as a police officer. He avoids any comments that would sound like criticism. It's important that the counselor stay with Jack. If he's feeling despair and hopelessness, then it's important for the counselor to convey to Jack that these feelings are being heard. If he is expressing guilt, it is important not to put a Band-Aid on the guilt, but to let Jack know that his feelings are being heard.

As was discussed at the beginning of the chapter, the impact of grief is determined in part by how the death occurs. It is likely that some who lost loved ones in the September 11 attacks may never reach acceptance or resolution, given the horrendous nature of this national tragedy. Many family members who had lost loved ones reported that pictures of the attack on the news or the scenes of Ground Zero were constantly retraumatizing them. In some instances, family members were harassed by sociopaths who wrote abusive letters because of the financial contributions and settlements they received. It seems that although the September 11 attacks brought out the best in those heroes who rushed to provide aide, they also seem to have brought out the worst in some people. This was best exemplified when 25 individuals were charged with having filed false claims of having lost a loved one in the September 11 attacks.

Based upon the *Assessment* that Jack is able to benefit from counseling, a Plan is agreed upon in which Jack *Commits* to attending individual counseling for the next 6 weeks and then will consider going into a group with other parents who have lost sons or daughters in the attacks.

Bereavement in Children: Crisis Intervention Case Example 3

Katie is 10 years old and is in the fifth grade at the Roosevelt Elementary School. Last month, Katie's mother died in a car accident. Katie's parents divorced when she was 4 years old, and her father moved out of state last year when his company transferred him to a new office. Katie was referred for counseling by her teacher, who noticed that her grades had fallen considerably and that she had been getting into fights with some of her classmates who had been her friends.

In this case example, the issue of bereavement in children is addressed. As discussed earlier, children and adolescents often grieve much differently than adults. Much of how a child grieves and copes with grief will be determined by how much preparation they may have received prior to the death and how the mourning is addressed after the death (Furman, 1974). Generally, it is thought that the older the child, the better his or her chances of understanding the permanence of death and, therefore, the better his or her overall adjustment. This naturally depends on how independent and emotionally stable the child is prior to the parent's death.

Coping will also be determined by how the child's questions and curiosities are handled. For example, if a child's questions are met with harshness or anxiety, his or her confusion will only increase. On the other hand, too much information can also be detrimental to overall adjustment. For example, Furman (1974) pointed out that children will often express concerns about losing the surviving parent by asking, "Will you die too, Mommy?" Although concerns about misleading or deceiving the child by replying, "No, mommy will not die" are valid, giving too much information about the unpredictability of life or our shared ultimate fate will only serve to increase anxiety. Similarly, even with younger children, when a parent dies from a terminal illness, it is best to properly label the disease, saying "Daddy is dying because of cancer" rather than "Daddy is sick." By not giving proper information, one runs the risk that the child will automatically associate all sickness with death. Sometimes, all of the details are not known. However, children seem to feel better when their parents tell them that details will be shared with them as they become known (Furman, 1974). Children naturally cannot deal with a flood of frightening details, but they can cope with the surviving parent's upset and tears. The child also benefits from reassurance that the family will remain together. There are often questions about whether a child should attend the wake or funeral service. With very young children, it is usually advised that they not attend the wake; however, older children can attend even an open-casket viewing provided that they are allowed to determine their distance from the casket and that they are accompanied by adults who will support and comfort them, as well as to respond to their questions and concerns. It is also important to recognize that the child's longing to be with the deceased parent is also part of the normal grief process, as are feelings of sadness and/or anger. Part of successful grieving in children (and adults for that matter) is the ability to withstand these feelings of longing or yearning to be with the deceased.

The counselor working with Katie begins by first establishing a connection with her, talking about things she likes, trying to get her to feel comfortable. Once a rapport has been established, the counselor will then try to get Katie to talk about her mother's death, even though she seems to be reluctant to do so, given the circumstances surrounding the referral. The counselor tries to roll with the resistance and not focus too much on Katie's grades or her recess behavior. In this *Listening* phase, the counselor hears about the car accident and how Katie was told of her mother's death. Katie begins to talk about going to the hospital with her maternal grandparents right after the accident and how she was able to see her mother just before she died. Katie has several recollections of seeing her mother in the emergency room and begins to cry as she tells the counselor about her mother's bruises, the tubes sticking out of her, the bloody bandages on the floor, her grandparents crying and holding her. The counselor *Assesses* that Katie is quite verbal and seems comfortable talking with her. The *Plan* is to encourage Katie to return for further counseling. The counselor makes certain before the session ends that Katie is composed enough to return to her classroom. She encourages Katie to return, even if they don't have a scheduled appointment, if she needs to talk.

Death of an Infant: Crisis Intervention Case Example 4

Marisol and Manuel are both 25 years old and have been married for 2 years. They were looking forward to having a baby and becoming parents. After having two miscarriages, Marisol finally gave birth to a baby boy. They were both ecstatic. However, they were then told that the baby had developed medical complications and was having difficulty breathing. A cardiac neonatologist was called to consult. She told Marisol and Manuel that the baby had major heart damage and was not expected to live. Their baby died when he was only 4 weeks old.

The death of a child is probably the singular most traumatic event that a parent can face. Similarly, the loss of a child that is put up for adoption or a child placed in long term foster care can often produce the same types of grief reactions. It is universally assumed that a child will outlive their parents. As Rando (1984) pointed out, when adults lose their parents they lose their past, but when they lose their children, they lose their future. The divorce rate for grieving parents is incredibly high. Some estimates suggest that the divorce rate for bereaved parents who do not receive any help is as high as 92% (Kanel, 2003). This can be attributed to a number of factors. First, after the tragic loss of the child, couples feel that they have profoundly changed. Second, parents will tend to grieve differently and because of this, they may feel frustration or anger with their partners. For example, if the husband (or male partner) views the death as something the couple can get over or that they can try to have another child, then his wife may perceive these thoughts as being cold and discounting of her feelings. Likewise, if the wife or female partner is experiencing tremendous grief, then the husband may feel that he is not doing enough or he may want his wife to move on so that they can resume their lives as a couple. Finally, since both husband and wife are experiencing grief, they often are unable to support one another through this process. They begin to feel isolated in their grief and disconnected.

In the case example described above, it is Marisol who seeks counseling approximately 4 days after their baby died. The couple's grief is compounded by their having experienced two miscarriages prior to the birth of their son. A miscarriage can be as devastating emotionally as any other tragic loss. Unfortunately, there have been only a few medical centers and crisis intervention providers who have been attuned to the need for some formal way to grieve the termination of a pregnancy by miscarriage or abortion. Some centers now provide grief counseling for those who have experienced a pregnancy loss. Some even provide grieving rituals, such as the planting of a tree in memory of the loss.

For the nurse or medical crisis counselor that would be working with Marisol and Manuel, the first step would be to express condolence and sympathy for their loss. It is important that the nurse or counselor be willing to *Listen* to their story of anticipating the birth and of being told that their infant son had medical complications. They may express anger towards the doctors or medical center for being unable to save their son or for being callous in how they communicated the baby's likelihood of death. It is best if the counselor listens to these feelings without offering some explanation or defending the doctors or center. Instead it is important to offer reassurance to Marisol and Manuel as a means of normalizing their grief.

In the *Assessment* phase it will be important to gain a sense of how each of them are coping with the loss. Do they differ in how they conceptualize the loss or in how they are reacting? For example, if the counselor has a sense at this point that Manuel is coping much differently than his wife, this may have both gender (men have to be strong) and ethnic (Latino men have to be even stronger) implications that may need to be explored later in the session. As the *Planning* process begins, it will be important to explore whether they would both be willing to return for either individual or group bereavement counseling. If both are willing to return, the counselor might comment that Manuel's willingness is a positive step. However, if he does not want to continue with counseling, this should not be interpreted negatively, and Marisol should not become disappointed or lose hope, even if he reneges on his agreement to join her. Towards the close of the first session, the counselor also tells Marisol about a couple of support groups for parents who have lost children. It seems that of all the treatments available for couples who have lost children, support groups are one of the most beneficial, because they allow for honest sharing with couples who have experienced the same loss and can therefore understand the same pain.

Death of a Pet: Crisis Intervention Case Example 5

Bertha is 75 years old and lives alone. Her husband died about 5 years ago from a massive heart attack. Bertha has three grown children who live in Atlanta and whom she sees every year during the summer and at the Christmas holidays. Bertha sought crisis counseling at the urging of some of her friends in the seniors group to which she belongs. Bertha explains that last week she had to have her dog, Jackie, put to sleep. Bertha and her husband had adopted Jackie from the local animal shelter when her husband retired about 10 years ago. Bertha feels that she has not only lost Jackie, but that she has lost her husband "all over again," as Jackie became a link to her past life with her husband.

In the case of Bertha, the issue of pet loss is addressed. Only recently were issues of pet loss recognized as necessitating grief counseling services. Today there are many support groups that solely address pet loss grief. In any card shop, along with other condolence cards there are also cards that offer condolences to those who have lost a pet. Pet loss can be just as hard on children as it is on adults. A pet often becomes an important member of the family and is perceived as "being there" through thick and thin, providing unconditional love. For Bertha, as with so many older individuals or people living alone, her pet became her family. For people living alone, pets are there when they come home and they provide a source of solace and companionship.

Bertha's situation not only demonstrates her grief over the loss of a pet, but also portrays how earlier losses can resurface in the face of a present loss. This is evident when Bertha exclaims, "It is like losing my husband all over again." In the initial crisis, it is important for the counselor to *Listen* to Bertha and to really tune into the grief that she is experiencing. It may be helpful to point out that, although grief seems never ending when it begins, eventually people do transcend their pain. The counselor may emphasize that there are things that Bertha can do to help ease her pain, such as talking about her loss. It would be helpful for the counselor to *Assess* what type of support network Bertha has available to her. In the *Planning* phase, it will be helpful to explore whether Bertha would be willing to seek further support through a bereavement counseling group or perhaps through individual counseling. Timing is important, though. For example, when referring Bertha to a pet loss support group, if the referral is made too quickly, Bertha might feel that she is being pushed off onto someone else. It is also helpful when making such a referral to have as much information about the group as possible and perhaps to have the name and phone number of a contact person in the group that Bertha could call to gather information about the group.

Grief and Divorce

Ray is a 54-year-old husband and father of two daughters, ages 20 and 17. He and his wife, Susan, had been married for 24 years. They met at work and were engaged for about a year. Ray thought that their relationship was solid. However, one day while going through some old e-mails on the computer, he came across one of Susan's files in which she had been communicating with an old high school boyfriend. In their e-mails to one another, there were details of their rendezvous and plans to be together once they were able to separate from their current marriages. Ray was devastated. When he confronted Susan, she denied the affair at first, but later admitted that everything in the e-mails was true. After going for some brief marital counseling, Ray realized that Susan no longer loved him, nor was she interested in salvaging the marriage. They decided to separate. Ray sought crisis counseling at the urging of his brother when he told him that he saw no reason going on with life, and that he was so depressed he had not been to work in 3 weeks.

In the case of Ray, a different type of loss is presented—separation and divorce. However, there are many who feel that the emotional pain associated with a divorce is tantamount to losing someone through death. In addition, just as there are hidden losses that one experiences when a loved one has died, so too do divorced individuals experience many tangential losses, for example loss of time with children, loss of income, loss of a home, loss of friends, loss of contact with in-laws, and loss of companionship. Even in the most amicable divorces, the sense of loss is tremendous and overwhelming. However, in the case of a contentious divorce, there may also be accompanying feelings of anger, rage, guilt, envy, and jealousy. When children are involved, the pain of loss often becomes greater. A friend and coworker who was going through a bitter custody battle over his son once remarked that after serving two tours in Vietnam as a combat infantryman, he was eventually able to watch movies such as *Platoon* (Daly & Gibson, 1986) and *Born on the 4th of July* (Stone & Ho, 1989) without breaking into a sweat. However, watching *Kramer vs. Kramer* (Jaffe, 1979) would reduce him to tears in seconds.

Scope of the Divorce Problem

Crises involving divorce are quite common, mostly because the United States has the highest rates of divorce (4.44 per 1,000) compared to other countries (United Kingdom, 2.97 per 1,000; Sweden, 2.40 per 1,000; and Germany, 2.07 per 1,000) (United Nations Secretariat, 1996). It is estimated that approximately 50% of marriages in the United States will end in divorce. There are several factors that are hypothesized as accounting for these extreme divorce rates. First, there is a greater acceptance of divorce in the United States. Marriage is not viewed as having the same permanence that it once had. Second, the roles of women have shifted. With more and more women in the workforce, they are no longer dependent on men and are therefore less willing to stay in unfulfilling marriages. Third, the sanctity of marriage as a religiously bound union is not as strongly accepted as it was years ago. Fourth, there has been a greater emphasis on seeking satisfaction of personal goals and higher expectations for marital happiness (Weitzman, 1985). Finally, people are living longer, so it is not unusual for people to divorce after their children have gone off to college or have married and moved away from home.

Overall, even in amicable separations, divorces tend to have a deleterious effect on one's mental health. Indeed divorce is associated with higher rates of depression (Anthony & Petronis, 1991; Gallo, Royall, & Anthony, 1993; Weissman, Bruce, Leaf, Florio, & Holzer, 1991); suicide (Cantor & Slater, 1995; Trovato, 1986); and substance abuse (Beck, Wright, Newman, & Liese, 1993). Granvold (2000) recommended that a thorough risk assessment be done when divorced individuals present for crisis intervention services because of these risk factors.

Crisis Intervention in Cases of Divorce

As discussed earlier in this chapter, bereavement reactions are often determined by the factors surrounding the death, such as cause of death, the survivor's relationship with the deceased, age, and ethnicity. So too do the events and factors surrounding a divorce play a role in the reactions of the individuals. For example, marital infidelity, physical violence, verbal and/or emotional abuse, alcoholism and substance abuse, physical and/or sexual abuse of the children, gambling, gross financial irresponsibility, and episodic violation of trust (e.g., lying, deceit) can lead to acrimonious divorces (Granvold, 2000). It is therefore important for crisis counselors to look for these other issues that surround a divorce when making their *Assessments* of a person in crisis. Whether the person in crisis is the one who perpetrates these problems or whether they are the victim, it will be important to address these issues as part of the crisis intervention *Plan.*

In the initial crisis intervention session, Ray is accompanied by his brother, Ted, who had become aware of Ray's veiled suicidal threats and his absence from work for several weeks. It is fortunate that his brother is attending the session with him, because Ted can help Ray make contacts and set up a few follow-up sessions to make certain that Ray is safe and beginning to make progress. It would be important for the counselor to explore some of the events leading up to the separation. In the *Listening* phase, the counselor would be attuned to Ray's emotional pain and disappointment. She would also be listening and asking about factors that might place Ray at high risk for suicide, such as whether he had attempted suicide before or whether he has a plan (these risk factors are covered in detail in chapter 7 or Weiss, 2001). The counselor may consider discussing a "no-suicide contract" with Ray. A "no-suicide contract" is something that many counselors use to help ensure the client's safety. While there are no guarantees that Ray would not act on impulse, the contract does specify a course of action that Ray agrees to take should he begin to feel suicidal again.

The counselor would also try to explore some alternatives with Ray. As was alluded to earlier, when someone is in the midst of intense grief reactions, it is usually not the best time to make major decisions. The *Plan* that they agree to may simply be for Ray to continue with counseling or to join a support group for men who are going through separations and divorces. If necessary, a referral for psychotropic medication may also be needed to help mobilize Ray. In some instances, an anti-depressant may be helpful on a short-term basis in order to get Ray functioning again. Finally, the session would conclude with Ray making a *Commitment* to the plan that had been agreed upon.

SOURCES OF CHAPTER ENRICHMENT

Print Sources

Boss, P. (1999). *Ambiguous loss: Learning to live with unresolved grief.* Cambridge, MA: Harvard University Press.

Bowlby, J. (1980). *Attachment and loss: Loss, sadness and depression* (Vol. III). New York: Basic Books.

Donnelly, K. F. (2001). *Recovering from the loss of a child.* New York: Dodd, Mead & Co.

Edelman, H. (1994). *Motherless daughters.* New York: Delta Press.

Gates, P. (1990). *Suddenly alone: A woman's guide to widowhood.* New York: Harper Perennial.

Huntley, T. (1991). *Helping children grieve.* Minneapolis, MN: Augsburg.

James, J. W., & Friedman, R. (2001). *When children grieve.* New York: Harper Collins.

Kubler-Ross, E. (1969). *On death and dying.* New York: Macmillan.

Kushner, H. S. (1981). *When bad things happen to good people.* New York: Avon Press.

Parkes, C. M., & Weiss, R. S. (1983). *Recovery from bereavement.* New York: Basic Books.

Rando, T. (1986) *Parental loss of a child.* Champaign, IL: Research Press.

Rando, T. (1984). *Grief, dying and death: Clinical interventions for caregivers.* Champaign, IL: Research Press.

Secunda, V. (2000). *Losing your parents, finding yourself.* New York: Hyperion.

Worden, J. W. (1982). *Grief counseling and grief therapy: A handbook for the mental health practitioner.* New York: Springer.

Internet Sources

Crisis, Grief & Healing (http://www.grohol.com/reviews/htm) This Web site is devoted to grief issues and provides information that helps people to better understand the grief process. There is also information pertaining to gender differences in grieving and many personal stories for others to read and share. This site is maintained by Tom Golden, LCSW. It can be accessed via Dr. Grohol's Web page, which also provides information and ratings on many other useful sites for crisis counselors.

Hospice Cares Links (http://hospice-cares.com/links/pages/Bereavement/) This Web site provides a link to many other bereavement-related Web sites, including on-line counseling services, on-line grief chat lines, and information on how a bereavement group can be run.

Maternal Grief (http://www.obgyn.net/women/loss/loss.htm) This Web site is devoted to women who have experienced pregnancy loss through miscarriage, stillbirth, neonatal death, sudden infant death, and infertility. This is an excellent resource that provides readers with articles and links to other related Web sites.

Bereavement Resources (http://www.members.tripod.com/~Tamy/links.html) This Web site provide links to many other grief resources including a Web site for teenagers experiencing grief, Web sites for maternal loss, Web sites for men, and links to Compassionate Friends, a self-help group for friends, families, and significant others who are grieving a loss.

GriefNet (http://www.GriefNet.com) This Web site provides a list of varied resources for those experiencing grief.

CHAPTER 9

Crisis Intervention in the Schools: When Teamwork Counts

Students at Middlewood Junior High overheard 14-year-old Max after school one day mumbling that he had "had enough" after Jim Michaels, his school counselor, notified him that he would have to repeat seventh grade the following year due to his ongoing pattern of academic failure. Earlier that same day, after storming out of Michaels's office upon hearing the news, Max passed a teacher on hall duty who overheard him vilifying Mrs. Carlton, his science teacher, for his woes, while yet another heard him faulting Michaels for "never giving him the time of day" to help him.

Three days later at the school's annual Spring Planting Day, a day for outdoor seasonal festivities for the student body, Max arrived at the periphery of the school soccer field, took a seat on a tree stump, and watched the student games as if he were a spectator at a sporting event. About 45 minutes into the gala, he approached the crowd carrying a .22 caliber pistol, which he had stolen from his uncle's house the night before. He opened fire about 50 feet from the gathering, sending students and staff members screaming and scrambling for cover. When he finished emptying the gun, two students lay dead and one wounded. Jim Michaels, who was supervising the students in the line of fire, was uninjured.

A post-mortem analysis of the event yielded this information: Max never seemed to have attracted as much attention from his classmates as he did the day before the shooting when he told a small group of students that he knew where he could get "a real gun with bullets." He also told one of the school custodians that the upcoming Spring Planting Day would "really be one to remember."

Defining School Crises

Considering the vast numbers of children, adolescents, and staff members who spend countless hours in the nation's schools, it stands to reason that all schools are at risk for crisis (Poland, Pitcher, & Lazarus, 1995). Poland (1994) observed that "any event that we could imagine today as too horrific to have ever occurred has already happened and a school has dealt with it." While multiple victim homicide events, such as in the case above, are on the increase, reports of non-lethal incidents are also on the rise. In a Metropolitan Life study (1999), 25% of students were considered to have been the victims of violent acts in or around school, while the number of teachers who reported being the victim of violence had increased from one in nine in 1994 to one in five in 1999. This same survey revealed that a significant number of students, teachers, and law enforcement officials think that violence in local public schools will increase in the near future.

School crises are not limited to violent events. The ripple effect of adolescent suicide, for example, which is considered to be the third leading cause of death for 15 to 24 year olds (*Understanding Violent Children,* 1998), can have a profound impact on a school community; the contagion factor lures others who identify with the victim to attempt self-injurious behaviors themselves.

Crises of Violence

The case of Max is a composite. His is a case that has many of the elements of actual school shootings—warning signs, risk factors, precipitating stressors, and access to a method. He and his shooting spree represent those well-documented school-based events that capture headlines, generate gun control discussions, and fill daytime and late-night talk shows with crisis survivors, crisis experts, and crisis reporters. Following are some of the cases that have reached the highest level of infamy.

- *Lake Worth, Florida, May 26, 2000:* A 13-year-old middle school student returned to school on the last day of the school year, even though he had been sent home for throwing water balloons. This time, however, he brought with him a .25 caliber pistol, which he used to kill one of his teachers for not allowing him to say goodbye to two friends. A single shot to the head felled the teacher in front of his class.
- *Flint, Michigan, February 29, 2000:* A 6-year-old first-grader, well known to school authorities due to several fighting incidents, took a .32 caliber semiautomatic weapon to school and fired a single shot at a fellow classmate that pierced her heart and killed her. Just before he pulled the trigger, he professed his dislike for her. This shooting took place in front of several students; the rest of the class was lined up in the hallway getting ready to attend computer class.
- *Littleton, Colorado, April 20, 1999:* Two Columbine High School students, members of the fringe group known less than affectionately as the "trenchcoat mafia," took an arsenal of weapons to school one day

and roamed throughout the building firing at students and staff members who were running away, hiding in corners, and huddled under tables. Before they turned the guns on themselves, they left 13 dead and 23 injured.

- *Springfield, Oregon, May 21, 1998:* A 15-year-old high school freshman killed his parents, then went to school and opened fire in the cafeteria, killing 2 students and wounding 23.
- *Jonesboro, Arkansas, March 24, 1998:* Two teenage middle school students fired their guns into a group of students who had left the building and entered an enclosed schoolyard for what all thought was a routine fire drill. Among the 5 killed was a sixth-grade teacher; 10 others were wounded.
- *West Paducah, Kentucky, December 1, 1997:* At the local high school's morning prayer circle, a freshman described as "a bit of a misfit" fired his gun into the 35-member group, killing three students and injuring five others.
- *Pearl, Mississippi, October 1, 1997:* A 16-year-old killed his 50-year-old mother at home, then drove to the local high school and gunned down two female students, one of whom he had dated. He randomly shot and wounded seven others.

Although there have been fewer school-associated violent deaths in recent years, multiple victim homicide events, such as those listed, have been on the increase (U.S. Department of Education and U.S. Department of Justice, 1999). Even in nonlethal incidents, juveniles' growing access to handguns has led to an alarming statistic; according to a U.S. Department of Education report (1999), in the 1997–1998 school year alone, a total of 3,930 students were expelled from school for bringing in firearms. Although 57% of these expulsions involved high school students, 33% were middle school students, and a full 10% were elementary school students. Another survey conducted by the Parent Resource Institute of Drug Education (1999) placed the number of school gun-toters at 800,000 6th through 12th graders in a single year.

Crises of Suicide and Sudden Death

The crisis that the family of a person who commits suicide experiences becomes the crisis of a school community as the act reverberates throughout the school corridors. Even during the best of times, students considered "at risk" can easily succumb to the lure of copying a suicidal act unless interventions are made. Sudden and unexpected death (of a student, a teacher, a principal, a troop leader) casts a similar pall on children in schools. Community-based disasters, such as industrial or vehicular accidents and natural disasters that destroy homes and families, also impact the lives of children. Alongside the lunches and books that they stuff into their backpacks, children bring to school the fears and anxieties attendant to these crises. Teachers, administrators, and counselors all must be ready to address students' crisis needs.

Crises in Our Schools Today: Causal Factors

Crisis intervention has come of age in today's schools. It has been formalized and systematized, as school buildings and their occupants are quite different today than were years ago. Crisis-prone students, once relegated to exclusionary special schools for a host of emotional and behavioral disabilities, now attend local public schools, supported by special services that include special education instruction, counseling, and myriad other services tailor-made to the unique needs of the student. Public Law 101-476, the Individuals With Disabilities Education Act (IDEA), enacted in 1992 and amended in 1997, serves as watchdog legislation, guaranteeing that all such students remain in the "least restrictive environment" of their home schools as long as possible.

The road to providing proper mental health services to people in need, particularly children, is filled with obstacles. Public funding for services is inadequate, and insurance coverage for these services is limited. In addition, changes in the delivery of mental health services to children via managed care policies has resulted in a needy and underserved population, leaving troubled children to fend for themselves and, in some cases, to find meaningful connections with a caring adults in schools that may blur any sense of community for them.

Compounding the problem is the instability and the mobility of the American family. Job changes lead to relocation. Newfound stock market riches in a booming economy take the Smiths to a better part of town. Families move into "starter" homes, planning with the unpacking of the first box to be on the pricier side of town within 5 years. Close to half of all marriages end up in divorce; as many as 50% of American children live in single-parent homes, resulting in an increase in unsupervised activity for children and adolescents. Rapid change leads to stress; stress leads to troubled children.

The boundaries between childhood and adulthood continue to be more permeable than ever before; young people continue to enter into territory once traversed only by adults. For example, the mass media bombards children with images and themes that once were the domain of only the adults in the household. Adolescent movie and sitcom heroes treat parents, adults, and teachers with little regard, modeling such behavior for whole generations of young people. Despite the obvious educational and recreational advantages of the Internet, it provides children and adolescents with the opportunity to access information of all sorts in the privacy of their computer rooms, taking them places once considered taboo for all but responsible adults.

Finally, children are exposed as never before to images of violence whenever they sit down to watch television: murder and mayhem, the perpetrator as hero, crime without punishment. Who can tell the good guys from the bad guys? The graphic violence in movies, television shows, music videos, and video games leads to increases in aggressive attitudes. Studies trace a strong link between television and movie violence and aggressive behavior in children and document children's resulting desensitization to violent acts of their own and to the pain and suffering of their victims. Aggressive children also tend to believe that others are motivated by a hostile intent and that aggression is an appropriate and an effective response to conflict.

National and Community Responses to School Crises

While forest fires take their toll on countless acres of a nation's woodlands, the nutrients left behind in the ashes that blanket the once verdant forest floor generate new growth—different from before, but hardy nevertheless. Similarly, the broken bone emerges from its plaster cast stronger than before. There can be no growth without trauma in these cases.

Erik Erikson (1963) represents those developmental theorists who believe that there can be no individual growth unless one is faced with crisis, or challenge. According to Erickson, by facing and resolving developmental crises, the individual is capable of reaching full maturity. Systems thinkers also view conflict/crisis as providing the dynamic by which systems become ever stronger; there can be no growth without tension, or crisis, that challenges the system.

Just as the charred forest floor nurtures new life, some of the nation's cruelest school shootings have prompted the national consciousness to focus on issues related not only to school violence but also to prevention and to the needs of victims and perpetrators alike. Even the meaning of the two Chinese symbols that comprise the term *crisis*—"opportunity blowing on an ill wind"—speak to this same notion. Although one neither welcomes nor anticipates crisis, crisis succeeds in creating an opportunity for examining environments that nurture crisis conditions and for fostering a call to action for prevention and intervention programs.

President Bill Clinton heeded this call to action when, in the wake of the triple murder in the West Paducah prayer group, he launched "a major initiative to produce for the first time an annual report card on school violence" (Clinton, 1997, p. 1993) in order to boost violence-prevention efforts. After yet another high school shooting in Springfield, Oregon, Clinton again directed the development of a document titled *Early Warning, Timely Response: A Guide to Safe Schools* (Dwer, Osher, & Warger, 1998) designed "to provide school communities with reliable and practical information about what they can do to be prepared and to reduce the likelihood of violence" (p. 8). "Responding to Crisis" was one of the Guide's eight topics.

The widespread appeal and acceptance of the Guide soon led to the development of a companion piece, *Safeguarding Our Children: An Action Guide* (Dwyer & Osher, 2000). The purpose of this latter guide was to provide its readers with practical, research-based recommendations for developing comprehensive violence prevention and response plans that can be customized to fit the structure and uniqueness of each school.

In addition to these federal directives to the nation's schools to be responsive to issues of violence and prevention, the National Organization for Victim Assistance (NOVA) has provided both direct on-site assistance in the aftermath of community crises of all types and training for organizations in crisis intervention. One such organization, the National Association of School Psychologists (NASP), sought this training following the bombing of the Alfred P. Murrah Federal Building in Oklahoma City in 1992. NASP developed its own National Emergency Assistance Team (NEAT) whose mission was "to develop policies and procedures, disseminate information, provide consultation and facilitate the training of school-based crisis teams in response to significant emergencies impacting children and adolescents" (Zenere, 1998). NEAT members received extensive NOVA training, and they followed NOVA's crisis response model (National Organization for Victim Assistance, 1998).

A Model of Crisis Intervention for the Schools

For purposes of the following discussion, the word *crisis* can be defined as "a perception of an event or situation as an intolerable difficulty that exceeds the resources and coping mechanisms of a person, group, or community" (Zenere, 1998). This definition is fitting for a discussion of school crises, since the notion of "community" suggests that even the crisis borne by an individual student impacts each of the interacting parts of the system within which the student lives. Other students, teachers, administrators, and support staff all feel the impact of the pain of a single member.

Since crisis intervention in schools can be a daunting task, considering the multiplicity of interacting individuals involved, adherence to a model should guide these efforts. For purposes of the following discussion, Gerald Caplan's (1964) crisis intervention model, which the NASP/NEAT crisis response team follows, will serve as the paradigm. Caplan's model consists of three components: primary, secondary, and tertiary prevention.

Primary Prevention

The goals of primary prevention, a philosophy more than a series of programs or activities, are to create an environment within which crises are less likely to occur, and if they do, to develop those skills which would enable individuals to cope with them. Primary prevention activities for myriad problems are well known to school districts throughout the nation. They are designed to impart to students those skills that will equip them with the ability to negotiate interpersonal conflict, avoid drugs, overcome test anxiety, express anger appropriately, and develop higher levels of self-esteem. Prevention programs are education programs and have been incorporated into the fabric of school curricula for many years. Some of the more prominent primary prevention programs include

- Students Against Drunk Driving,
- anger management,
- stress management,
- conflict resolution,
- social problem solving,
- suicide prevention,
- drug/alcohol use prevention,

- AIDS prevention/safe sex,
- communication training,
- assertiveness training, and
- smoking cessation.

In an ideal world, if Max (see introductory case) had been through an anger management program, for example, it might have provided him with the skills to express his dismay over his retention in seventh grade in more prosocial ways than through the use of violence. Although no complex act can be reduced to such a singular cause and effect connection, the purpose of primary prevention programs is to impart prosocial skills to children and adolescents and to create a humanistic environment that is incompatible for some, but not all, crises. Such activities always take place *before* the onset of crisis. This level will be known simply as *prevention* for the rest of this chapter.

Secondary Prevention

Secondary prevention comprises those efforts designed to minimize the harmful effects of a crisis *once it has already occurred* and to keep it from spiraling out of control. What was the response of Max's school in the immediate aftermath of the shooting? This question and many others are "grist for the mill" for secondary prevention. Since schools tend to view crisis intervention only on this level (Poland, 1994), the remainder of this chapter will refer to the secondary prevention level simply as *intervention*.

Tertiary Intervention

Once the crisis has passed, steps taken to provide long-term follow-up care for those most affected by the crisis comprise the tertiary intervention level of prevention. For example, what was the long-term response of Max's school once the funerals were over and all the students were back in class? What, if anything, was planned for the first anniversary of the event? What to do and whom to do it with are the subjects of the tertiary intervention level. Crisis intervention activities that occur in the long-term aftermath of the crisis event will heretofore be referred to as *postvention*.

Applying the Model: Prevention

Prevention activities seem to be common sense: brushing one's teeth daily prevents tooth decay, going for an annual medical exam prevents a disease from advancing unchecked, changing a car's oil every 3,000 miles prevents the transmission from grinding to a halt before its time. People hardly smack themselves on the forehead and shout "Eureka" when they hear these bits of advice. This is also the case with some of the basic school-related prevention practices. *Safeguarding Our Children: An Action Guide* (Dwyer & Osher, 2000) describes four components that are very basic and practical in a common sense sort of way. The *Action Guide* considers the following factors to be part of a comprehensive and effective school-wide plan responsive to all children and preventive of school violence.

- *Create a caring school community in which all members feel connected, safe, and supported.* Particularly in large and diverse schools, establishing a supportive relationship between students and staff allows for the mentoring of young people in an environment that encourages children to share, among other things, safety concerns with adults.

- *Teach appropriate behaviors and social problem-solving.* In addition to mastering the three Rs, students also must also learn how to act appropriately with peers and how to resolve emotionally charged conflicts nonviolently. School staff and faculty can teach social skills through structured lessons or by integrating topics into various aspects of the curriculum. Banning aggressive or violent encounters via standard disciplinary channels without offering guidance in more positive prosocial behaviors tends to be counterproductive and futile.

- *Implement positive behavior support systems.* Effective school-wide discipline systems must be simple and positive; everyone, both staff and students alike, should understand these rules and the consequences for violating them. Behaviors should be stated in positive rather than negative terms ("Remain in your seat" instead of "Don't get out of your seat"). Providing incentives and rewards for appropriate behavior is more effective than punishments for negative behavior.

- *Provide appropriate academic instruction.* In order to eliminate as much as possible the disruptive and out-of-control behaviors generated by academic frustration and failure, instruction should be meaningful and should provide students with opportunities for success. Although numerous interventions exist to address the needs of individual students who have difficulty learning, there also is a need for effective instructional interventions for entire school systems. Among these school-wide programs, according to the *Action Guide,* are class-wide peer tutoring, cooperative learning, and direct instruction.

Despite their simplicity, these components of prevention are not always utilized in some schools. And simple things yield great benefits when applied consistently throughout the system.

Developing a School Crisis Plan

If educators were able to predict crises the way meteorologists predict hurricanes, school administrators would be able to get students out of the line of fire long before the arrival of a perpetrator, counselors would be lined up in advance of a traumatic event, and parents would be notified in advance to expect the arrival of the unexpected. However, crises do not lend themselves to prediction. Even meteorologists who must factor into their predictions the vagaries of suddenly changing wind patterns are in a much better position to foretell with some degree of success the next sunny day or blustery nor'easter. The role of school-based crisis workers, therefore, is not to predict crises, but rather to anticipate that the unexpected will indeed occur in their schools one day and to develop a system that can be activated when needed to cope with whatever comes.

One must remember that the key component of this chapter's working definition of *crisis intervention* is the notion that crisis victims should be restored to a level of functioning enjoyed before the onset of the crisis. Just as intervention cannot make the crisis event disappear, prevention also cannot keep it from happening. In the field of crisis intervention, a more appropriate term for *prevention* is *preparedness*. Two of the most important prevention/preparedness issues for crisis intervention in schools are developing a school crisis plan and forming a crisis team.

Before the onslaught of multiple-victim shootings in recent years, most school districts treated with benign neglect the possibility that such horrors could occur in their corridors. "The less we do, the better" and "If we plan for it, it might happen to us too," seemed to be the prevailing wisdom. Fearful of being faulted for creating crises or for overseeing a school within which such things could happen, school administrators tended to leave the emotional aftermath of the crisis to the families and to the community-based mental health practitioners who learned by doing, rather than by training, to attend to the emotional needs of children in crisis.

However, the seemingly endless media coverage of school shootings has made school administrators crisis savvy and knowledgeable enough about the topic to know that they must have a plan available to cope with these events. The arrival of the *Early Warning Guide* and the *Action Guide* at every school district in the country emphasized the federal government's role in encouraging all school districts to come to terms with the growing need to prepare for the unexpected. Likewise, there has been a glut of crisis information made available via workshops, conferences, and mailings to all professional organizations that have roles in schools: teachers, parents, psychologists, social workers, guidance counselors, drug and alcohol counselors, principals, vice principals, school superintendents, and school board members.

Garnering administrative support for the crisis plan is critical. The task, however, of instilling an awareness of school crisis planning in the administration of a school district should not be a difficult one, given the aforementioned information available already. Central to school crisis intervention is the development of a written crisis plan. This plan should be brief, practical, and clear in terms of its intentions and the roles to be carried out by the district and community members involved. Following are the four guiding principles for developing a crisis plan suggested by the National Education Association (NEA):

1. The plan should be a collaborative effort among all members of the school community: teachers, support staff, administrators, law enforcement, mental health agencies, parent-teacher organizations, and other community partners.
2. The plan's goal should be to support students and staff.
3. The plan should provide strategies for informing all school staff, parents, and broader community members of the plan's purpose, process, and assignment of responsibilities. All staff should be aware of these plans and what they should do in the event of different kinds of crises.
4. Plans should be updated and practiced by all participants on a regular basis.

A committee consisting of both school and community members should develop the plan itself, which should include the following items:

- a mission statement drafted with input from various sectors of the community;
- encouragement of participation in the plan by teachers and other staff, parent groups, local police and fire departments, clergy, and the mental health community;
- a warning system for notification of troubled students who may pose a threat;
- adequate communication system for reporting threats or suspicious incidents;
- adequate communication system during a crisis;
- two-way communication to the school's main office in every room;
- adequate visitor registration and sign-in procedures;
- implementation of dispute resolution training for both students and teachers;
- a memorandum of understanding with law enforcement and rescue crews;
- distribution of the plan to involve agencies and school staff;
- mechanism for the police to notify the school of critical incidents impacting schools, such as the death of a child or school employee or a significant event (murder, suicide, accident, natural disaster) that would impact the students;
- procedures for gathering and disseminating factual information about the crisis;
- a plan for providing support and counseling for students and staff;
- a plan for attending to long-term needs in the aftermath of the crisis; and
- development of a crisis team.

School districts, depending upon size, location, and other factors, will have items specific to their own circumstances that they will have to include in their plans. However, as long as these crisis committees have members who are representative of the entire community, all salient points should be covered. However, one of the most important elements of all plans is development of the crisis team.

Developing a School Crisis Team

Considering the vast numbers of students, staff, support personnel, parents, community members, and ultimately the media who are drawn into a crisis event, it becomes nearly impossible to attend to the overwhelming tasks that present themselves during times of chaos and confusion. Although chief school administrators may be declared in charge of school activities on a typical school day, it would be a Herculean task for one person to be able to manage the avalanche of demands during crisis. Responsibilities for taking care of these demands must be distributed among a group of people, each with a particular specialty area. Thus, perhaps the most critical component of the crisis plan is the crisis team.

School crisis teams will consist of those members to whom certain carefully circumscribed tasks will be delegated in an attempt to organize as much as possible the multitude of tasks that must be done. It is important that these teams be neither too big (not much of an improvement in the chaos) nor too small (too many responsibilities falling on one set of shoulders). Pitcher and Poland (1992) suggested that teams of four to eight members are advisable. The team members would be able to attend to the core medical, security, parental, and emotional issues of the crisis. In addition, the school administrator (principal if the team is specific to a particular school, or superintendent if the team covers a school district) would be responsible for chairing the team, and an additional two members, at most, could be added to handle related crisis tasks.

Although it may be reasonable to assume that such individuals as the school nurse, school psychologist, school social worker, school counselor, or drug and alcohol counselor should sit on the crisis team, the title of the professional position is not as important as the personality style and temperament of the individual.

Most urban and suburban schools are large enough to form crisis teams that consist of members who work within the individual school buildings. Team members should know the students and staff well. The nurse knows those students with chronic medical problems, those on medication, and those whose somatic ailments may mask other problems related to depression and anxiety. The school principal knows students who are chronically referred for discipline problems, while the school psychologist and the school counselor tend to know those at-risk students who may be in the midst of their own crises. Additionally, these in-building staff members have ready access to other sources of information regarding students (i.e., teachers, tutors, etc.).

Although it is a bit more difficult to organize and maintain than an in-building team (Pitcher & Poland, 1992), some school districts prefer to form

BOX 9.1

Who Is Best Suited to Serve As a Crisis Team Member?

Crisis is chaos. Crisis is high emotion. Crisis is the trauma of the unexpected. Crisis intervention is not a task for everyone.

Those who come to serve on crisis teams should not come because they have been assigned to do so as a professional responsibility by the school administrator, nor should they come because they are looking for another source of income (if school districts pay a fee for its team members, that is). Likewise, finding crisis events exciting is no reason to participate, nor is the appeal of the "voyeur" to get behind the scenes of a newsworthy event. Individuals with their own "rescue fantasies" also need not apply, and the omniscient—those who have all the answers—should leave the crisis work to others. Individuals whose communication styles are marked by more than a 2:1 ratio of talking to listening (author's formula) probably are not well suited either.

Pitcher and Poland (1992) also added a short list of personality quirks that contraindicate an effective crisis worker:

- the need to be a hero;
- the need to be in control;
- difficulty tolerating unhappiness or strong emotions in others;
- taking on too much responsibility for the organization;
- discomfort with consultation, indirect roles; and
- the need to have things go perfectly.

Those individuals who *are* effective as crisis team members are those who can accept their roles as facilitators rather than as experts, who can tolerate the lack of closure, even after their intervention, and who can see themselves as providing comfort and support instead of advice. Those who can refrain from being judgmental and morally righteous about difficult issues such as suicide possess appropriate qualities for crisis work as well. Being able to deal with emotionally charged situations and issues (e.g., premature death, suicide) is another plus. Other personality traits that may be independent of training (Wilson & Sigman, 1996) include the ability to

- function well in confused, chaotic environments;
- "think on your feet" and have a common-sense, practical, flexible, and often improvisational approach to problem solving;
- handle changing situations well and function with role ambiguity, unclear lines of authority, and minimal structure;

- monitor and manage their own stress;
- handle the sights and sounds of physical trauma; and
- enjoy people and maintain a solid confidence level.

district-wide crisis teams consisting of staff members from each of the schools throughout the districts. In district-wide crisis teams, where the team is composed of representatives from different schools, one or more of the team members will hail from the school that is involved in a particular crisis. This configuration of a team, however, is best suited to those districts that consist of small to medium-sized schools that don't have enough appropriate staff members to comprise a full team. Disadvantages, of course, with this model include not being able to control the availability of a crisis team member from another location in the district when a crisis presents itself. Staffers from outside the crisis-affected building also will not be familiar with the students, staff, or procedures of the school to which they are responding.

Probably the most practical format for small and for rural school districts is a *community team* consisting of both school and non-school personnel. The latter group might include local police, fire, medical, or mental health representatives (Pitcher & Poland, 1992). Members of the local clergy also may be appropriate. However, as with the district team format, there is no controlling the availability of an outside participant, nor are they familiar with the students in the school; deciding upon this type of crisis team would be the responsibility of those developing the overall crisis plan for the district. Different circumstances in these small, rural communities will dictate who should sit on the team.

Roles of Crisis Team Members

Once organized, the team must decide what each member's role will be. These roles can be changed and modified from time to time, but it is advisable that these changes be made at periodic meetings of the team rather than during the tumult of the crisis. Although team members will vary from school to school, the roles of the team members will remain constant; these roles will consist of the following (Poland & McCormick, 1999):

- crisis coordinator,
- counseling liaison,
- medical liaison,
- media liaison,
- parent/family liaison,
- campus/staff liaison, and
- security liaison.

CRISIS COORDINATOR The school principal will serve as the crisis coordinator. In most crisis situations, the principal is the first one notified of the event. His or her primary responsibility, then, would be to take charge of the situation. First, if needed because of an emergent violent event, he or she would notify the local police. Then, he or she would communicate knowledge of the situation to the central administration and to the school board. He or she would immediately summon the crisis team, present the members with the facts, as they are available at the time, and instruct the members to carry out their roles and functions.

The principal should be ever present throughout the crisis, as his or her presence will provide some sense of comfort for the student body, particularly those on the elementary level. He or she also should be the conduit of accurate information from outside sources to the school staff and crisis team members, updating the crisis conditions factually and dispelling any rumors that persist. In most crisis events, the principal should be the liaison with the press, particularly if news crews descend on the school or if reporters simply call to ascertain the extent and the type of crisis being experienced. Having multiple responders to reporters' questions only adds to the confusion and guarantees that inaccurate and misleading information will be dispersed.

COUNSELING LIAISON School psychologists, counselors, and social workers are the logical team members to provide those services for which they were trained: counseling and comfort to those students and staff affected by the crisis. It is said that the ability to tolerate ambiguity is an important trait for those in the psychology/counseling field. This trait is most critical under crisis conditions. Ambiguity and lack of clarity reign in crises, particularly during the initial stages when facts often are not known and when emotions control the intellect. Therefore, trained psychologists and counselors must be prepared to provide solace and support in the midst of confusing conditions.

Flexibility also is required of these team members; they must be prepared to be available on a moment's notice. In the immediate aftermath and in the more prolonged postvention period, the mental health professional should remain quite visible and accessible to the students. Seeking out close friends of the deceased and any other students known to the counselor as at risk (having the potential to be affected more than others by the unsettling and tragic news) also is an important task for this team member. Since it will be unlikely in most situations that the counselor will know each student in the school who qualifies as at risk, consulting with faculty members, school disciplinarians, and other support staff in order to ascertain the identities of such students will surely yield names for the counselor to keep in mind.

When the crisis involves the death of a student, especially via suicide, the team counselor should perform outreach service to the following groups of students considered generally to be at risk (Underwood & Dunne-Maxim, 1997):

- close friends of the deceased;
- students on teams, in clubs, or involved in activities with deceased;
- friends or siblings of the deceased;

- "enemies" of the deceased;
- students who have experienced losses that may be reactivated by the current death;
- vulnerable students (e.g., those with drug/alcohol problems, emotional problems, previous suicide ideation or attempts);
- students preoccupied with death or suicide;
- students identified by peers, faculty, or parents as at risk; and
- students who self-identify.

MEDICAL LIAISON   The school nurse is usually responsible for administering first aid to those in need and for making sense of the medical information pertinent to the crisis, to update it as new information is available, and to provide it to the school principal/team coordinator. Nurses also are in the unique position in schools to know the medically involved children as well as those lonely, sad, anxious, and forlorn students whose visits to the nurse's office are cries for attention under the guise of assorted medical woes. News of trauma is particularly distressing to such students.

MEDIA LIAISON   As the chief administrator for the affected school, the school principal is the logical choice to serve as the liaison between the school and the local media. The primary function of this individual is to keep the media informed as to the state of the crisis, either through formal press conferences or via periodic telephone interviews. Having more than one person perform this role can only lead to misinformation and rumor. Some crisis teams, however, delegate all media contact to one person besides the school principal, thereby freeing him or her up to attend to all other facets of the event. Still others utilize central office public relations personnel for this purpose.

PARENT/FAMILY LIAISON   Due to the potentially sensitive nature of this assignment, a psychologist, counselor, or social worker would be the appropriate person to fulfill the responsibilities of this role. In those crises involving violence, this liaison may have to deliver news of injury, or even death, to parents. However, in all crises, regardless of type, this liaison would be the primary source of information for parents who may call or visit the school for information. Keeping abreast of the developments of the crisis as they unfold and communicating them consistently to the parents are two of the primary functions of this role.

CAMPUS/STAFF LIAISON   This individual will communicate the details of the crisis to the school staff and will assign them as needed to assist in some part of the crisis management. This person also will consult with the staff as to how each of them can respond to those students who have particular questions about the event. Keeping a finger on the "pulse" of the staff and student body as the crisis unfolds and communicating these impressions to the crisis coordinator also are important functions of this position. For these reasons, a psychologist, social worker, or counselor should serve in this capacity.

SECURITY LIAISON   If the school has a security officer, he or she would be the appropriate person for this role. If not, then a member of local law enforcement (who ideally was part of the development of the crisis plan) would suffice. This team member would secure the crime scene, if needed, and would serve as a security person who could monitor the building for well-intentioned intruders, such as the media and other community members, whose presence would just serve to confuse things. Such visitors, particularly the media, should be ushered to a central location and not allowed unrestrained access to all parts of the school building.

Training the Crisis Team

Training is a critical component of the development of any crisis team. Those chosen to serve on the team need appropriate training to be able to fulfill their prescribed roles effectively. However, it is important to note that crisis work is not for everyone. See Box 9.1 on page 212 for a discussion of the types of individuals best suited for crisis work.

Once the team is chosen, training must begin. Crisis training should cover many topics, which fall into any one of the following four categories: crisis principles, crisis skills, prerequisite knowledge of children, and practical considerations during a crisis (see Table 9.1). Lichtenstein, Schonfeld, and Kline (1994) stressed the importance of both content and process in crisis training. Content-level training refers to instruction in those topics listed in Table 9.1, while process-level training involves facilitating crisis team building and communication. This level of training is accomplished through specific small-group exercises designed to apply the crisis model to hypothetical crisis situations. This latter procedure allows team members to problem-solve as a team and to practice individual roles that they will carry out one day under realistic crisis conditions.

IN VIVO TRAINING: CRISIS DRILLS   Schools conduct fire drills as frequently as once a month to prepare for the eventuality that fire might strike the building; potential bomb scares are handled in much the same way. However, having a board-approved crisis plan in a three-ring binder on the principal's office shelf, its pages yellowing with age, and a printed roster of content-trained team members might not be sufficient to maintain a level of preparedness for the arrival of a crisis. Static crisis plans and 3-year-old training leaves the district wanting. What about the team member who retired last year? Or who took another position out of state? Or who replaced the juvenile officer as the local police department's school liaison when he was promoted to chief of police? And which team member will take responsibility for outreach during a crisis in the new wing of the building, constructed after the initial crisis plan was written?

In order to answer these questions and more regarding a district's crisis plan, the team must be ever alert and adaptive to policy, personnel, and other day-to-day changes. One of the best ways to do this is to conduct crisis drills in much the same manner as the schools conduct their fire drills (Poland, 1994; Pitcher & Poland, 1992; Poland, Pitcher, & Lazarus, 1995). Crisis drills add a new dimension to crisis planning, and they make the plans themselves more meaningful for both team members and the larger school community. Crisis drills should follow certain guidelines, as described in the following sections.

Notification   First before the team conducts the first drill, all parents should be informed by the administration that the district's crisis plan calls for periodic crisis drills to be conducted in each of its schools; this notification can best be done through the mail. Alerting parents to this policy, as well as to the approximate timing of the drills throughout the year, will go a long way toward avoiding frantic phone calls from parents whose children return home from school talking about the strange goings-on in school that day. Engaging the local media in publishing articles about the importance of crisis drills also serves as notification and as a "sales pitch" for their worth. Similarly, notification should be given to local agencies regarding these drills, and whatever precautions are necessary should be followed to keep from unduly alarming the students themselves prior to the drill.

TABLE 9.1
Crisis Team Training Goals

Crisis Principles

- A thorough understanding of the district-approved crisis plan and of the team's organization and chain of command during crisis
- An appreciation of the role and function of each of the team members whenever the team is activated
- An awareness of the realistic goals of the crisis team during times of crisis
- A knowledge of the crisis theory that guides the team and how it applies to a school setting
- Types of school crises
- An ability to distinguish between those crises that merit a full crisis team response and those that do not (i.e., child abuse, drug/alcohol abuse, episodes of bullying, physical altercations among students)

Crisis Skills

- Communication skills: active listening, demonstrating empathy and support, etc.
- Knowing the importance of providing students and staff with the facts in order to dispel rumors
- Being able to allow for a wide range of emotions in those affected by crisis
- Being prepared for vast differences in the experiences of crisis, as past involvement with loss and with other unresolved issues will reawaken dormant emotions in some individuals more than others
- Knowing that the type, intensity, and duration of the crisis event will have a lot to do with how individuals are affected by it
- Being able to remain nonjudgmental regarding atypical behaviors and to avoid making value judgments of the person in crisis
- Coming to terms with one's own feelings of loss and tragedy in one's life before undertaking the crisis role

(Continues)

TABLE 9.1
Crisis Team Training Goals *(Continued)*

Prerequisite Knowledge of Children

- An appreciation of children's developmental stages, particularly as they apply to the understanding of death and to the experience of tragedy
- Knowledge of the emotional, cognitive, and behavioral manifestations of crisis in children and the role development plays in them as well
- Being able to consult with parents and with teachers regarding their children's needs for post-crisis understanding and support
- Being aware of the contagion factor in the aftermath of suicide and the need, as a result, for performing outreach to other individuals

Practical Considerations During Crisis

- Appreciating the importance of ongoing communication among all team members, including the need to meet frequently in order to evaluate the progress of crisis management
- Making sure that the school is kept open in order to provide a place of support for families and community members
- Developing a checklist of crisis steps to guide the team's actions
- Developing organizational aides, such as a telephone chain, to enable the administrator to alert school personnel to a crisis so that they can begin planning

Planning the Drill   Once the crisis team has assembled, it should conduct a paper and pencil activity in which the team chooses as many as five different crisis situations. These cases can be culled from the front pages of local or national newspapers, or they can be created as prototypical cases by the team. The members then will use these situations as discussion points. First, they would write down the tasks that they would perform during these crises, and discussion would follow. The goal for this particular activity is the refining and/or restructuring of the team members' roles and the general fine tuning of the crisis intervention plan. Once the team completes this step, it would then choose one crisis scenario per semester to reenact in school.

The Crisis Reenactment   Just as in a standard fire drill, the crisis drill will involve large numbers of students and staff in a simulation of a potentially life-threatening event. However, certain precautions must be taken in order to keep from unnecessarily alarming students and staff members. Of course, it must be made clear to the staff long before the first live-action crisis drill that drills will be conducted periodically throughout the year; the crisis plan itself should include a statement of the arrangements for crisis drills.

One of the precautions that crisis drills should consider is the avoidance of high drama (i.e., no realistic-looking handguns, no simulated shots fired, no ketchup posing as blood). Posting signs that label the crisis scene clearly as a drill will alert uninformed passers-by, both inside and outside the school, that a simulation is taking place. Team members also must be ready to reach out to those members of the school community who, for reasons of absence, newness to the school, or mere forgetfulness, don't realize that they are in the middle of a reenactment, rather than a genuine crisis event. Finally, crisis drills are most effective if they include the practice of moving staff and students to a safe location.

Since the purpose of the drills is to help the team to practice and to fine tune its intervention skills, it would be critical for the team to receive feedback regarding its performance in the simulated crisis. One of the most efficient ways for this feedback to be gathered is to have an objective, uninvolved crisis team member from another school building visit the crisis scene and observe its functioning. This observer then would meet with the entire team upon the conclusion of the simulation to provide feedback about the day's event. Based upon this feedback, as well as the team's discussion of the reenactment, the crisis plan and/or the roles of the team members may be modified in some way.

Applying the Model: Secondary Prevention (Intervention)

Schools tend to view the real business of crisis intervention as a secondary prevention activity (Poland, 1994). Schools implement intervention activities at this level *in the immediate aftermath of the crisis.* The following sections will illustrate those intervention activities that would be utilized in the aftermath of three prototypical case examples, the first of which was introduced at the beginning of this chapter.

School Crisis Intervention Case Example 1

Recall from the beginning of this chapter that 14-year-old Max stole a pistol from his uncle's house and on the following day, opened fire on a crowd of students who were participating in his school's annual outdoor event, Spring Planting Day. Two students were killed and one was wounded. During those rare instances when violence results in loss of life during the school day and on school grounds, managing the first hour of the chaos is critical. In a case such as this one, the six tasks that must be tended to first (Poland & McCormick, 1999) include the following:

1. Address human safety and provide medical assistance.
2. Summon help.
3. Secure the crime scene and contain the media.
4. Verify the facts and prepare a crisis fact sheet.
5. Deliver injury/death notifications.
6. Communicate with parents/other family members.

As Max fired on his classmates, the last thing that those under siege probably thought of was the location of the crisis coordinator, the school principal.

However, in this case, he happened to be present at the school's annual event, and he knew that the first order of business was simple: safety first!

In the few seconds it took Max to discharge the six shots from his handgun, the principal and the other supervising faculty members scurried about trying to get each of the students in the line of fire to lie down on the soccer field. Although no one, including school staff, is under a legal mandate to sacrifice his or her own physical safety when confronting an armed assailant, it is those spontaneous heroic actions that often result in lives saved. In the West Paducah shooting, a classmate was able to intervene and to convince the shooter to put down the gun, while a teacher sacrificed her own life to save another student in the Jonesboro nightmare. In this case however, Max threw his emptied gun to the ground and ran back into the woods after the deed, thereby leaving the scene entirely. The principal was then able to make a quick assessment of the injuries with the assistance of the other present faculty members.

The principal then assigned a teacher to go into the school building and to call local police and medical emergency personnel while he remained with the injured. The school nurse, the medical liaison, also had been summoned and was with the principal by this time. The remaining faculty members were directed to take the uninjured children back into the building and to their regularly scheduled classrooms for that class period. Getting the students back into some semblance of classroom routine with a familiar teacher allows for close, small-group supervision of the students and also provides a better forum for assisting the students in beginning to come to terms with what happened.

It is in just such a setting that the counseling liaisons will begin their work. Even though the crisis coordinator was unable to call a formal crisis team meeting due to the chaos of the last twenty minutes, he was able to assign the counseling liaisons to begin their work in the classrooms. The counselors first visited those classrooms with students who had been involved in the shooting, and they then made themselves available to all classes, both for students and staff alike. However, at this time, before any medical or other news has been confirmed, it is important that *only that information which has been determined to be fact be communicated.* Questions related to the extent of the injuries, the identities of the dead and wounded, and the reasons for the carnage may still be speculative at this point, so it is permissible to let everyone know that certain information has not yet been verified. Once this information is known, the crisis team will arrange for a fact sheet to be distributed. The main function of the counseling liaisons at this time is simply to provide emotional support and to try to keep the students and staff calm.

Once the police arrived at the site of the tragedy, they took over the management of the crime scene, thereby allowing the crisis coordinator/principal to attend to other tasks. After providing his own eyewitness account to the police, he re-entered his building and continued to assign responsibilities to the appointed crisis team members. With the medical and counseling liaisons already engaged in their tasks, he assigned the security liaison to prepare for the onslaught of both parents and media personnel and the media liaison to ready herself for media briefings.

The security liaison secured a specific location for the media to assemble; the chosen spot was in the district's administrative offices across the street from the school. The media, it was determined, could be sufficiently accommodated in the conference rooms that the building provided. Although media folks hungry for the story are entitled to cooperation from the school, they are not entitled to unlimited access throughout the building during the confusion of the immediate aftermath of a crisis. Unhappy with this arrangement, the visiting reporters and news people registered their complaints with the security liaison, but the plan remained in effect.

The media liaison was able to confirm via the school nurse much of the medical information that had been verified from the hospital. The crisis coordinator, the principal, originally had delegated one of the crisis team members to manage these media responsibilities, but after several briefings with the media were handled by the liaison, he took a shared role in this capacity himself. It is appropriate eventually for someone "in charge" to disseminate factual information to the media.

When the parent/family liaison realized after the first several phone calls from parents that the sheer number of calls would be too overwhelming for her alone, the crisis coordinator assigned two school secretaries and one faculty volunteer to take the incoming calls from parents. However, she also briefed them beforehand regarding the manner in which they were to answer questions about the incident: only facts, no speculation, and no names of the dead or wounded without prior notification of the family. The campus liaison also maintained a steady flow of information for the faculty.

Many of the parents who had arrived at school questioned whether or not they could take their children home. The crisis coordinator decided to allow the younger children to go home to be with their primary caretakers, while he explained to the parents of the older children that their children's physical and emotional needs would be just as well served by allowing them to stay in school for the remainder of the day. The adherence to some routine, the familiarity with classmates and teachers, and the availability of a group forum to process what happened actually favored the students remaining in school. He agreed, however, to let the very insistent parents take their children home.

AFTER THE DUST SETTLES: LATER IN THE DAY   Once the immediate impact of the trauma had passed, there were numerous tasks that had to be accomplished. First, since the crisis coordinator was not able to do so during the first 2 hours of the ordeal, he called a formal meeting of the crisis response team. The team made a quick assessment regarding the collective emotional state of both students and staff and reassigned the functions of some of the team members. For example, the team decided that a sixth-grade class that included an older sister of one of the deceased was much more distraught than the other classes; the crisis team assigned an additional counselor to the class. Additionally, the team also summoned other crisis teams from its own district schools and alerted another team from a neighboring school district to stand by to assist with these special needs.

Other tasks that the team addressed at its meeting included

- *completion of a crisis fact sheet.* This document was a factual, ever-changing account of the day's events; sufficient copies were made to distribute to parents, teachers, media personnel, and any other interested parties.
- *planning for the afternoon faculty meeting.* The purpose of the meeting was not to provide an update only to the staff, but rather to allow the staff to process the day's events. Allowing time at this meeting to express their feelings about the tragedy better prepared them to provide comfort for the students the following day. The team's counseling liaison decided to facilitate this meeting.
- *planning the schedule for the following day.* Since the return to routine is helpful after a crisis such as this one, the team decided to follow a regular class schedule the next day. However, at another faculty meeting the next morning, teachers were encouraged to make academics secondary to the students' needs to continue to talk about and work through the shooting. Teachers also were given information regarding children's emotional and behavioral reactions to trauma. Additional counselors were made available to each of the classrooms as part of the follow-up plan.
- *planning for the evening parent meeting.* An important component for any crisis response is the parent/community meeting. This meeting was well publicized via intense media coverage. Letters notifying parents of the meeting also were distributed to all students prior to their departure from school, and the time and location of the meeting were posted on the school's Web site. The entire crisis team attended the meeting, along with a representative of the police department. The counseling liaison facilitated much of the meeting so that parents were able to process in this forum the myriad emotional issues experienced in the tragedy. They also were given information about children's reactions to traumatic events and suggestions for dealing with them at home.
- *planning follow-up for the next day.* The crisis team decided that the counseling liaison would devote much of the day after the shooting to providing outreach to those thought to be most needy, including students who were on the field in the immediate vicinity of the gunfire, friends and siblings of the deceased, and the students who expressed guilt over hearing Max's veiled threat before the shooting and disbelieving it. The team also enlisted the support of some of the members of the counseling staff to follow the deceased students' schedules for the entire day to help their fellow students process the tragedy. It also was agreed that the next day would begin with an early morning faculty meeting to discuss the day's schedule.
- *scheduling regular crisis team meetings.* In order to allow the team to continue to function as efficiently as possible, regular meetings were deemed essential to allow the team to continue to keep pace with the

changing demands in the days and weeks following the crisis. As team members requested, roles and responsibilities were changed at the team meeting the next day; one of the counseling liaisons asked for reassignment to a different role due to his sense of being overwhelmed with the emotional reactions of the first 24 hours.

It was several weeks before the school really settled into something that even remotely resembled a familiar routine. As Max was brought to court, emotions ran high again at the realization that he might not be charged as an adult and might serve only a few years in a detention facility. Other reminders kept emotions high during the ensuing months: the birthdays of the deceased, graduation day, anniversaries of the event, discussion of an appropriate memorial for the tragedy, and the inevitable news articles about how it all could have been prevented.

School Crisis Intervention Case Example 2

Mrs. Monaco, a third grade teacher at Little Valley Elementary School, had just arrived at school. She exited the main office after signing in and was en route to her classroom to make ready for the arrival of her students. Before she reached her room, she was approached by a frantic, inconsolable parent of one of her students, with the equally inconsolable student in tow. The parent asked Monaco if she had heard anything about the school bus accident. Did she know which bus it was? Which students were on it? Which ones were killed?

Before Monaco could even make her way back to the office for some answers, hordes of students began to enter the building crying, all of them having just heard of the tragedy as they got off their own buses. School bells rang, signaling the beginning of homeroom, but crowds of weeping students, parents, and staff milled about the main corridor trying to come to terms with this unconfirmed news. Dr. Silver, the school principal, tried to restore some sense of order by ushering the students to their assigned locations while also attempting to gather some facts.

When Dr. Silver found herself confronted with the unconfirmed report of a school bus accident resulting in fatalities of some of her students, she was in a much different situation than the one experienced by Max's principal. In her case, the reported accident and loss of life occurred off campus, and the details, as a result, were rumors only. There were no eyewitnesses. There were no police reports as yet. There was only panic and speculation fueling the ever-expanding rumor of the accident.

Unlike Max's story, there were no safety issues for Silver to tend to, since the off-campus site of the crash was being managed by local police and medical emergency personnel. However, the first challenges for Silver were to ascertain the veracity of the crash reports and to call together her school's crisis response team.

Since her staff members were already on their way into school that day, Silver simply posted a notice by the faculty sign-in sheet that there would be a crisis meeting immediately upon arrival in the building. She also alerted the school secretary to notify each of the team members verbally about the meeting. Anticipating a rash of calls from the community as the report spread, Silver assigned the secretary and two clerical aids in the front office to answer telephone questions truthfully: that the reports were unconfirmed at that time and that the school would share all information upon its confirmation.

Silver then telephoned her contact with the police, a juvenile officer who had participated in the development of the school's crisis plan, in an attempt to collect the facts pertinent to the report of the crash. Within minutes, everyone's worst nightmare was realized; the officer confirmed that a school bus had been struck by a car at a busy intersection, injuring nine children and killing one, all of them students in Silver's school.

The crisis team sprang into action at that point. They developed a crisis fact sheet that would be distributed to each of the teachers to be read to the class. It must also be noted that while the team was working out the responsibilities of its members, Silver and her administrative assistant stayed in the school's main corridor encouraging all students and staff to move, as per the typical daily routine, to their homerooms. Despite some tears and looks of anguish, she refrained from confirming any of the facts in such a busy, frenetic main hallway, yet assured everyone that information would be forthcoming soon.

Meanwhile, in the crisis meeting, the assigning of responsibilities went smoothly.

- The counseling liaison decided to request the assistance of the crisis teams from the three other district schools. The plan was for counseling personnel to visit each of the injured and deceased student's classes and to remain with them for as long as they thought appropriate. Their goal was to help students process the news and express their reactions in the supportive and familiar milieu of their own classrooms. The other counseling staff members would remain very visible by circulating within the building and offering assistance to students and staff when needed.

- The school nurse was to remain in steady contact with the local hospital, where all the children had been taken, and to keep the team, particularly Silver, the crisis coordinator, updated on the medical conditions of the children.

- The liaisons for both the staff and parents fulfilled similar roles: keeping both groups abreast of all the details. Small groups of parents were taken into the school cafeteria to inform them of the accident. When the liaison explained to them what the school crisis team's plans were for the remainder of that day and for subsequent days, most parents agreed to let their children remain in school. However, those who insisted on removing their children for the day were allowed to do so, particularly if they were kindergartners or first-graders.

- Considering the size of the school and the fact that there was crisis team assistance from other schools, Silver recommended that he also serve in the capacity as the media liaison. He was able to manage most of the media's telephone inquiries regarding the school's response to the accident. Those on-site media visitors, however, were ushered to a central location, the school auditorium, by the crisis team's security liaison and kept from wandering unescorted through the school corridors.

As had also been done in Max's case, an after-school faculty meeting was held, as was a meeting for parents in the evening. Concerns from both groups were quite similar: Would the school follow a regular schedule the next day? What services would be available to the children and staff during the next few days or weeks to help them process the crash? What if the children developed fears of riding a school bus again?

The crisis coordinator who chaired each of these meetings stressed for both groups the importance of returning to a routine as quickly as possible. A regular school day was planned for the next day, although counselors would continue to be available throughout the day to continue to provide support for the students and staff. Counselors also planned to ride on the school buses for the next several days to assist the drivers with the emotional aftermath. It was made clear to both faculty and parents that they were to keep in close contact with the crisis team in the days following the incident in order to report on those individual students whose particularly strong reactions to the crash called for special outreach services from the counseling liaisons.

Parents also received a special information sheet describing not only the cognitive, emotional, and behavioral indicators of crisis in their children, but also a list of helpful hints for them to use with their children at home. Referrals to local mental health centers and private practitioners were made available to parents, as was the telephone number for the team's parent liaison.

School Crisis Intervention Case Example 3

Flossie was an active, outgoing first-grader who was known to most teachers in her small primary school. She and her brother, Grant, a third-grader in the same school, were severe asthmatics. Flossie was a frequent visitor to the school nurse's office, and during a particularly bad allergy season, she was in nurse Walker's office at least three times daily. One night after suffering a serious asthma attack with both her parents out of the house for the evening, Flossie died. News spread quickly, and the next day those students who came to school could do nothing but talk about her death. Nurse Walker also noted a significant increase in the number of student visitors to her office with asthma-related questions and from asthmatics themselves, although none of them severe, looking for reassurances that they would not die.

The advantage (if indeed there can be an advantage in the death of a child) for the crisis team from Flossie's school was that her death occurred in the evening at home, allowing the team to receive notice of the death in time to plan its course of action. One of the local emergency medical personnel who was called to the house to administer to Flossie and who knew that she had died called the school principal at his home to report the news. The principal then activated the crisis team's telephone chain, passing along the request that the team meet the next morning approximately 90 minutes prior to the arrival of the students.

Unlike the unpredictability and the chaos in which the two previous cases unfolded, Flossie's death was more of a private matter that attracted little of the media attention that the others did and impacted a smaller segment of the community than did the others. Therefore, the crisis team had the opportunity to plan its activities in a more rational, measured manner than the previous two teams.

At the early morning meeting, the crisis team, having had the time to confirm the facts of Flossie's death, wrote its crisis fact sheet and made enough copies for the staff and for other interested parties (community members in particular). It also developed a carefully worded statement that was given to each teacher to be read during the homeroom period. The team decided that a counselor would be present in each of the first grade classrooms (Flossie's grade) throughout most of the morning; the counselor and the teacher from each class then would decide on the ongoing need for the counselor's full-time presence.

Since Flossie died due to complications from asthma, the school nurse played a key role in targeting those special needs students for some counseling intervention, particularly other asthmatic students who frequented her office during the day for medication or for regular use of their inhalers. Joey was the first visitor to the nurse late that morning who acknowledged that he was an asthmatic "just like Flossie." The nurse was able to provide a list of eighteen such students; they then became the first group on which the counseling liaison focused his attention. Rather than single out these students needlessly, the counselor instead decided to alert each of their teachers to be mindful of any strong reactions that they might observe over the course of the ensuing weeks. In case Flossie's death did make some of them more conscious of their mortality than others, the counselor decided to spend the latter part of the day in the nurse's office, in case they felt the need to visit her. The crisis team also decided to call the parents of the asthmatic students to alert them to their children's increased vulnerability to having a greater anxiety reaction to Flossie's death.

Flossie's classroom teacher made a request of the crisis team that one of its members read the announcement of the death to the class and to take a major role in processing the event with her students, explaining that she would not be able to do so without becoming emotionally overwrought in front of the class. The team agreed with her assessment and assigned one of the counselors to take over these duties. It is important to note that even though it would have been very appropriate for Flossie's teacher to exhibit grief in front of her students, it would have been too traumatic for the children if her emotional reaction were so strong that it terrified them. The children needed someone in control of her own emotions in order to draw some reassurances from her that all would be well; the presence of an inconsolable teacher would not have provided them with this reassurance.

One of the first questions that the crisis team members asked the teachers as they received the sheet to read to their classes was whether or not they could do it without being overwhelmed with grief; if not, a team member volunteered to do it. Only Flossie's teacher admitted that she would be unable to do it. However, her comfort level in addressing this issue of loss increased as she sat quietly in the classroom observing the counselor talking with her students about the death. By the end of the day, she sent the crisis team member on her way and expressed a greater sense of comfort in handling the class herself.

Although the school received a number of phone calls from community members regarding Flossie, the team decided that an evening parent meeting was not essential. The crisis coordinator instead decided to contact the family and to make a visit to the home to offer assistance. However, an after-school faculty meeting was held in order to process the day's events and to determine additional needs for the following day. The teachers were assured at this meeting that there would be a counseling presence in the building for the next day and for as long as it was deemed necessary. Teachers also reported on the activities initiated by the students to honor Flossie: creating their own cards to send to the family, planting flowers in her honor, making a donation to charity.

The crisis team's response to Flossie's death was different than it was for Max or for Dr. Silver's school bus deaths. Unlike the high profile status that each of these two cases shared, Flossie's death was more of a private matter. The hordes of media and community members that the other cases would attract was not so with Flossie. Children whose own school grounds were violated by violence or who shared a common experience (riding the school bus) would have experienced a different level of anxiety than Flossie's classmates, since they would have identified more closely with the victims. However, Flossie's asthma was not a common experience shared by most of her classmates, so it would have marked her as "not like me" for most students. As a result, it would have created some distance between her and her peers to help soften the blow of her death. Physical illness also makes death appear to be a more understandable phenomenon than random violence or life-ending accidents.

Because of the various kinds of crises that can impact schools, individual crisis teams will respond differently. Schools will access different levels of resources, depending on the crisis type, the age of the children involved, the size and setting of the school, the age and experience level of the faculty, and the community needs. Crisis intervention doesn't really end; the follow-up services required over the long term extend well beyond the immediate resolution of the crisis.

Applying the Model: Tertiary Prevention (Postvention)

Even after the tsunami devastates the shore, the waters behind it remain turbulent for some time. Postvention refers to those activities that take place even long after the tsunami of the crisis event has passed, because the disruption lingers. Crisis team members must be prepared to continue to provide services to children, their families, and to staff for a period of time which will be determined only by the needs of these groups and by the manner in which they experienced the crisis. The typical routines of the school day may have to be put on hold for a period of time, depending on many of the factors listed previously.

The counselor from the crisis team should be prepared to continue to support, counsel, or monitor those students most affected by the crisis. If this proves to be too daunting a task for the available counselor(s), then referrals should be made to other local mental health services. Coordinating these needs for the survivors is a critical function for the team. The counselor, in conjunction with the appropriate teachers and family members, will determine the level of services the children need.

A designated team member, usually the parent/community liaison, should also maintain ongoing meetings with interested and needy parents. Whether these meetings should be scheduled on a weekly or monthly basis will depend upon the unique demands of the situation. A practical approach would include weekly meetings for several weeks that fade into monthly ones. However, if a parent has far more needs than what these ongoing consultations can accommodate, then a referral to the appropriate community resource would be a better course of action. When a crisis reawakens old wounds or creates the final stressor in an already overburdened family system, then weekly school meetings do not comprise the proper forum to address these issues. However, in all circumstances, the counseling liaison must remain a staunch advocate for and supporter of these parents.

A thorough postvention program must also provide follow-up services to the teaching staff. With the needs of students tending to be the primary focus of crisis intervention in the schools, it is not unusual to lose sight of the sense of loss, for example, that Flossie's teachers felt after her death. In order to monitor their progress following the crisis, the crisis team should keep in close touch with them, particularly those most affected. An additional benefit derived from this close follow-up is the opportunity to obtain feedback regarding the function of the crisis team during the crisis. It is only with this kind of input that the team will be able to revise its roles or functions in order to better prepare for the next crisis.

A Postvention Ritual: Memorials

Renaming school buildings. Planting a tree. Erecting a monument. Holding school assemblies. Writing a song. The ways in which children and adolescents choose to memorialize their friends whose lives were lost to crisis are limitless. Memorials represent an important step in recovering from such a loss, as they signal both closure to the process of grieving and a time to move on to routine activities shattered, for a time, by trauma (Payne, 1999). Schools should not prevent such memorial activities. In fact, their participation in the planning of these efforts would go a long way toward assisting in the healing of the student body.

Some of the more familiar formats for memorializing students include memorial services, permanent memorials, activity-based memorials, and fundraising. When a service is planned, some of Payne's (1999) suggestions include the following:

- Keep the memorial short: 15 to 20 minutes for elementary students, 30 to 40 minutes for secondary.
- Involve students in the planning of the memorial, particularly those who were close to the deceased.
- Include music, particularly student performances.
- Have several brief speakers. If students have written poems or other tributes, students themselves or staff can read samples.
- Invite family members.
- Involve all students as much as possible.
- Plan the activity to occur within a week of the death, if possible.

Allowing the passage of time and some emotional distance from the crisis before planning a permanent memorial structure is advisable. Otherwise, the discrete park bench by the baseball field with an engraved plaque honoring the deceased might have been an archway over the entrance to school, if it had been planned immediately after the crisis event. Planning such structures too quickly doesn't leave the opportunity for reason and insight and can leave a school regretting such obtrusive remembrances of the victim months after their construction. The best memorial is one that students may visit on their own and which does not confront them daily.

It is not unusual for students, particularly adolescents, to decide to take a proactive stance in commemorating a death: opening a school chapter of Students Against Drunk Driving, handing out leaflets for gun control, or lobbying local government for a traffic light at the scene of a fatality. Schools can encourage these approaches in lieu of a permanent memorial, although the students themselves should assume the primary responsibility for organizing them. Finally, fundraising for things such as medical expenses for a surviving family or for the establishment of a scholarship in the deceased's honor can be a powerful way of harnessing the passion of adolescents in particular to make some sense out of the crisis.

A Caveat: When the Death Is a Suicide

Before planning a memorial of any kind, the school must consider first the cause of death; if the cause of death was suicide, the victim *should not be memorialized in any way* (Peterson & Straub, 1992; Poland & McCormick, 1999; Underwood &

Dunne-Maxim, 1997). Drawing an inordinate amount of attention to the victim of suicide suggests that he or she was more valued in death than in life and can lead to suicide "contagion," the copying of a suicidal act by others, especially those close to the victim or considered at risk for other reasons.

The American Association of Suicidology (American Association of Suicidology, 1998) provides suicide postvention guidelines, including the following:

- Don't dedicate a memorial to the deceased.
- Don't encourage funeral attendance during school hours.
- Don't hold an assembly to notify the school of the death.
- Give the facts to the students, but downplay the method.
- Emphasize that no one is to blame for the suicide.
- Emphasize that suicides can be prevented and that help is available.

The challenge a crisis team faces after a suicide is to continue to provide outreach services for the two most vulnerable groups mentioned previously. Being ever vigilant in the days and weeks following the suicide is crucial; alerting teachers to monitor the well-being of their students and to report to the counselors any concerns they may have over even subtle changes in their students' behavior is of utmost importance. Memorials, however, and other well-intentioned attempts to dramatize the death are strictly taboo.

SOURCES OF CHAPTER ENRICHMENT

Print Sources

Bonilla, D. (Ed.). (2000). *School violence.* Washington, DC: H.W. Wilson Co.

Brown, B., & Merritt, R. (2002). *No easy answers: The truth behind death at Columbine.* New York: Lantern Books.

Dwyer, K., Osher, D., & Warger, C. (1998). *Early warning, timely response: A guide to safe schools.* Washington, DC: U.S. Department of Education.

Dwyer, K., Osher, D., & Warger, C. (2000). *Safeguarding our children: An action guide.* Washington, DC: U.S. Department of Education.

Johnson, K. (1998). *Trauma in the lives of children.* Alameda, CA: Hunter House Publishers.

Osofsky, J. D. (Ed.). (1998). *Children in a violent society.* New York: Guilford.

National Organization for Victim Assistance. (1997). *Community crisis response team training manual* (2nd ed.). Washington, DC: Author.

Internet Sources

National Association of School Psychologists (http://www.nasponline.org) In addition to providing a wide range of information related to children, adolescents, and families regarding both school and other issues, this organization devotes part of its Web site to the National Emergency Assistance Team (NEAT), a partnership with the National Organization for Victim Assistance to help children, schools, families, and communities cope with crises.

American School Counselor Association (http://www.schoolcounselor.org) This organization provides numerous resources for coping with school-related crises.

National Education Association (http://www.nea.org/crisis) The NEA offers its own "Crisis Communications Guide and Toolkit" via its Web site.

National Organization for Victim Assistance (http://www.try-nova.org) NOVA, the oldest victim assistance and advocacy organization in the country, provides a great variety of resources related to crisis and crisis victims, as well as numerous opportunities for interested professionals and lay people to obtain NOVA-sponsored crisis training.

CHAPTER **10**

Community Responses to Crisis

In the early morning hours of September 11, 2001, American Airlines Flight 11 and United Airlines Flight 175 left Boston for distant destinations. Within hours, a group of terrorists crashed Flight 11 into the north tower of New York City's 110-story World Trade Center. Flight 175 hit the south tower 18 minutes later. It will never be known exactly how many people died at impact or in the minutes immediately after in the incinerating heat of the jet fuel-fed fireballs, but we do know that the dying did not end there. As hundreds of firefighters struggled valiantly to help thousands of office workers get out of the buildings, both of the towers collapsed in an avalanche of concrete and steel. Across America and the world, shocked and despairing friends and relatives of the victims, and millions more, watched the entire spectacle unfold right before their eyes on TV. Just before the first tower collapsed, American Airlines Flight 77 crashed into the Pentagon in Washington, DC. United Airlines Flight 93 never reached its likely intended target, the White House, being forced to the ground by the passengers themselves in a struggle with the terrorists. The human toll that horrific morning reached nearly 3,000 casualties.

Hurricane Andrew, the most destructive U.S. hurricane of record, hit southern Florida on August 24, 1992, with winds peaking at 164 miles per hour. More than 2 million people in Florida and Louisiana were evacuated as Andrew approached. The high winds and intense rainfall (7 inches) in three states resulted in $26.5 billion in property damage and in the deaths of 26 people in the United States and another 3 in the Bahamas; indirect loss of life attributable to Andrew, however, totaled 65. These figures do not begin to describe the devastation. Miles and miles of residential neighborhoods in southern Florida were wiped out. Many victims needed rescuing and/or immediate medical attention. Neighbors and family members called for help on cell phones, but with street signs blown away, with debris everywhere, and with trees, power lines, and telephone poles down, rescue and emergency medical teams had great difficulty finding them. For

> weeks, residents sifted through the rubble of their destroyed homes, searching for remnants of cherished possessions. Many went for days without food, water, or shelter as they wandered aimlessly through the destroyed neighborhoods.

*T*he same basic questions arise about each of these community-wide disasters:

- How does any individual, group, community, or nation go about responding to a disaster event of such enormity?
- Where does one begin to address the needs of the community?
- Who will help?
- Is crisis intervention different for large-scale crises than for individual crises?

In order to answer these questions, this chapter will focus on how larger systems respond to catastrophic events similar to the ones described above. It will explore the public agony of whole communities of people attempting to rise from the rubble of a widespread disaster event. It will also examine the workings of a community-wide movement of helpers—lay people and professionals, the trained and the untrained, the blood donor and the counselor—who play a role in lifting a community of victims from its pain and anguish.

Poet John Donne (1624/1952) stated it poignantly when he wrote in "Meditation XVII"

> No man is an island, entire of itself; every man is a piece of the continent, a part of the main. ... any man's death diminishes me, because I am involved in mankind, and therefore never send to know for whom the bell tolls; it tolls for thee. (p. 441)

The word *system* refers to a complex of interacting and interdependent parts that comprise a united whole; changes to even one of the individual parts most certainly affect other parts of the system. The serious illness of a young child, for example, generates waves of concern, not just among family members, but also among classmates, teachers, and other community members who may only have been remotely acquainted with the child. Similarly, the high-profile death of a single celebrity from the entertainment industry sparks strong reactions of grief from individuals around the country. In the case of a disaster such as 9/11, it would be difficult to find anyone in the country who was not affected.

From the loosely knit grassroots level to the more structured organizational level, this chapter also will examine the larger community's response to such crises. Whether it's a local youth group selling candy to raise money for dis-placed homeowners after Hurricane Andrew or the hundreds of millions of dollars donated to the families of 9/11 victims through the Red Cross, commu-nity responses to crisis are broad and all-encompassing.

A Light Among the Rubble

Perhaps some of the most enduring images embedded in the consciousness of the television-viewing public in the aftermath of the terrorist attacks on New York City's Twin Towers were those of the many thousands of volunteers who manned everything from food booths to crisis centers to bucket brigades haul-ing debris from the site, which will always be known as Ground Zero. Contributing also to these images were the local residents who opened their homes to stranded city workers and the pleasure boaters who repeatedly fer-ried commuters across the water to the shores of New Jersey in the absence of a functional mass transit system. The horror of the Tower fireballs eventually was mitigated in some small, yet reassuring way by the school and community groups, formal organizations, loosely knit friendship groups, survivors and their family members, and total strangers who were committed to providing aid and comfort to anyone affected by the tragedy. The evening news programs and the morning talk shows highlighted these acts of selflessness by lay people who contributed considerable effort to relief and recovery.

We begin this chapter by highlighting the manner in which individuals, community groups, government agencies, and professional organizations respond to crisis. These are, of course, overlapping and interacting efforts, none of which can exist independently of the others. The volunteer force heeds gov-ernment appeals for service and sacrifice, while professional organizations pro-vide training and other resources, not only to implement government initiatives, but also to train and mobilize the eager and motivated volunteer corps.

Volunteers: Grassroots Response to Crisis

Volunteerism has long been at the forefront of community response to tragedy. A cadre of volunteers in each community toil alongside one another to per-form even the most menial of tasks to contribute to the common good during trying times. Volunteers traditionally have provided all types of services to both private and public organizations, particularly those plagued by budget constraints and by economic downturns, resulting in reduced workforces who could not manage the myriad tasks needed to keep things afloat. They have provided numerous and ongoing acts of service, including companionship for the lonely, tutoring for the illiterate, counseling for the troubled, healthcare for the sick, mentoring for those in need of role models, and shelter for the trou-bled and homeless. Among the mental health community, they have been a highly visible component of many crisis centers and counseling agencies, while the 24-hours-a-day, 7-days-a-week demands of suicide hotlines, particularly those in major cities, utilize the greatest number of volunteers for their round-the-clock services (James & Gilliland, 2001).

National surveys have estimated that, on average, nearly half (44%) of adults in the United States volunteer for 3.6 hours per week. One survey developed a methodology to calculate the monetary value of time spent in volunteering, estimating that the dollar value of volunteers' efforts in 1994 was worth approximately $16.05 per hour, with the total value nationwide reaching $239 billion per year, the equivalent of 9 million full-time employees (Independent Sector, 1994). Many assume that this figure is bound to increase with the relaxing of government programs and services for the underprivileged and needy (Penner & Finkelstein, 1998). Other estimates place the number of American adults who provided regular volunteer services at just more than 89 million, with approximately 23.6 million of them volunteering for 5 or more hours each week (Clary et al., 1998).

Opportunities for volunteer service appear to be practically limitless; in fact, the *Encyclopedia of Associations: National Organizations of the U.S.* (2004) lists under "Voluntarism" a total of 210 programs or organizations available to those individuals interested in donating their time and energy. The number of charities, social welfare organizations, and religious groups that consider volunteering as central to their ability to serve their communities has reached 1.23 million, while a full 85% of nonprofit groups and 92% of religious organizations report the need for even more volunteers with specific skill sets (Independent Sector, 2002). Still countless other grassroots organizations exist throughout the country, but are not yet included in this reference book.

Although the commitment to volunteerism is not specific to America, the events of September 11, 2001, thrust into the spotlight the collective efforts of all Americans in responding to this crisis. Television viewers from around the world began to assign different meaning to the images of the attacks, to the terms *9/11* and *ground zero,* and to the status of the uniformed services, particularly the New York firefighters and policemen and women. Yet even prior to the attacks on the Twin Towers and the Pentagon, volunteerism had become increasingly popular in the United States. The United Way of America, in its 2001 State of Caring index, documented a 10% rise in volunteerism over the previous decade, reaching a 12-year high. However, calamitous events such as 9/11 tend to lead to immediate increases in social/community involvement, particularly via volunteer activity. More than half of the 1,000 Americans polled in the immediate aftermath of the Twin Towers attacks reported giving money to charities, while 70% acknowledged some other charitable involvement (Independent Sector, 2002). Thus, the United States may see one of the greatest surges in volunteerism since the attack on Pearl Harbor more than 60 years ago. Even though this "spike" in interest in volunteerism may be only temporary, the ongoing threat posed by the terrorist network held responsible for the attacks will likely sustain this increase.

Who Volunteers?

The casual observer responds to this question with the answer that everyone volunteers in a crisis. The number of blood donors skyrocketed after 9/11, leading New York City-based medical personnel to request that volunteer fervor be demonstrated in other ways besides giving blood, since the flood of donations quickly began to surpass the ability to test the blood and store it properly. New York City even had to refuse all but the most skilled and essential volunteers, considering the vast numbers who appeared. Individuals baked cakes and donated canned goods to survivors and to rescue workers, while others simply reported to locations of their own choosing in an attempt to determine what it was they could do during the crisis. There was a similar response in the aftermath of the bombing of the Murrah Federal Building in Oklahoma City and Hurricane Andrew.

The poet-philosopher sees the origins of volunteerism as the individual's response to a felt need. Just as a sense of loneliness compels us to reach out and engage others in some social encounter, so too, does a sense of aimlessness and emptiness lead individuals to look beyond their own needs and make a positive contribution to the larger community. For some, however, embracing service to the community is a much surer way of dispelling loneliness than just finding a social group. As Moore (1999) proclaims, "The volunteer chooses to cross the border between the surface delights of the protected life and the inner beauty of raw human existence. ... The reward is immeasurable because it fills the heart and soul rather than the wallet or the ego" (p. 10). However, others look at the phenomenon of volunteering from a more empirical perspective.

The root of the word "volunteer" is from the Latin word *velle*, meaning "to will, to wish." That an individual would "wish" to sacrifice time and effort for another person, oftentimes a stranger, has long been a topic of social psychological research. Much of this research, however, has focused on those immediate, short-term, and short-lived acts of helping, and has even differentiated *volunteerism* from *helping*. Researchers have considered these two activities to be separate, defining volunteerism as "planned helping" and helping itself as "spontaneous helping" (Clary et al., 1998). These same researchers delineate the differences between these two acts in the following way:

Helping (Spontaneous Helping)	Volunteerism (Planned Helping)
When a potential helper is faced with an unexpected need for help.	When someone actively seeks out the opportunity to help others.
When the context calls for an immediate decision to act.	When someone deliberates and decides to become involved.
When the opportunity provides only one relatively brief act of helping.	When someone commits to an ongoing helping relationship at some personal cost.

The "helper" in this paradigm is the person who assists a stranded motorist with a ride to a service station or with the changing of a flat tire, or the person who comes to the aid of a victim during the commission of a crime. The help tendered is quick, immediate, and of relatively short duration. There is no intention to return to the scene of the helping act, to repeat the act, or to follow up with any long-term assistance. The act also is not mediated cognitively by the helper, but rather is carried through to fruition as an impulsive act elicited by a number of situational characteristics. Volunteerism, however, presents several features not found in helping. By definition, volunteerism must be a more voluntary and sustained act: the college student who has answered telephones at the local women's emergency shelter twice a week for 3 years; the 20-year little league coach; and the person who organizes the food booth at the annual Special Olympics competition.

Researchers know more about spontaneous acts of helping than volunteering. Research journals are replete with studies of those factors, both internal and external to the individual, that influence the decision to help another in an emergency. The impetus for this research has been such front page newspaper stories as the repeated stabbing of Kitty Genovese in front of approximately 38 silent, passive, and unresponsive witnesses in New York City in 1963. In general, this research was designed to explain exactly what aspects of a situation either encouraged or discouraged prosocial acts, known as bystander interventions. The team of John Darley and Bibb Latane pioneered this research in the 1970s; they found that the number of bystanders (crowded vs. non-crowded areas) and the anonymity of the bystander, among other factors, contributed significantly to the likelihood of a prosocial response. The more bystanders present, the less likely they were to help, the researchers claimed. They called this phenomenon the "bystander effect," which results from the diffusion of responsibility (giving over responsibility to the larger group rather than maintaining it individually) and the bystander's contingent decision-making regarding whether or not the situation really requires some kind of prosocial response.

These findings spawned considerable research in other disciplines as well. Sociologists looked at the depersonalization of urban life as a contributing factor to the lack of response in the Genovese story, while others explored the existential void and cultural decay as possible explanatory factors. Despite the wealth of research into this particular form of helping (or nonhelping) behavior, there exists a real dearth of research and of theoretical models that attempt to explain volunteerism (Penner & Finkelstein, 1998). More is known about why people help in sudden, immediate situations than why they engage in continuous acts of helpfulness.

Some researchers have posited the idea that specific personality characteristics breed volunteerism (Penner, Fritzsche, Craiger, & Freifeld, 1995). These researchers have suggested that those with a prosocial personality orientation are inclined toward volunteerism; the tendency to be concerned about others, to think about their welfare, and to act in a way that benefits them are the hallmarks of this personality type. Empathy and helpfulness also are two correlated factors with the prosocial personality. A conceptual cousin to this construct is a cluster of behaviors known as organizational citizenship behavior (OCB) (Organ, 1994). These behaviors include those that are specifically intended to improve the well-being of an organization or of the individuals who work within it; an important component is the notion that these behaviors are neither rewarded nor requested by others. Like the research on volunteerism, OCB involves long-term, purposeful behavior that is self-initiated and that is not a response to another's command or request.

Although the act of volunteering may serve different functions for different people, research (Clary et al., 1998) has proposed six functions served by volunteerism. They include:

1. the opportunity to express values related to altruism and humanitarian concerns for others;
2. opportunities for new learning experiences and for the chance to exercise knowledge, skills, and other abilities that might otherwise go unpracticed;
3. opportunities to be with friends or to be viewed favorably by important others;
4. ability to obtain career benefits;
5. opportunities to reduce guilt over being more fortunate than others and to address one's personal problems; and
6. individual growth and development.

The Government's Role in the Volunteer Effort

Out of crisis comes resolve.
From the ashes of tragedy rise the wings of resilience and repair.

The federal government has long promoted the cause of volunteerism among its citizenry. Whether in times of war or peace, the government has always championed an involved corps of civilian volunteers. During World War II, Americans waged war of their own at home via their efforts at gasoline and food rationing, tin foil drives, victory gardens, and buying war bonds. Even Hollywood celebrities modeled duty-bound selflessness by entertaining troops abroad, selling war bonds, and encouraging rationing drives. Although the current government's relatively recent foray into the volunteerism initiative (see later sections) predated the Twin Towers attack on September 11, 2001, this major crisis event provided a significant impetus for the presidential call for volunteers. The purpose of the Towers-related support for volunteers was to keep Americans engaged in the "war on terrorism," to keep the national spirit up, and to provide a role for Americans who wanted to display their patriotism by doing more than just hanging a flag over their front porch. The government basically decided to join forces with the volunteer spirit and to create a nationwide pool of volunteers who would answer the call to service.

In 1993, President Bill Clinton was in the vanguard of government-sponsored initiatives when he drafted the legislation that lead to the creation of the

Corporation for National and Community Service (CNCS), an umbrella organization chartered by Congress that oversees millions of citizens who work on social and disaster relief projects nationwide. Since its inception, the CNCS essentially has connected Americans with opportunities to engage in voluntary service; estimates suggest that more than 2 million Americans are involved each year. The three main programs of the CNCS include AmeriCorps, Senior Corps, and Learn and Serve America.

AMERICORPS More than 50,000 Americans have been serving their communities for between 20 and 40 hours a week through AmeriCorps. Its members serve through more than 2,100 nonprofits, public agencies, and faith-based organizations, and they serve with local and national organizations such as Habitat for Humanity, the American Red Cross, Teach for America, Big Brothers/Big Sisters, and the Boys and Girls Clubs. Some of their functions involve building affordable housing, cleaning parks and streams, running after-school programs, tutoring and mentoring youth, and helping communities respond to disasters. In exchange for a year of service, AmeriCorps members earn an education award that can be used to pay for college or to pay back student loans. Approximately half of its members also receive a small living allowance and health benefits. AmeriCorps funnels three-quarters of its funds through various state-appointed commissions to local causes and to different nonprofit groups, while a competitive grants process assists with the distribution of the remainder of the funding.

SENIOR CORPS This program consists of a network of volunteer opportunities that tap the experience and talents of citizens ages 55 and older by placing them in community service projects. Its three primary activities include Foster Grandparents (serving as tutors and mentors to young people with special needs), Senior Companions (helping homebound seniors and others to enable them to maintain independence in their own homes), and the Retired and Senior Volunteer Program (RSVP). This latter group of volunteers assists law enforcement with safety patrols, provides educational services to children and adults, and responds to natural disasters.

LEARN AND SERVE AMERICA This component of the CNCS initiative provides grants to schools to link classroom studies with community service and volunteerism in order to assist teachers with lesson planning and instructional ideas. Called "service learning," this approach is intended to engage students in a long-term commitment to volunteer activities via a structured educational/classroom component in conjunction with active student participation in specific service areas. A class of fifth graders, for example, studies the importance of good nutrition in a series of health class activities while also sponsoring and staffing a food drive for needy families in the community. Learn and Serve America issues $43 million in grants each year to schools, colleges, and community organizations to promote similar activities;

it also sponsors a recognition program and a scholarship program for outstanding community service.

The CNCS, in conjunction with the U.S. Department of Education, developed a guidebook entitled *Students in Service to America* to help classroom teachers develop academic lessons for formal service projects. This resource includes research, instructional strategies, and classroom ideas for service learning. Approximately 130,000 public and private elementary and secondary schools, home schools, and after-school programs throughout the country received copies of the guidebook and a companion CD-ROM.

Crisis Services of Volunteer Organizations

For many years, loosely knit groups of volunteers and grassroots organizations, both large and small, public and private, tended to function independently of one another. The result was that victims of crises ran the risk of being at the receiving end of a haphazard delivery of services, leading to the duplication of some and the neglect of others. Volunteers during a crisis event could find the drop-off site for food donations, but they were not nearly so clear about how to provide for other physical, psychological, or emotional needs. In general, the overall coordination of services and information regarding crisis/disaster needs was negligible. Adding to the confusion were the difficulties encountered by different government agencies whose financial and jurisdictional constraints stymied them in their quest to provide proper disaster responses for each community.

Considering the potential "quagmire" posed by these problems, it was only a matter of time before an organizational response to the myriad volunteers who came forward to play a role in the midst of crisis was formed. The federal government saw to this need for coordination by establishing the Federal Emergency Management Agency (FEMA) in 1979 (discussed further later in this chapter). In the meantime, a slow, inexorable movement among individual leaders of various volunteer organizations resulted in a united call for better articulation among their groups as well as a more efficient way of providing services.

Spurred on by a representative of the American Red Cross, representatives of seven volunteer organizations came together in 1970 and formed National Voluntary Organizations Active in Disaster (NVOAD). The purpose of this all-volunteer group was to coordinate the disaster-specific efforts of many volunteer groups. NVOAD does not provide direct services itself, but rather merely encourages cooperative relationships among its independent members in providing relief and recovery to crisis victims in an efficient response mode while avoiding duplication of effort. NVOAD currently has 35 member organizations, with 52 state and territorial VOADs and a growing number of local VOADs. Among the more prominent member groups are the *American Red Cross* and the *National Organization for Victim Assistance (NOVA)*.

American Red Cross

What better way to continue an examination of the role of organizations' responses to crisis than to look at the role played by the American Red Cross (ARC), one of the first volunteer disaster-relief agencies. In the aftermath of the battle of Solferino in 1859, which left 6,000 dead and 30,000 wounded, the idea for the ARC was born. A visitor to the battlefield, Swiss businessman Henri Jean Dunant, horrified at what he had seen, organized a group of local women to tend to the needs of the wounded who had been left to die where they lay. Determined to provide for the suffering from that day on in a consistent and organized manner, he set about gathering a volunteer corps to assist in this regard. Within the next five years, Dunant and a handful of colleagues established the forerunner of the ARC, the International Committee for Relief to the Wounded, and drafted the first Geneva Convention, a humanitarian code of conduct for the battlefield. "Red Cross" was added to its name in 1875.

The International Committee for the Red Cross currently governs 137 national societies worldwide, with more than 250 million members (Moorehead, 1998). One if its societies, the American Red Cross (ARC), operates with an annual budget of approximately $3 billion and responds to 67,000 disasters annually. Although not a government agency, the ARC received a charter from Congress in 1900 to "carry on a system of national and international relief in time of peace and apply the same in mitigating the sufferings caused by pestilence, famine, fire, floods, and other great national calamities, and to devise and carry on measures for preventing the same" (http://www.redcross.org/museum/charters.html). In short, the ARC focuses on meeting the needs of victims of crisis or disaster. Whether the crisis is looming or striking, the ARC sees to the provision of the basic human needs of food, shelter, and clothing. Added to its mandate also are the mental health needs of those in need.

Contributing training in disaster mental health services to its repertoire of crisis responses, the ARC entered into a Statement of Understanding with the American Psychological Association (APA) to provide mental health services to disaster victims, their families, and to the relief workers themselves. The APA and the American Counseling Association also have joint agreements with the Red Cross for disaster mental health training. This training takes the form of a two-day Disaster Mental Health Services course after the completion of a brief preliminary Introduction to Disasters course. The entry-level course usually is offered on a frequent basis at most local Red Cross chapter offices, while the more advanced course is offered with less regularity, generally in conjunction with a partner organization. Additionally, the Red Cross has been the organization designated by the National Transportation Safety Board, as per federal mandate, to provide for the emotional needs of victims, survivors, and rescue workers in the aftermath of any aviation disaster.

National Organization for Victim Assistance

Another member organization of NVOAD, NOVA is a private, nonprofit group of "victim and witness assistance programs and practitioners, criminal justice agencies and professionals, mental health professionals, researchers, former victims and survivors, and others committed to the recognition and implementation of victim rights and services." Founded in 1975 by a group of victim advocates from rape crisis centers, law enforcement agencies, and other community-based organizations, NOVA stands today as the oldest group of its kind in the victims movement. NOVA's four stated purposes are as follows:

1. National advocacy:
   - Lobbying state governments to expand compensation programs for crime victims
   - Lobbying successfully for the department of justice to use federal funds to help victims of terrorism and mass violence
   - Working to allow victims' statements to be used at sentencing and parole hearings in virtually every state
   - Helping with passage of the victims of crime act and the violence against women act, freeing up more money to rehabilitate crime victims
   - Lobbying for a bill of rights for crime victims in state legislatures (29 states have passed such an amendment)
   - Helping to establish a "national victim's rights week"
2. Direct services to victims:
   - Developing training materials for staff and volunteers in crisis intervention and victim advocacy (see the section on the National Crisis Response Teams)
   - Serving as the conduit between needy victims and resources available to them through any one or more local community service agencies
   - Instituting the National Crime Victim Information and Referral Hotline (1-800-TRY-NOVA)
   - Creating the concept of multidisciplinary teams (National Crisis Response Teams) dispatched to the scenes of major crimes, disasters, and accidents
   - Working toward the development of an international manual on victim assistance for the United Nations' Commission on Crime Prevention
3. Assistance to professional colleagues:
   - Providing training via more than 500 workshops and seminars to members of the helping professions
   - Organizing national and regional conferences on victims' issues

- Establishing multi-level training programs in crisis intervention
4. Membership activities and services:
   - Becoming the recognized umbrella group for national organizations with an interest in victim issues
   - Convening an annual conference that attracts international interest and presenters

NATIONAL CRISIS RESPONSE TEAM   NOVA's Crisis Response Team (CRT) made its first appearance in 1986 in the aftermath of the Edmond, Oklahoma disaster when a postal worker killed 14 people before killing himself. Appearing within 24 hours of this crisis, a team of seven experienced crisis interveners made its way to Edmond where it provided crisis intervention to the survivors and to assorted community members. Since that event, the NOVA CRT has responded to more than 100 communities in a variety of crisis situations. The key concept of CRT intervention, however, is that the response is for the entire community rather than for just the individual(s).

Rather than descend upon the crisis location like rescuers, the CRT members arrive for a short period of time in order to mobilize local relief providers to respond to the community's distress. In the chaos of the moment, local caregivers tend to be stymied in their attempts to help community members through the crisis. Until they are able to follow through with a plan of action effectively, the CRT provides information and suggestions on how to proceed. That is, the CRT members are consultants to local groups on a temporary basis only; once the crisis has passed and the community caregivers are able to resume a caregiving function, the CRT departs. It functions just as a family therapist conducts therapy, not by prescribing a remedy for the family, but rather by becoming a part of the family system and facilitating, not directing, the system to return to some sense of equilibrium. The CRT also does not intrude into a crisis location; it responds only to requests for assistance, and it responds within 24 hours.

The members of a typical CRT may vary from disaster site to disaster site, since the demographics of each individual community will dictate, to some degree, the membership of the team. Generally, however, the members have all completed the NOVA CRT training, and they tend to include mental health practitioners, victim advocates, public safety individuals, members of the clergy, and other related professionals. NOVA reports that its CRTs perform the following three primary tasks:

1. helping local decision-makers identify all the groups at risk of experiencing trauma;
2. training the local caregivers who are to reach out to those groups after the CRT has left; and
3. leading one or more group crisis intervention sessions ("debriefings") to demonstrate how these sessions can help victims start to cope with their distress.

Approximately 4,000 crisis responders have received the NOVA training. Members of this group have responded to crisis locations around the globe: Oklahoma City after the Murrah building bombing; New York City after the Twin Towers attacks; southern Florida in the wake of Hurricane Andrew; Kobe, Japan after a killer earthquake claimed 7,000 lives; and Costa Rica after the shooting deaths of two American tourists. The training provided by NOVA consists of a 40-hour basic CRT training program that highlights organizational planning for responders as well as basic crisis intervention techniques for victims of trauma. Only upon the conclusion of this level of training is the CRT trainee eligible for the second level of advanced training, a 3-day course totaling 24 hours.

The days immediately following the terrorists attacks on September 11, 2001, saw NOVA CRTs employing their training at multiple sites related to the attacks. In Washington, DC, NOVA established a drop-in crisis center for members of the military suffering from the effects of the airplane crash into the Pentagon. Directly across from the Twin Towers, in Jersey City, New Jersey, NOVA provided crisis intervention and general support to the family members of the hundreds of dead, wounded, and missing. A NOVA CRT also worked with the flight attendants at Boston's Logan Airport, the point of departure for the two Towers-bound airplanes. For all of its work with crisis victims, NOVA was chosen as one of the "Best Human Services Charities" in the December, 2001, edition of *Worth Magazine*.

Governmental Crisis Services

This section will highlight the roles and contributions of three different government agencies during times of crisis and disaster: the Federal Emergency Management Agency (FEMA), the National Institute of Mental Health (NIMH), and the Center for Mental Health Services (CMHS).

Federal Emergency Management Agency

The Federal Emergency Management Agency (FEMA) was born out of an attempt to coordinate the many fragmented emergency and disaster activities with which state and local governments had to cope after a local disaster. For example, after hazards of nuclear power plants and the transportation of hazardous materials had been added to the list of possible disasters, there were more than 100 federal agencies involved at some level of a disaster response. In the 1970s the National Governors Association sought to decrease the number of agencies with which state and local governing bodies had to coordinate services. Due in part to their efforts, President Jimmy Carter in 1979 merged many of these disparate disaster-related responsibilities and functions by creating a new Federal Emergency Management Agency (FEMA).

An independent federal agency with more than 2,600 full-time employees, FEMA reports to the president of the United States and is charged with responding to, planning for, recovering from, and mitigating against disaster. It provides a broad range of services to locations declared disaster areas by the president of the United States. Whenever the size and extent of a disaster overwhelms the ability of state and local governments to respond effectively, the governor can request of the president that he make a disaster declaration in order to ensure federal intervention. Since 1979 FEMA has made a total of 906 disaster declarations, an average of 34 per year. Depending upon the disaster type, the decision regarding this declaration may take several hours or weeks. The intervention falls into two major categories: public assistance and individual assistance.

Public assistance programs generally consist of financial aid to state and local governments to pay for part of the cost of rebuilding the damaged infrastructure of affected communities. In addition to this repair and replacement function, FEMA's public assistance also includes prevention-oriented services. For example, after a devastating natural disaster, FEMA will assist in making replaced homes more flood or earthquake-resistant or in relocating those in chronically flood-ravaged areas.

FEMA's individual assistance programs generally include temporary disaster housing for those individuals displaced from their damaged or destroyed homes, cash grants for up to $14,800, low interest loans for homeowners or business owners for property loss and/or economic injury, and disaster grants for significant disaster-related needs or expenses not covered by other aid programs. Another disaster aid program is crisis counseling. According to FEMA, this counseling is provided "to help relieve any grieving, stress, or mental health problems caused or aggravated by the disaster or its aftermath." The help takes the form of supplemental funds to state and local mental health agencies and is available to the eligible survivors of presidentially declared major disasters.

FEMA also adopted, expanded, and supported the Community Emergency Response Team (CERT) concept, originally developed by the Los Angeles City Fire Department in 1985. Originally designed as a mode of disaster intervention for natural disasters such as fires and earthquakes, CERT underscored for FEMA the importance of preparing citizens to help out in just such crises. As a result, in 1993, FEMA adopted and expanded CERT training, making it available nationally; to date, 28 states and Puerto Rico have conducted CERT training. This training consists of seven weekly two-and-a-half hour sessions. Although most of the sessions are devoted to responding to the physical and safety needs of natural disaster victims, the sixth training session covers "Disaster Psychology and Team Organization." The training manual addresses the importance of "psychological first aid" for disaster-induced stress and trauma in those victims encountered at disaster sites. Toward that end, this component of CERT training covers the following areas:

- phases of a crisis;
- post-event psychological and physiological symptoms;
- humanizing the rescue operation;

- emotional first aid for rescuers; and
- emotional first aid for victims.

Trainees instructed in the last topic learn specific counseling techniques: establishing rapport, listening, empathizing, and providing confidentiality.

National Institute of Mental Health

A specialty division within the National Institute of Health, the National Institute of Mental Health (NIMH) is generally considered to be the gatekeeper of medical and behavioral research for the country. Since its formal establishment in 1949 via the National Mental Health Act (signed by President Truman), NIMH has had as its mission the diminishing of the burden of mental illness through research in basic neuroscience, behavioral science, and genetics. Ultimately, it sees as its goal the prevention of mental illness. Although a research branch of the federal government, NIMH has collaborated with FEMA in responding to community disasters by providing instruction, consultation, and expertise in the affected areas (James & Gilliland, 2001). This help included the provision of trained crisis counselors.

Center for Mental Health Services

The Center for Mental Health Services (CMHS) is a component of the Substance Abuse and Mental Health Services Administration (SAMHSA) of the Department of Health and Human Services. Since its inception in 1992, CMHS has become the federal government agency that leads the national efforts to promote mental health and to prevent mental illness. Its goal is to provide those treatment and support services for children and adults with serious emotional and mental disorders; CMHS administers programs and distributes funding for the delivery of theses services.

CMHS is organized into five divisions, including the Division of Prevention, Traumatic Stress, and Special Programs; among the many constituencies served by this division are those individuals affected by disasters and terrorism. Its Emergency Services and Disaster Relief Program recognizes that crisis counseling is just as important at a crisis site as is clearing debris and rebuilding property. Through an interagency agreement with FEMA, CMHS trains crisis counselors in presidentially declared disaster areas to provide immediate, short-term crisis counseling and ongoing support after federal relief workers leave the crisis/disaster site. This collaboration lead to the development of the *Field Manual for Mental Health and Human Services Workers in Major Disasters* (Department of Health and Human Services, 2000). Both agencies have administered a program based on this manual, also known as the Crisis Counseling Program (CCP), since 1974. The bombing of the Murrah Federal Building in Oklahoma City resulted in a shift in focus of the CCP, however, to one of planning and preparation for incidents of mass criminal victimization. This crisis event lead the CMHS to sign an agreement with the

Department of Justice's Office for Victims of Crime to coordinate training and technical assistance related to mass criminal incidents; the development of training curricula and other publications came out of this agreement. Additionally, the CMHS has increased its involvement with the U.S. Department of Education to assist with a coordinated federal response to school shootings and other violent events.

The events of September 11, 2001, also spawned the recovery project known as Project Liberty, a New York State program designed to aid individuals and families in coping with the aftereffects of the World Trade Center disaster. Sponsored by both FEMA and CMHS and administered by the New York State Office of Mental Health, Project Liberty is an illustrative example of a government-supported, collaborative effort among local and national government and local provider organizations. The range of services needed as a result of the Twin Towers attacks included individual and group counseling services, education services, and referrals to agencies or mental health professionals. LifeNet, a 24-hour, 7-day-a-week mental health information and referral hotline was a key component of Project Liberty.

Thus far, we have presented information about various governmental agencies and their roles in responding to national crises. We would be remiss however, if we didn't mention all of the local first responders who often risk their lives in dealing with the initial impact of a disaster. Local, county, and state police; firefighters; emergency medical services technicians; and emergency room personnel are often the first helpers to arrive on the scene of a major disaster, and in many instances they may be the only professionals available to help for several days, depending on the nature and scope of the disaster.

Crisis Services of Professional Organizations

It would be difficult, if not impossible, to determine the number of professional organizations involved in some way in crisis services. The American Red Cross (ARC) alone lists no less than 89 partner organizations comprising religious, community, business, and professional organizations. The ARC provides everything from training to information dissemination to consultation only to its partner groups. Other organizations provide training and crisis services of their own to their members and other interested parties. The following sections will examine just a few of those professional organizations and their crisis response services.

American Psychological Association

In recognition of the potentially devastating impact that crises or disasters of any type can have on the psychological well-being of individuals, the American Psychological Association (APA) determined that psychological intervention in the immediate aftermath of a traumatic event was critical in minimizing the long-term consequences of a crisis event. The APA responded to this need by developing its Disaster Response Network (DRN), the mechanism through which psychologists are able to respond to local and national disasters. Since the development of the DRN in 1992, more than 3,000 psychologists have volunteered their time and expertise to individuals and to communities in crisis.

Initially, the American Red Cross's disaster response capability did not include a mental health component. Prior to the development of any formal mental health training component, the ARC tended to utilize licensed mental health professionals to provide these services as part of its own disaster response. However, in December of 1991, the APA helped the ARC address this need by becoming the first national mental health organization to sign a joint Statement of Understanding with the agency, agreeing to collaborate with it in providing disaster mental health services to both disaster victims and relief workers. Thus, the primary function of the DRN was to facilitate joint disaster-related activities with the ARC. In the aftermath of Hurricane Andrew alone, more than 200 DRN psychologists assisted the Red Cross.

As part of this formal agreement, any psychologist choosing to participate is required to complete the ARC's Disaster Mental Health Services (DMHS) course for certification. This course, developed in consultation with the APA and other mental health organizations, also presumes that participating psychologists have some previous training via internships and other supervised experiences in mental health disorders. The DMHS course focuses primarily on basic Red Cross disaster operations and on the application of prior experience to a disaster response setting. Additional training, recommended but not required by the ARC, can be obtained either through university graduate courses or through other organizations such as NOVA. Other areas of training recommended by the APA include debriefing techniques, crisis intervention, traumatic stress reduction, death notification, and services to diverse and special needs populations.

American Counseling Association

In the same manner in which the APA forged its collaborative relationship with the Red Cross, the American Counseling Association (ACA) also signed a Statement of Understanding with the agency in 1994 for training for its membership and for coordination of mental health services during times of crisis. ACA members also would take the ARC's Disaster Mental Health Services course prior to volunteering their services at the disaster scene.

National Association of Social Workers

In 1997 the National Association of Social Workers (NASW) signed a 5-year partnership agreement with the ARC to provide disaster mental health services to victims, rescue workers, military personnel and their families, and refugees. Considering that the ARC's statistics indicated that social workers comprise the largest group of ARC disaster mental health-trained volunteers (40%) (American Red Cross, 2000), it would appear that this partnership has been productive.

National Association of School Psychologists

In the aftermath of the Murrah Federal Building bombing in Oklahoma City, the National Association of School Psychologists (NASP) decided to be proactive and to make a commitment to assist children, schools, and communities in coping with crisis events; the concurrent spate of school shootings also reinforced this commitment. Toward this end, NASP developed its own group to spearhead this process. This crisis-specific group became known as the National Emergency Assistance Team (NEAT), a group of seven nationally certified school psychologists who represent different regions of the country. While school-related traumatic events generally can be managed effectively internally (see chapter 9), some crisis situations require outside help. NEAT members respond to requests for assistance to this type of crisis. NEAT's intervention varies from situation to situation, ranging from consultation to direct involvement on the crisis scene, but only when invited. NASP has utilized NOVA's extensive training model for the development of its school Crisis Response Teams, considering the NOVA model to be a comprehensive one.

NASP's approach to crisis planning and intervention adheres to Caplan's (1964) model of "preventive psychiatry." That is, there are three different levels of response to crisis: *primary prevention,* involving the prevention of and preparation for crises; *secondary prevention,* involving the immediate response to crisis events; and *tertiary prevention,* involving the long-term and follow-up treatment of traumatized individuals (Brock, 2002; see chapter 9 for additional discussion of these levels).

Crisis Intervention With Groups

Crises are affecting an ever-increasing number of businesses, schools, and communities, and mass disasters are becoming virtually epidemic (Everly, Lating, & Mitchell, 2000). The Twin Towers attacks underscore the extent of the horror and chaos that a single event can generate, as well as the need for formalized crisis intervention programs, not for the individual victim of crisis, but for those large groups of crisis victims who are the focus of this chapter.

The group crisis intervention model, which is generally considered to be the most widely used model in the world for community-wide disasters (Everly, Lating, & Mitchell, 2000), is the model proposed by Mitchell (1983), himself a Maryland firefighter and paramedic. The model originally was designed to deal only with emergency responders, but it is now applied to individuals who have been the victims of some form of trauma. Mitchell's model is essentially a two-tier model encompassing *critical incident stress management*

(CISM), a comprehensive, integrative, multi-component crisis intervention system (Everly, Lating, & Mitchell, 2000), and *critical incident stress debriefing* (CISD), a group intervention that is one of the more important components of CISM. Although there are now several debriefing models, they all involve the same basic elements of Mitchell's model, therefore this section will highlight his model only. The Red Cross's model of disaster response also has been adapted from Mitchell's work.

Despite the criticisms of the single-session CISD model, which will be discussed in the next section of this chapter, single-session debriefing has been standard clinical practice after traumatic events (van Emmerik, Kamphuis, Hulsbosch, & Emmelkamp, 2002). As crisis intervention has evolved over the last 50 years, more sophisticated multi-component systems also have emerged (Everly, Flannery, & Eyler, 2002). CISM is an example of just such a crisis intervention model, born out of the belief that crisis intervention must be multi-faceted in order to be as effective as possible (Everly & Mitchell, 1999).

Critical Incident Stress Management

CISM is a comprehensive system of crisis intervention, encompassing the entire temporal spectrum of a crisis from the pre-crisis phase through the acute phase to the post-crisis phase (Everly, Lating, & Mitchell, 2000). Thus, the continuity of crisis services is consistent with Caplan's model (1964), covering primary, secondary, and tertiary interventions. Given the vast numbers of people who are impacted by the types of community-wide crises discussed in this chapter, the CISM approach also is comprehensive in that any of its components can be applied to large groups, organizations, or even communities.

CISM consists of the following seven core components. Each one of the following is designed to be conducted in either a large or small group format.

1. Pre-crisis preparedness training
   - This training is offered to emergency care providers within the community (e.g., police chiefs, health department officials, fire and rescue chiefs, hospital and community mental health representatives). It is somewhat similar to the school crisis team concept, but applied to the larger community. The training includes
     - the provision of information regarding the nature of stress and the nature of psychological trauma;
     - setting expectations regarding common types of crises and the stressors faced;
     - teaching about the most common signs of psychological distress;
     - teaching and rehearsing stress management and other coping techniques; behavioral rehearsal is key.
2. One-on-one individual counseling/psychological support

- Depending on the nature and severity of the crisis, this component calls for one to three contacts with an individual in crisis, with each contact lasting 15 minutes to 2 hours; if the individual remains unstable, referral to family, community, or other medical resources are appropriate.

3. Demobilization/decompression

- Designed for large groups, this component involves removal from the disaster site, food and rest in an informal setting, informational briefings, town meetings, and facilitating access to mental health resources.

4. Critical incident stress debriefing

- Critical incident stress debriefing (CISD) is a core component of the CISM system. In debriefing, specially trained crisis counselors gather a group of crisis victims together and encourage them to talk about their crisis experiences in a supported and controlled setting (see the section on CISD at the end of the chapter for elaboration). Debriefing sessions typically last 1 to 3 hours; they are provided 24 to 72 hours after the crisis.

5. Defusing

- Defusing sessions involve group discussion, and are a shortened version of CISD sessions; defusing sessions are only 20 to 45 minutes in duration. They are advisable immediately after a crisis (within 12 hour), and may eliminate the need for a formal debriefing session later. The purpose of defusing sessions is assessment, triage, and mitigation of acute symptoms.

6. Family crisis intervention

- In many instances, the entire family may be impacted by a particular disaster, and therefore, crisis counseling would be provided to the family as a whole.

7. Follow-up and referral component

- Referrals are made to psychological, medical, religious, legal, career, or other human services providers.

The CISM developers have emphasized that this approach, although an all-encompassing model of crisis intervention utilizing several technologies, is neither psychotherapy nor a substitute for it. Rather, it can more accurately be considered a "form of psychological first aid" (Everly, Lating, & Mitchell, 2000). It utilizes a systems approach and involves the individual, the family, community members in large groups, and other resources. CISD, on the other hand, is one component within this umbrella program, albeit the most widely used part of CISM. CISD, the generic term, has been replaced by the term CISM. Given the prominence of CISD as at least a crisis intervention step since 1983, the following section will analyze its components.

Critical Incident Stress Debriefing

One of the components of the broader array of services that are part of CISM is CISD. The debriefing usually involves two trained members of the response team, and the debriefing session generally takes from 1 to 3 hours to complete. It consists of seven phases during which crisis victims are allowed to talk about their crisis experiences in a supported, yet controlled setting. CISD's purpose is to mitigate the psychological impact of the traumatic event, restore homeostasis and equilibrium, prevent Posttraumatic Stress Disorder (PTSD), and identify people who require additional mental health follow-up beyond the session. The CISD session provides a structure that allows for the flow from cognitively mediated processing of the crisis event to a more emotionally involved experiencing of it, and then back again to a more educational, cognitive process. The structured educational component in particular is contraindicative of a psychotherapeutic process; CISD is not to be construed as therapy. The format for the session is described in the following sections.

PHASE 1: INTRODUCTION Critical for setting the tone and for the eventual success of the session, the team members will introduce themselves and of the purpose of the session. In addition to presenting an overview of the process, it is important to assure the participants of confidentiality and to explain to them the guidelines for the session. These guidelines or session "rules" should include:

- no outsiders allowed in the session;
- speak only for yourself;
- no interruptions in the session due to phone calls, etc.;
- no one is required to speak—participation is voluntary; and
- questions are welcomed at any time.

PHASE 2: FACT FINDING Description of the facts only is expected in this phase. Since facts are not emotionally laden and are only a direct recounting of the events, they are a relatively "safe" vehicle for the participants to use to talk about the crisis itself (Everly, Lating, & Mitchell, 2000; James & Gilliland, 2001). Participants are encouraged, though in no particular order and with no coercion at all, to tell the group what they saw, heard, or experienced during the crisis. Session leaders set the stage with a statement such as the following:

> Our team was not present during the crisis, so we only have a sketch of what happened. It would be helpful if you would fill us in on what happened, so that we can get an idea of what took place. Tell us who you are, what your role was during the event, and what happened from your point of view. We'll start over here, but if anyone prefers not to talk at this time, that's alright, too.

PHASE 3: THOUGHTS   The CISD leaders now move the participants to a more personal level, as they are asked to share their initial or most poignant thoughts about what happened (James & Gilliland, 2001). The transition from impersonal facts in the previous phase to more personal and emotional descriptions of these thoughts in this phase allows for emotions to surface.

PHASE 4: REACTION   Typically the most emotionally powerful of all the phases, the reaction phase should proceed naturally from the first three phases. Participants speak spontaneously in this phase and follow no particular order; the discussion is open-ended. Some possible leaders' questions that generate most of the discussion include the following:

- What was the worst thing about this situation for you personally?
- If you could erase one part of the situation, what part would it be?
- What aspect of the situation causes you the most pain?

Leaders will serve more as passive facilitators at this point, as the participants speak on their own to the questions posed (Mitchell & Everly, 1995).

PHASE 5: SYMPTOMS   The transition at this point is back toward more cognitive, rather than emotional, discussions. It should be noted that the end result of all debriefings is to bring the participants back to the cognitive level. The leaders question the group members regarding their affective, behavioral, cognitive, or physical experiences related to the crisis, focusing on any symptoms they can recall. The purpose behind this symptom-sharing is to demonstrate the universality of the crisis experience and the commonalities they all might share in the aftermath of the crisis.

PHASE 6: TEACHING   Once participants have shared their symptoms with the group, it is the role of the leaders in this phase to reaffirm to the group that what they described were typical and normal reactions to the crisis they had just encountered. Leaders also caution the group members about the possibility that they might develop other symptoms as time passes, thus preparing them for future concerns. Other topics of discussion that the leaders should introduce are those stress management techniques and other coping strategies for the members' present and future crisis-related symptoms. Once again, the instructional aspect of this phase moves the discussion further away from the emotional and into the cognitive realm.

PHASE 7: REENTRY   Possibly the most important phase of the formal debriefing process, it is the final opportunity to summarize the session and to bring closure to all of the issues that have been discussed. Leaders will answer questions, provide reassurance to the members, and make summary comments of the session. Participants also may be provided with additional information and feedback in the form of handouts. Group leaders should offer referral sources as deemed appropriate for follow-up assessment and therapy, and they should end the session by each providing summary statements of the session experience; appropriate ending comments would include words of encouragement, support, and direction. Finally, one way to achieve closure in a positive, uplifting way is for the leaders to provide feedback to the group about the common themes heard throughout the members' descriptions of their experiences, suggesting the universality of their stress reactions (Everly, Lating, & Mitchell, 2000).

There has been some criticism levied against the use of single-session debriefing as a response to the victims of crisis, suggesting that this procedure is at least ineffective, if not harmful (The Cochrane Library, 2002, 2001). Some mental health researchers fear that one-time debriefing sessions that educate people about their symptoms and encourage them to vent their emotions while offering no specific coping strategies could put crisis sufferers at risk by sending them out into the world without the ability to manage the psychological sequelae of the traumatic event. Additionally, considering the fact that most post-crisis symptoms, such as sleep disturbances, irritability, startle reactions, and great sadness, are normal reactions to traumatic events and will fade with time, even without treatment, debriefing may not be necessary.

Mitchell himself, the president of the International Critical Incident Stress Foundation, has supported the use of the CISM model, while emphasizing the fact that the single-session CISD is only one element of the multi-dimensional "umbrella" model, CISM. Criticism of the one-session model is congruent with Mitchell's belief that additional interventions must also be made for the intervention to be successful. He also attributed the poor outcome of these studies to the fact that some of these single-session debriefings either were conducted by poorly trained counselors or were thrust upon crisis victims without prior consent. Nevertheless, group debriefing sessions, whether part of a more inclusive crisis intervention model or not, continue to be utilized as an efficient means of reaching vast numbers of trauma victims and responders.

SOURCES OF CHAPTER ENRICHMENT

Print Sources

Erickson, K. (1994). *A new species of trouble: Explorations in disaster, trauma, and community.* New York: W.W. Norton & Company.

Gist, R. (1989). *Psychosocial aspects of disaster.* Hoboken, NJ: John Wiley & Sons.

Haddow, G., & Bullock, J. (2003). *Introduction to emergency management.* St. Louis, MO: Butterworth-Heineman.

Landesman, L. (2001). *Public health management of disaster: The practice guide.* Washington, DC: American Public Health Association.

Lee, R., & Lee, M. (1995). *Everything you need to know about natural disasters and post-traumatic stress disorder.* New York: Rosen Publishing.

Rosenbloom, D., & Williams, M. (1999). *Life after trauma: A workbook for healing.* Guilford Press.

Wright, T. (1993). *Wright's complete disaster survival manual: How to prepare for earthquakes, hurricanes, tornadoes, floods, wildfires, thunderstorms, tsunamis, and volcanic eruptions.* Charlottesville, VA: Hampton Roads Publishing.

Internet Sources

Federal Emergency Management Agency (http://www.fema.gov) FEMA provides a broad range of disaster services to any area of the country declared a disaster by the president of the United States.

American Red Cross (http://www.redcross.org) Each year, the American Red Cross responds to more than 67,000 disasters of all types. Although not a government agency, it provides shelter, food, and physical and mental health services to take care of basic human needs.

Substance Abuse and Mental Health Services Administration (http://www.mental-health.samhsa.gov) SAMHSA and FEMA coordinated the production of the *Field Manual for Mental Health and Human Services Workers in Major Disasters,* which can be ordered from this Web site.

National Organization for Victim Assistance (http://www.try-nova.org) This private, nonprofit agency provides advocacy and services for victims of violence and disaster. It provides disaster training nationwide for organizations.

National Voluntary Organizations Active in Disaster (http://www.nvoad.org) Although it does not provide direct disaster services itself, the organization coordinates the efforts and services of more than 35 other organizations that do.

REFERENCES

Administration for Children and Families. (2002). *How to report suspected child maltreatment*. Washington, DC: U.S. Department of Health and Human Services.

Aguirre-Molina, M., & Molina, C. (1994). Latino populations: Who are they? In C. W. Molina & M. Aguirre-Molina (Eds.), *Latino health in the U.S.: A growing challenge* (pp. 3–22). Washington, DC: American Public Health Association.

Allen, N. H. (1983). Homicide followed by suicide: Los Angeles, 1970–1979. *Suicide & Life Threatening Behavior, 13,* 155–165.

American Association of Suicidology. (1998). *Suicide postvention guidelines: Suggestions for dealing with the aftermath of suicide in the schools*. Washington, DC: Author.

American Counseling Association. (1995). *Code of ethics and standards of practice*. Alexandria, VA: Author.

American Medical Association. (1991). *Report of the Council of Scientific Affairs: Violence Against Women*. Proceedings of the House of Delegates, Chicago, IL.

American Psychiatric Association. (1994). *Diagnostic and Statistical Manual of Mental Disorders* (4th ed.). Washington, DC: Author.

American Psychiatric Association. (2000). *Diagnostic and Statistical Manual of Mental Disorders* (4th ed., text revision). Washington, DC: Author.

American Red Cross. (2000, August). *Disaster mental health services: Technical Update*. Washington, DC: Author.

Ammerman, R. T. (2000). Etiological models of child maltreatment: A behavioral perspective. *Behavior Modification, 14,* 230–254.

Ammerman, R., & Patz, R. (1996). Determinants of child abuse potential: Contribution of parent and child factors. *Journal of Clinical Child Psychology, 25,* 299–307.

Anderson, R. N. (2001). Deaths: Leading causes for 1999. *National Vital Statistics Report, 49*(11), Hyattsville, MD: National Center for Health Statistics. Available at http://www.cdc.gov/nchs/data/nvsr/nvsr49/nvsr49_11.pdf.

Andrews, J. A., & Lewinsohn, P. M. (1992). Suicidal attempts among older adolescents: Prevalence and co-occurrence with psychiatric disorders. *Journal of the American Academy of Child & Adolescent Psychiatry, 31,* 655–662.

Anthony, J. C., & Petronis, K. R. (1991). Suspected risk factors for depression among adults 18–44 years old. *Epidemiology, 2,* 123–132.

Anthony, J. C., Warner, L. A., & Kessler, R. C. (1997). Comparative epidemiology of dependence on tobacco, alcohol, controlled substances, and inhalants: Basic findings from the National Comorbidity Survey. In G. A. Marlatt & G. R. VandenBos, (Eds.) *Addictive behaviors: Readings on etiology, prevention and treatment* (pp. 3–39). Washington, DC: American Psychological Association

Appel, A., & Holden, G. (1998). The co-occurrence of spouse and physical child abuse: A review and appraisal. *Journal of Family Psychology, 12,* 577–579.

Avnet, J. (Producer), & Greenwald, R. (Director). (1984). *The burning bed* [TV movie]. United States: Tisch/Avnet Productions.

Barbaree, H. E. (1990). Stimulus control of sexual arousal: Its role in sexual assault. In W. L. Marshall, D. R. Laws, & H. E. Barbaree (Eds.), *Handbook of sexual assault: Issues, theories, and treatment of the offender* (pp. 115–142). New York: Plenum Press.

Barbaree, H. E. & Marshall, W. L. (1991). The role of male sexual arousal in rape: Six models. *Journal of Consulting and Clinical Psychology, 59,* 621–630.

Batemen, E. (1991). The context of date rape. In B. Levy (Ed.), *Dating violence: Young women in danger* (pp. 94–99). Seattle, WA: Seal.

Baumeister, R. F., Catanese, K. R., & Wallace, H. M. (2002). Conquest by force: A narcissistic reactance theory of rape and sexual coercion. *Review of General Psychology, 6*(1), 92–135.

Beautrais, A. L., Joyce, P. R., & Mulder, R. T. (1996). Prevalence and comorbidity of mental disorders in persons making serious suicide attempts: A case control study. *American Journal of Psychiatry, 153*, 1009–1014.

Beck, A. (1967). *Depression: Clinical, experimental and theoretical aspects.* New York: Harper & Row.

Beck, A. (1986). Hopelessness as a predictor of eventual suicide. *Annals of the New York Academy of Science, 487*, 90–96.

Beck, A., Brown, G., & Steer, R. (1989). Prediction of eventual suicide in psychiatric inpatients by clinical ratings of hopelessness. *Journal of Consulting and Clinical Psychology, 57*, 309–310.

Beck, A., & Steer, R. (1989). Clinical predictors of eventual suicide: A 5- to 10-year prospective study of suicide attempters. *Journal of Affective Disorders, 17*, 203–209.

Beck, A. T. (1991). Beck Scale for Suicide Ideation. San Antonio, TX: Psychological Corporation.

Beck, A. T. (1993). Beck Hopelessness Scale. San Antonio, TX: Psychological Corporation.

Beck, A. T. , Wright, F. D., Newman, C. F., & Liese, B. S. (1993). *Cognitive therapy of substance abuse.* New York: Guilford Press.

Beebe, D. K., & Walley, E. (1991). Substance abuse: The designer drugs. *American Family Physician, 43*, 1689–1698.

Bell, J. L. (1995). Traumatic event debriefing: Service delivery designs and the role of social work. *Social Work, 40*, 36–43.

Benson, R. T., & Sacco, R. L. (2000). Stroke prevention. *Neurologic Clinics of North America, 19*, 309–320.

Bergen, R. (1996). *Wife rape: Understanding the response of survivors and service providers.* Thousand Oaks, CA: Sage Publications.

Berglas, S. (1985). Why did this happen to me? *Psychology Today*, 44–48.

Bernard, J. L., & Bernard, M. L. (1984). The abusive male seeking treatment: Jekyll and Hyde. *Family Relations, 33*, 543–547.

Blader, J. C., & Marshall, W. L. (1989). Is assessment of sexual arousal in rapists worthwhile? A critique of current methods and the development of a response compatibility approach. *Clinical Psychology Review, 9*, 569–587.

Blumenreich, P. E., & Lewis, S. J. (1993). *Managing the violent patient: A clinician's guide.* Philadelphia, PA: Brunner/Mazel.

Bohen, S. (2002, June). Psychiatric emergencies. Seminar and workbook offered by PESI HealthCare LLC, Eau Claire, WI.

Bohner, G. (1998). *Rape myths.* Landau, Germany: Verlag Empirische Pädagogik.

Bowlby, J. (1980). *Attachment and loss: Loss, sadness and depression* (Vol. III). New York: Basic Books.

Bradford, J. M. W., Greenberg, D. M., & Motayne, G. G. (1992). Substance abuse and criminal behavior. *Psychiatric Clinics of North America, 15*, 605–622.

Bradley v. State of Mississippi, (1824). 1 Miss. 156

Brammer, L. M. (1985). *The helping relationship: Process and skills* (3rd ed.). Englewood Cliffs, NJ: Prentice-Hall.

Brecher, M., Wang, B. W., Wong, H., & Morgan, J. P. (1988). Phencyclidine and violence: Clinical and legal issues. *Journal of Clinical Psychopharmacology, 8*, 397–401.

Brehm, S., Kassin, S., & Fein, S. (2002). *Social psychology* (5th ed.). Boston: Houghton Mifflin Co.

Bridges, J. S., & McGrail, C. A. (1989). Attribution of responsibility for date and stranger rape. *Sex Roles, 21*, 273–286.

Brock, S. (2002). Crisis theory: A foundation for the comprehensive crisis prevention and intervention team. In S. Brock, P. Lazarus, & S. Jimerson (Eds.), *Best Practices in School Crisis Prevention and Intervention* (pp. 5–17). Bethesda, MD: NASP Publications.

Bronfenbrenner, U. (1979). *Ecology of human development.* Cambridge, MA: Harvard University Press.

Brown, S. L., & Forth, A. E. (1997). Psychopathology and sexual assault: Static risk factors, emotional precursors, and rapist subtypes. *Journal of Consulting and Clinical Psychology, 65*(5), 848–857.

Brownmiller, S. (1975). *Against our will: Men, women, and rape.* New York: Simon & Schuster.

Bureau of Justice Statistics. (2001). National Crime Victimization Survey. Washington, DC: U.S. Department of Justice, Office of Justice Programs. Data available at http://www.ojp.usdoj.gov/bjs/cvict.htm.

Burgess, A. W., & Holmstrom, L. L. (1974). Rape trauma syndrome. *American Journal of Psychiatry, 131*, 981–986.

Burnam, M. A., Stein, J. A., Golding, J. M., Siegel, J. M., Sorenson, S. B., Forsythe, A. B., & Telles, C. A. (1988). Sexual assault and mental disorders in a community population. *Journal of Consulting and Clinical Psychology, 56,* 843–850.

Campbell, A. (1993), *Men, women and aggression.* New York: Basic Books.

Campbell, R., & Raja, S. (1999). Secondary victimization of rape victims: Insights from mental health professionals who treat survivors of violence. *Violence and Victims, 14,* 261–275.

Cantor, C. H., & Slater, P. J. (1995). Marital breakdown, parenthood, and suicide. *Journal of Family Studies, 1,* 91–104.

Caplan, G. (1964). *Principles of preventative psychiatry.* New York: Basic Books.

Capuzzi, D., & Golden, L. (Eds.). (1988). *Preventing adolescent suicide.* Muncie, IN: Accelerated Development, Inc.

Capuzzi, D. (1994). *Suicide prevention in the schools: Guidelines for middle and high school settings.* Alexandria, VA: American Counseling Association.

Carkhuff, R. (1969). *Helping and human relations: A primer for lay and professional helpers.* New York: Holt, Rinehart, & Winston.

Carkhuff, R. R., & Berenson, B. G. (1977). *Counseling and psychotherapy: Theories and interventions.* Englewood Cliffs, NJ: Prentice-Hall.

Castro, F. G., Proescholdbell, R. J., Abeita, L., & Rodriquez, D. (1999). Ethnic and cultural minority groups. In B. S. McCrady & E. E. Epstein (Eds.), *Addiction: A comprehensive guidebook.* Oxford: Oxford University Press.

Cavaiola, A. A., & Schiff, M. (1988). Behavioral sequelae of physical and/or sexual abuse in adolescents. *Child Abuse & Neglect, 12,* 181–188.

Cavaiola, A. A., & Lavender, N. (1999). Suicidal behavior in chemically dependent adolescents. *Adolescence, 34,* 735–744.

Centers for Disease Control and Prevention. (1998). Suicide among black youths— United States, 1980–1995. *MMWR, 47*(10).

Chu, J. A. (1999). Trauma and suicide. In D. G. Jacobs (Ed.), *The Harvard Medical School guide to suicide assessment and intervention* (pp. 332–354). San Francisco: Jossey-Bass.

Clark, R. & Clark, J. (2001). *The encyclopedia of child abuse* (2nd ed.). New York: Facts on File.

Clary, E., Snyder, M ., Ridge, R., Copeland, J., Stukas, A., Haugen, J., & Miene, P. (1998). Understanding and assessing the motives of volunteers: A functional approach. *Journal of Personality and Social Psychology, 74,* 1516–1530.

Clayton, P. J., Desmarais, L., & Winokur, G. (1968). A study of normal bereavement. *American Journal of Psychiatry, 125,* 64–74.

Clinton, W. J. (Pres.). (1997, December 15). The President's Radio Address. *Weekly Compilation of Presidential Documents, 33*(50), 1993–2031. Washington, DC: Office of the Federal Registry.

Cochrane Database of Systematic Reviews. (2002). *Psychological debriefing for preventing post traumatic stress disorder (PTSD).* Available from http://www.ncbi.nim .nih.gov/entrez/query.fcgi

Coffin, C. (Ed.) (1952). *The complete poetry and selected prose of John Donne.* New York: Modern Library.

Copeland, A. R. (1985). Dyadic death— revisited. *Journal of the Forensic Science Society 25,* 181–188.

Crisis Prevention Institute. (1999). Nonviolent crisis intervention: A practical approach for managing violent behavior (training materials). *Violence Prevention Resource Center,* www.crisisprevention.com

Cross, T. L., Bazron, B. J., Dennis, K. W., & Isaacs, M. R. (1989). *Toward a culturally competent system of care.* Washington, D. C.: Georgetown University Child Development Center.

Crowley, T., Chesluk, D., Dilts, S., & Hart, R. (1974). Drug and alcohol abuse among psychiatric admissions. *Archives of General Psychiatry, 30,* 13–20.

Cull, J. G., & Gill, W. S. (1989). *Suicide Probability Scale.* Los Angeles, CA: Western Psychological Services.

Currens, S., Fritsch, T., Jones, D., et al. (1991). Homicide followed by suicide: Kentucky 1985–1990. *MMWR, 40,* 652–653, 659.

Daly, J., Gibson, D., Kopelson, A. (Producers); Stone, O. (Director) (1986) *Platoon,* Cinema 86

Dana, R. H. (1993). *Multicultural assessment perspectives for professional psychology.* Boston: Allyn & Bacon.

Davidson, M. W., Wagner, W. G., & Range, L. M. (1995). Clinician's attitudes toward no-suicide agreements. *Suicide & Life Threatening Behavior, 25,* 410–414.

Davis, D. I. (1984). Differences in the use of substances of abuse by psychiatric patients compared with medical and surgical patients. *Journal of Nervous and Mental Diseases, 172,* 654–657.

Davison, G., Neale, J., & Kring, A. (2004). *Abnormal psychology* (9th ed.). New York: John Wiley & Sons, Inc.

Decker, K. P., & Ries, R. K. (1993). Differential diagnosis and psychopharmacology of dual disorders. *Psychiatric Clinics of North America, 16,* 703–718.

Dinwiddie, S. W. (1994). Abuse of inhalants: A review. *Addiction, 89,* 925–929.

Dorpat, T. L. (1966). Suicide in murderers. *Psychiatry Digest, 27,* 51–55.

Doweiko, H. E. (1998). *Concepts of chemical dependency* (4th ed.). Belmont, CA: Wadsworth/Brooks/Cole.

Dutton, D. G. (1995). *The batterer: A psychological profile.* New York: Basic Books.

Dutton, D. G. (1996). *The Domestic Assault of Women.* Vancouver: UBC Press.

Dutton, D. (1998). *The Abusive Personality.* New York: Guilford Press.

Dwyer, K., & Osher, D. (2000). *Safeguarding our children: An action guide.* Washington, DC: U.S. Departments of Education and Justice, American Institutes for Research.

Dwyer, K., Osher, D., & Warger, C. (1998). *Early warning, timely response: A guide to safe schools.* Washington, DC: U.S. Department of Education.

Dyer, J., & Kreitman, N. (1984). Hopelessness, depression and suicidal intent in parasuicide. *British Journal of Psychiatry, 144,* 127–133.

Edleson, J. L., & Tolman, R. M. (1992). *Intervention for men who batter.* Newbury Park, CA: Sage Publishers.

Edwards, S. M. (1989). *Policing domestic violence: Women, the law and the state.* London: Sage.

Eckhardt, C., Barbour, K., Davison, G. (1998). Articulated thoughts of martially violent and nonviolent men during anger arousal. *Journal of Consulting and Clinical Psychology, 66,* 229–269.

Egan, M. P. (1997). Contracting for safety: A concept analysis. *Crisis, 18,* 17–23.

Eisen, S. V., Grob, M. C., & Dill, D. L. (1987). *Substance abuse in a generic inpatient population* (McLean Hospital Evaluative Service Unit, Report No. 71). Belmont, MA: McLean Hospital.

Eisen, S. V., Grob, M. C., & Dill, D. L. (1988). *Substance abuse in an inpatient population: A comparison of patients on Appleton and generic units* (McLean Hospital Evaluative Service Unit, Report No. 75). Belmont, MA: McLean Hospital.

Ellis, A. E., & Ratliff, K. (1986). Cognitive characteristics of suicidal and nonsuicidal psychiatric patients. *Cognitive Therapy and Research, 1,* 625–634.

Encyclopedia of Associations (Vol. 1, Pt. 3, 41st ed.). (2004). Farmington Hills, MI: Thomson Gale.

Ensink, B., & Van Berlo, W. (2000). Problems with sexuality after sexual assault. *Annual Review of Sex Research, 11,* 235–257.

Erikson, E. (1963). *Childhood and society* (2nd ed.). New York: Norton Press.

Evans, P. (1992). *The verbally abusive relationship.* Holbrook, MA: Adams Media Corporation.

Evans, W. N. (1998). Assessment and diagnosis of the substance use disorders (SUDs). *Journal of Counseling & Development, 76,* 325–333.

Everly, G., Flannery, R., & Eyler, V. (2002). Critical incident stress management (CISM): A statistical review of the literature. *Psychiatric Quarterly, 73,* 171–182.

Everly, G., Lating, J., & Mitchell, J. (2000). Innovations in group crisis intervention. In A. Roberts (Ed.), *Crisis intervention handbook* (2nd ed., pp. 77–97). New York: Oxford University Press.

Everly, G., & Mitchell, J. (1999). *Critical incident stress management: A new era and standard of care in crisis intervention* (3rd ed.). Ellicott City, MD: Chevron.

Fawcett, J., Scheftner, W., Fogg, L., Clark, D., Young, M., Hedeker, D., & Gibbons, R. (1990). Time-related predictors of suicide in major affective disorder. *American Journal of Psychiatry, 147,* 1189–1194.

Federal Bureau of Investigation. (2000). Uniform Crime Reports. Washington, DC: U.S. Department of Justice. Data available at http://www.fbi.gov/ucr/ucr.htm.

Feeney, J., & Noller, P. (1996). *Adult attachment.* Thousand Oaks, CA: Sage Publications.

Finkelhor, D., & Korbin, J. (1988). Child abuse as an international issue. *Child Abuse and Neglect, 12,* 3–23.

Fischer, D., Halikas, J., Baker, J., & Smith, J. (1975). Frequency and patterns of drug abuse in psychiatric patients. *Diseases of the Nervous System, 36,* 550–553.

Fitch, F. J., & Papantonio, A. (1983). Men who batter: Some personality characteristics. *Journal of Nervous and Mental Disease, 171,* 190–192.

Foa, E. B., & Rothbaum, B. O. (1998). *Treating the trauma of rape: Cognitive behavioral therapy for PTSD.* New York: Guilford Press.

Foa, E. B., Rothbaum, B. O., Riggs, D. S., & Murdock, T. B. (1991). Treatment of posttraumatic stress disorder in rape victims: A comparison between cognitive-behavioral procedures and counseling. *Journal of Consulting and Clinical Psychology, 5* for doing crisis intervention and brief therapy from a process view. *Crisis Intervention and Time-Limited Treatment, 4,* 159–177.

Frazier, P. A. (1990). Victim attribution and post-rape trauma. *Journal of Personality an Social Psychology, 59*(2), 298–304.

Frierson, R. L., Melikian, M., & Wadman, P. C. (2002). Principles of suicide risk assessment. *Postgraduate Medicine, 112*(3), 69–71. Available at www.postgradmed.com /issues/2002/09_02/frierson4.htm

Furman, E. (1974). *A child's parent dies: Studies in childhood bereavement.* New Haven, CT: Yale University Press.

Gallo, J. J., Royall, D. R., & Anthony, J. C. (1993). Risk factors for the onset of depression in middle age and later life. *Social Psychiatry & Psychiatric Epidemiology, 28,* 101–108.

Gardner, R. (1987). *The parental alienation syndrome and the differentiation between fabricated and genuine child sex abuse.* Cresskill, NJ: Creative Therapeutics.

Garrison, C. Z., McKeown, R. E., & Valois, R. F. (1993). Aggression, substance use and suicidal behaviors in high school students. *American Journal of Public Health, 83,* 179–184.

Geffner, R., Mantooth, C., & Franks, D. (1989). A psychoeducational, conjoint therapy approach to reducing family violence. In P. L. Caesar & L. K. Hamberger (Eds.), *Treating men who batter: Theory, practice and programs* (pp. 103–133). New York: Springer.

Geffner, R., & Pagelow, M. D. (1990). Mediation and custody issues in abusive relationships. *Behavioral Science & the Law, 8,* 151–159.

Gilmartin, P. (1994). *Rape, incest, and child sexual abuse: Consequences and recovery.* New York: Garland Publishing, Inc.

Gladding, S. (1999). *Counseling: A comprehensive profession* (4th ed.). New York: Prentice-Hall.

Golan, N. (1978). *Treatment in crisis situations.* New York: Free Press.

Goldberg, L. (Producer), & Rubin, J. (Director). (1991). *Sleeping with the enemy* [Motion Picture]. United States: Twentieth Century Fox.

Granvold, D. K. (2000). The crisis of divorce: Cognitive-behavioral and constructivist assessment and treatment. In A. R. Roberts (Ed.) *Crisis intervention handbook: Assessment, treatment and research.* New York: Oxford University Press.

Greenstone, J., & Leviton, S. (1993). *Elements of crisis intervention.* Belmont, CA: Brooks/Cole Publishing.

Group for the Advancement of Psychiatry. (1989). *Suicide and ethnicity in the United States* (GAP Report 128). Formulated by the Committee on Cultural Psychiatry, Washington, DC.

Haft, S., Witt, P. J., & Thomas, T. (Producers); Weir, P. (Director) (1989) *Dead Poets Society,* Touchstone Pictures.

Hall, G. C. N. (1989). Sexual arousal and arousability in a sexual offender population. *Journal of Abnormal Psychology, 98,* 145–149.

Hall, G. C., & Hirschman, R. (1991). Toward a theory of sexual aggression: A quadripartite model. *Journal of Consulting and Clinical Psychology, 59,* 662–669.

Hamberger, L. K., & Barnett, O. W. (1995). Assessment and treatment of men who batter. In L. VandeCreek & S. Knapp (Eds.), *Innovations in clinical practice: A source book* (Vol. 14, pp. 31–54). Sarasota, FL: Professional Resource Press.

Hamberger, L. K., & Hastings, J. (1986). Personality correlates of men who abuse their partners: A cross validation study. *Journal of Family Violence, 1,* 323–341.

Hanzlick, R., & Koponen, M. (1994). Murder-suicide in Fulton County, Georgia, 1988–1991. *American Journal of Forensic Medical Pathology, 15,* 168–173.

Hare, R. D. (1993). *Without conscience: The disturbing world of psychopaths among us.* New York, NY: Guilford Press.

Harwood, H. J., Napolitano, D. M., Kristiansen, P. L., & Collins, J. J. (1984). *Economic costs to society of alcohol and drug abuse and mental illness: 1980* (Publication No. RTI/2734/00001FR). Research Triangle Park, NC: Research Triangle Institute.

Herman, J. (1997). *Trauma and recovery: The aftermath of violence—From domestic abuse to political terror.* New York: Basic Books.

Horton, C. (1995). Best practices in the response to child maltreatment. In A. Thomas & T. Grimes (Eds.), *Best practices in school psychology III* (pp. 963–976). Washington, DC: National Association of School Psychologists.

Horton, C., & Cruise, T. (1997). Child sexual abuse. In G. Bear, K. Minke, & A. Thomas

(Eds.), *Children's needs II: Development, problems, and alternatives* (pp. 719–727). Bethesda, MD: National Association of School Psychologists.

Hotaling, G. T., & Sugarman, D. B. (1986). An analysis of risk markers in husband to wife violence: The current state of knowledge. *Violence & Victims, 1,* 101–124.

Hymen, S. E., & Cassem, N. H. (1995). Alcoholism. *In Scientific American medicine.* (Rubenstein, E., & Federman, D. D., eds.). New York: Scientific American Press.

Individuals With Disabilities Education Act of 1997, Pub. L. No. 105–17, S 1 et seq.

Independent Sector. (1994). *Giving and volunteering in the United States: Findings from a national survey.* Washington, DC: Author.

Independent Sector. (2002, February 15). *Giving and volunteering in the United States.* Retrieved February 15, 2002, from http://www.independentsector.org/media/voltime02PR.html

Jaffe, S. R. (Producer); Benton, R. (Director) (1979) *Kramer vs. Kramer,* Columbia Pictures

Jacobson, N. & Gottman, J. (1998). *When Men Batter: New Insights into Ending Abusive Relationships.* New York: Simon and Schuster.

James, R. & Gilliland, B. (2001). *Crisis intervention strategies* (4th ed.). Belmont, CA: Wadsworth/Brooks Cole.

Johnson, V. (1980). *I'll quit tomorrow: A practical guide to alcoholism treatment.* San Francisco, CA: Harper Collins.

Johnston, L. D., O'Malley, P. M., & Bachman, J. G. (1995). National survey results on drug use from the Monitoring the Future Study, 1975–1994: Vol. 1. Secondary school students. (NIH Publication No. 95–4026). Washington, DC: Government Printing Office.

Kachur, S., Potter, L., James, S., & Powell, K. (1995). *Suicide in the United States, 1980–1992* (Violence Surveillance Summary Series, No. 1). Atlanta: Centers for Disease Control and Prevention, National Center for Injury Prevention and Control.

Kanel, K. (2003). *A guide to crisis intervention* (2nd ed.). Pacific Grove, CA: Brooks/Cole Publishing.

Kassinove, H. (Ed.). (1995). *Anger disorders.* Washington, DC: Taylor Francis.

Kaufman, J. & Ziegler, E. (1987). Do abused children become abusive parents? *American Journal of Orthopsychiatry, 57,* 186–192.

Kendall, P., & Hammen, C. (1998). *Abnormal psychology: Understanding human problems.* Boston: Houghton Mifflin Co.

Kessler, R. C., McGonagle, K. A., Ahzo, S., Nelson, C. H., Hughes, M., Kovacs, M. (1996). Children's Depression Inventory. Los Angeles, CA: Western Psychological Services.

Kilpatrick, D. G., Best, C. L., Veronen, L. J., Amick, A. E., Villeponteaux, L. E., & Ruff, G. A. (1985). Mental health correlates of victimization: A random community survey. *Journal of Consulting and Clinical Psychology, 53,* 866–873.

Kilpatrick, D. G., Edmunds, C. N., & Seymour, A. K. (1992). *Rape in America: A report to the nation.* Arlington, VA: National Victim Center.

Kilpatrick, D. G., Saunders, B. E., Veronen, L. J., Best, C. L., & Von, J. M. (1987). Criminal victimization: Lifetime prevalence, reporting to the police, and psychological impact. *Crime and Delinquency, 33,* 479–489.

Kim, S., McLeod, J. H., & Shantzis, C. (1992). Cultural competence for evaluators working with Asian American communities: Some practical considerations. In M. A. Orlandi, R. Weston, & L. G. Epstein (Eds.), *Cultural competence for evaluators* (pp. 203–260). Washington, DC: Office of Substance Abuse Prevention.

Klassen, D., & O'Connor, W. A. (1988). A prospective study of predictors of violence in adult male mental health admissions. *Law & Human Behavior, 12,* 143–158.

Klein, A. (1996). Re-abuse in a population of court-restrained male batterers: Why restraining orders don't work. In E. S. Buzawa & C. G. Buzawa (Eds.), *Do arrests and restraining orders work?* (pp. 192–213). Thousand Oaks, CA: Sage Publications.

Kleinman, A. (1991, April). *Culture and DSM-IV: Recommendations for the introduction and overall structure.* Paper presented at the National Institute of Mental Health Conference on Culture and Diagnosis, Pittsburgh, PA.

Klingbeil, K. S., & Boyd, V. D. (1984). Emergency room intervention: Detection, assessment and treatment. In A. R. Roberts (Ed.), *Battered women and their families: Intervention strategies and treatment programs* (pp. 7–32). New York: Springer.

Koss, M. P. (1993). Rape: Scope, impact, interventions, and public policy responses. *American Psychologist, 10,* 1062–1079.

Koss, M. P. & Harvey, M. R. (1991). *The rape victim: Clinical and community interventions.* Newbury Park, CA: Sage Publications.

Koss, M. P., Woodruff, W. J., & Koss, P. (1991). Criminal victimization among primary care medical patients: Prevalence, incidence, and physician usage. *Behavioral Sciences and the Law, 9,* 85–96.

Kubany, E. S., Leisen, M. B., Kaplan, A. S., & Kelley, M. P. (2000). Validation of a brief measure of posttraumatic stress disorder: The distressing event questionnaire. *Psychological Assessment, 12,* 197–209.

Kubler-Ross, E. (1969). *On death and dying.* New York: Macmillan.

Labell, L. (1972). Wife abuse: A sociological study of battered women and their mates. *Victimology, 4,* 258–267.

Lachkar, J. (1998). *The many faces of emotional abuse.* Northvale, NJ: Jason Aronson.

Lanceley, F. (1999). *On scene guide for crisis negotiators.* Boca Raton, FL: CRC Press.

Lehmann, N., & Krupp, S. (1984). Alcohol-related domestic violence: Clinical implications and intervention strategies. *Alcoholism Treatment Quarterly, 1,* 111–115.

Lehman, L. B., Pilich, A., & Andrews, N. (1994). Neurological disorders resulting from alcoholism. *Alcohol Health & Research World, 17,* 305–309.

Lerner, M. J. (1980). *The belief in a just world: A fundamental delusion.* New York: Plenum.

Levinson, D. J. (1978). *The seasons of a man's life.* New York: Alfred A. Knopf.

Lewis, D. C. (1997). The role of the generalist in the care of the substance-abusing client. *Medical Clinics of North America, 81,* 831–843.

Lichtenstein, R., Schonfeld, D., & Kline, M. (1994). How to respond to and prepare for a crisis. *Educational Leadership, 52,* 79–83.

Lidell, H. G., & Scott, R. (1968). *The Greek-English lexicon.* Oxford: Clarendon Press.

Lindemann, E. (1944). Symptomotology and management of acute grief. *American Journal of Psychiatry, 101,* 141–148.

Linehan, M. M. (1999). Standard protocol for assessing and treating suicidal behaviors for patients in treatment. In D. G. Jacobs (Ed.), *The Harvard Medical School guide to suicide assessment and intervention* (pp. 146–187). San Francisco: Jossey-Bass.

Litwack, T., Kirschner, S., & Wack, R. (1993). The assessment of dangerousness and prediction of violence: Recent research and future prospects. *Psychiatric Quarterly, 64,* 245–273.

Lonsway, K. A. & Fitzgerald, L. F. (1994). Rape myths: In review. *Psychology of Women Quarterly, 18,* 133–164.

Loos, M., & Alexander, P. (1997). Differential effects associated with self-reported histories of abuse and neglect in a college sample. *Journal of Interpersonal Violence, 12,* 340–360.

Lowenthal, B. (2001). *The educator's guide to the identification and prevention of child abuse.* Baltimore, MD: Paul H. Brookes Publishing.

Mahoney, P., & Williams, L. (1998). Sexual assault in marriage: Prevalence, consequences and treatment of wife rape. In J. Jasinski & L. Williams (Eds.), *Partner Violence: A Comprehensive Review of 20 Years of Research* (pp. 113–162). Thousand Oaks, CA: Sage.

Malamuth, M. A. (1996). The confluence model of sexual aggression: Feminist and evolutionary perspectives. In D. M. Buss & N. M. Malamuth (Eds.), *Sex, power, conflict: Evolutionary and feminist perspectives* (pp. 269–295). New York: Oxford University Press.

Malamuth, N. M. (1981). Rape proclivity among males. *Journal of Social Issues, 37,* 138–157.

Malamuth, N. M. (1998). The confluence model as organizing framework for research on sexually aggressive men: Risk moderators, imagined aggression, and pornography consumption. In R. G. Geen & E. Donnerstein (Eds.), *Human aggression: Theories, research, and implications for social policy* (pp. 230–247). San Diego: Academic Press.

Malamuth, N. M., & Check, J. V. P. (1983). Sexual arousal to rape depictions: Individual differences. *Journal of Abnormal Psychology, 92,* 55–67.

Malley, P. B., Kush, F., & Bogo, R. J. (1994). School-based adolescent suicide prevention and intervention programs: A survey. *The School Counselor, 42,* 130–136.

Maltsberger, J. T. (1992). The psychodynamic formulation: An aid in assessing suicidal risk. In R. W. Maris, A. L. Berman, J. T. Maltsberger, & R. T. Yufit (Eds.), *Assessment and prediction of suicide* (pp. 362–380), New York: Guilford Press.

Margolin, L. (1992). Rape: The facts. *Women: A Journal of Liberation, 3,* 19–22.

Marin, G., & Marin, B. V. (1991). *Research with Hispanic populations.* Newbury Park, CA: Sage Publications.

Maris, R. W. (1992). The relationship of nonfatal suicide attempts to completed suicides. In R. W. Maris, A. L. Berman, J. T. Maltsberger, & R. T. Yufit (Eds.) *Assessment and prediction of suicide* (pp. 362–380), New York: Guilford Press.

Martin, P., & Hummer, R. (1989). Fraternities and rape on campus special issue: Violence against women. *Gender and Society, 3*, 457–473.

Marzuk, P. M., Tardiff, K., & Hirsch, C. S. (1992). The epidemiology of murder-suicide. *Journal of the American Medical Association, 267*, 3179–3183.

Mayer, N. (1978). *The male mid-life crisis: Fresh starts after 40.* Oxford: Doubleday.

Maxmen, J. S., & Ward, N. G. (1995). *Essential psychopathology and its treatment* (2nd ed.). New York: W. W. Norton & Co.

McCrady, B. S., & Epstein, E. E. (1999). *Addictions: A comprehensive guidebook* Oxford, England: Oxford University Press.

McNeil, D., & Binder, R. (1991). Clinical assessment of risk of violence among psychiatric inpatients. *American Journal of Psychiatry, 148*, 1317–1321.

Meadows, R. J. (1998). *Understanding violence and victimization.* Upper Saddle River, NJ: Prentice Hall.

Meloy, J. (1987). The prediction of violence in outpatient psychotherapy. *The American Journal of Psychotherapy, 41*, 38–45.

Metropolitan Life Survey of the American Teacher. (1999). *Violence in America's public schools: Five years later.* Retrieved December 8, 2002, from http://metlife.com /Applications/Corporate/WPS/CDA/Pag eGenerator.html.

Miller, D. (1994). *Women who hurt themselves.* New York: Basic Books.

Miller, M. C. (1999). Suicide-prevention contracts: Advantages, disadvantages and an alternative approach. In D. G. Jacobs (Ed.) *The Harvard Medical School guide to suicide assessment and intervention* (pp. 463–481). San Francisco: Jossey-Bass.

Milzman, D. P., & Soderstrom, C. A. (1994). Substance use disorders in trauma patients. *Critical Care Clinics, 10*, 595–612.

Mitchell, J. (1983). When disaster strikes … The critical incident stress debriefing process. *Journal of Emergency Medical Services, 8*, 36–39.

Mitchell, J., & Everly, G . (1995). *Critical incident stress debriefing: An operations manual.* Ellicott City, MD: Chevron.

Molin, R. S. (1986) Covert suicide and families of adolescents. *Adolescence, 21*, 177–184.

Monahan, J. (1995). *The clinical prediction of violent behavior.* Northvale, NJ: Jason Aronson.

Mooney, J. (2000). *Gender, violence, and the social order.* New York: Palgrave.

Moore, T. (1999). In B. O'Connell & R. Taylor (Eds.), *Voices from the heart: In celebration of America's Volunteers* (pp. 8–11). San Francisco: Jossey-Bass Publishers.

Moorehead, C. (1998). *Dunant's dream: War, Switzerland, and the history of the Red Cross.* Berkeley, CA: Publisher's Group West.

Mosher, D., & Tomkins, S. (1987). Scripting the macho man: Hypermasculine Socialization and Enculturation. *Journal of Sex Research, 25*, 60–84.

Motto, J. A. (1999). Critical points in the assessment and management of suicidal risk. In D. G. Jacobs (Ed.), *The Harvard Medical School guide to suicide assessment and intervention* (pp. 224–238). San Francisco: Jossey-Bass.

Mulvey, E., & Lidz, C. (1995). Conditional prediction: A model for research on dangerousness to others in a new era. *International Journal of Law & Psychiatry, 8*, 129–143.

Murphy, S. A., & Johnson, C., & Cain, K. C. (1998). Broad spectrum group treatment for parents bereaved by the violent deaths of their 12–28-year-old children: A randomized controlled trial. *Death Studies, 22*, 209–235.

Myer, R. (2001). *Assessment for crisis intervention.* Belmont, CA: Brooks/Cole.

National Center on Child Abuse and Neglect Information. (2003). *About the federal child abuse prevention and treatment act.* Washington, DC: U.S. Department of Health and Human Services.

National Crime Victimization Survey. (2003). *Crime and victims statistics.* Washington, DC: U.S. Department of Justice, Bureau of Justice Statistics.

National Highway Traffic Safety Administration. (1998). *Alcohol traffic safety facts 1997.* Washington, DC: US Department of Transportation.

National Institute of Mental Health. (2002). Suicide facts and statistics. Retrieved April 8, 2002 from http://www.nimh.nih .gov/suicideprevention/suifact.cfm.

National Organization for Victim Assistance. (1998). *Community crisis response team training manual* (2nd ed.). Washington, DC: Author.

National Violence Against Women Survey. (2000). *Findings from the National Violence Against Women Survey.* Washington, DC: U.S. Department of Justice, Bureau of Justice Statistics.

New York Times (September, 2001). *After the attacks: Counseling; Some therapists fear services could backfire.*

Nietzel, M., Speltz, M., McCauley, E., & Bernstein, E. (1998). *Abnormal psychology.* Needham Heights, MA: Allyn & Bacon.

Nock, M. K., & Marzuk, P. M. (1999). Murder-suicide: Phenomenology and clinical implications. In D. G. Jacobs (Ed.) *The Harvard Medical School guide to suicide assessment and intervention* (pp. 188–209). San Francisco: Jossey-Bass.

Oates, R. K. (1996). *The spectrum of child abuse: Assessment, treatment, and prevention.* New York: Brunner/Mazel, Inc.

Odem, M. E., & Clay-Warner, J. (1998). *Confronting rape and sexual assault.* Wilmington, DE: Scholarly Resources, Inc.

Oliver, J. E. (1993). Intergenerational transmission of child abuse: Rates, research, and clinical implications. *American Journal of Psychiatry, 150,* 1315–1325.

Organ, D. (1994). Personality and organizational citizenship behavior. *Journal of Management, 20,* 465–478.

Osofsky, J. (Ed.). (1998). *Children in a violent society.* New York: The Guilford Press.

Paget, K. (1997). Child neglect. In G. Bear, K. Minke, & A. Thomas (Eds.), *Children's needs II: Development, problems, and alternatives* (pp. 729–740). Bethesda, MD: National Association of School Psychologists.

Palmer, S., & Humphrey, J. A. (1980). Offender-victim relationships in criminal homicide followed by offender's suicide, North Carolina, 1972–1977. *Suicide & Life Threatening Behavior, 10,* 106–118.

Parent Resource Institute for Drug Education. (1999). *Pride questionnaire report.* Retrieved August 10, 2001, from http://www.pridesurveys.com/main/supportfiles/natsum99.pdf

Parkes, C. M. (1970). "Seeking" and "finding" a lost object: Evidence from recent studies of the reaction to bereavement. *Social Science & Medicine, 4,* 187–201.

Parkes, C. M., & Weiss, R. S. (1983). *Recovery from bereavement.* New York: Basic Books.

Patterson, W. M., Dohn, H. H., Bird, J. et al. (1983). Evaluation of suicidal patients: The SAD PERSONS scale. *Psychosomatics, 24,* 343–349.

Payne, C. (1999). Tragedy response and healing—Springfield unites. In A. S. Canter & S. A. Carroll (Eds.), *Crisis prevention and response: A collection of NASP resources* (pp. 187–190). Washington, DC: National Association of School Psychologists.

Penner, L., & Finkelstein, M. (1998). Dispositional and structural determinants of volunteerism. *Journal of Personality and Social Psychology, 74,* 525–537.

Penner, L., Fritzsche, B., Craiger, J., & Freifeld, T. (1995). Measuring the prosocial personality. In J. Butcher & C. D. Spielberger (Eds.), *Advances in personality assessment* (pp. 147–163). Hillsdale, NJ: Erlbaum.

Peters, K. D., Kochanek, K. D., Murphy, S. L. (1998). Deaths: Final data for 1996. *National Vital Statistics Report, 47*(9), Hyattsville, MD: National Center for Health Statistics. Available at http://www.cdc.gov/nchs/data/nvsr/nvsr47/nvs47_09.pdf

Petersen v. State of Washington, Wash. 2d 421, 671 P.2d 230 (1983) (en banc).

Peterson, S., & Straub, R. (1992). *School crisis survival guide.* West Nyack, NY: The Center for Applied Research in Education.

Petronis, K. R., Samuels, J. F., & Moscicki, E. K. (1990). An epidemiological investigation of potential risk factors for suicide attempts. *Social Psychiatry & Psychiatric Epidemiology, 35,* 193–199.

Pitcher, G., & Poland, S. (1992). *Crisis intervention in the schools.* New York: The Guilford Press.

Poland, S. (1994). The role of school crisis intervention teams to prevent and reduce school violence and trauma. *School Psychology Review, 23,* 175–189.

Poland, S., & McCormick, J. (1999). *Coping with crisis: Lessons learned.* Longmont, CO: Sopris West.

Poland, S., Pitcher, G., & Lazarus, P.(1995). Crisis intervention. In A. Thomas & J. Grimes (Eds.), *Best practices in school psychology—III* (pp. 445–458). Washington, DC: The National Association of School Psychologists.

Pollard, P. (1992). Judgment about victims and attackers in depicted rapes: A review. *Journal of Social Psychology, 31,* 307–326.

Pope, H. G., & Katz, D. L. (1990). Homicide and near-homicide by anabolic steroid users. *Journal of Clinical Psychiatry, 51,* 28–31.

Pope, H. G., & Katz, D. L. (1994). Psychiatric and medical effects of anabolicandrogenic steroid use: A controlled study of 160 athletes. *Archives of General Psychiatry, 51*, 375–382.

Prater, C. D., Miller, K. E., & Zylstra, R. G. (1999). Outpatient detoxification of the addicted or alcoholic patient. *American Family Physician, 60*, 1175–1183.

Quackenbush, R. L. (1989). A comparison of androgynous, masculine sex-types, and undifferentiated males on dimensions of attitudes towards rape. *Journal of Research in Personality, 23*, 318–342.

Rape, Abuse, and Incest National Network. (2001). RAINN Statistics Archive. http://www.rainn.org/statistics.html

Rando, T. (1984). *Grief, dying and death: Clinical interventions for caregivers,* Champaign, IL: Research Press.

Rando, T. (1986) *Parental loss of a child.* Champaign, IL: Research Press.

Reed, B. J., & May, P. A. (1984). Inhalant abuse and juvenile delinquency: A control study in Albuquerque, New Mexico. *International Journal of Addictions, 19*, 789–803.

Rein, M., Jacobs, N., & Quiram, J. (Eds.). (2001). *Child abuse: Betraying a trust.* Wylie, TX: Information Plus.

Reinecke, M. A. (2000). Suicide and depression. In F. M. Dattilio & A. Freeman (Eds.), *Cognitive-behavioral strategies in crisis intervention* (pp. 84–125). New York: Guilford Press.

Remley, T. P., & Herlihy, B. (2001). *Ethical, legal and professional issues in counseling.* Upper Saddle River, NJ: Merrill/Prentice Hall.

Resick, P. A. (1992). Cognitive treatment of crime-related post-traumatic stress disorder. In R. Peters, R. McMahon, & V. Quincy (Eds.), *Aggression and violence throughout the life span* (pp. 171–191). Newbury Park, CA: Sage.

Reynolds, W. M. (1991). Adult Suicidal Ideation Questionnaire. Odessa, FL: Psychological Assessment Resources Inc.

Reynolds, W. M. (1992). Suicidal Ideation Questionnaire. Odessa, FL: Psychological Assessment Resources Inc.

Reynolds, W. M., & Mazza, J. J. (1993). Suicidal Behavior History Form. Odessa, FL: Psychological Assessment Resources Inc.

Rhodewalt, F., Madrian, J. C., & Cheney, S. (1998). Narcissism, self-knowledge organization, and emotional reactivity: The effect of daily experience on self-esteem and affect. *Personality and Social Psychology Bulletin, 24*, 75–87.

Richards, J. (1993). *Therapy of substance abuse syndromes.* Northvale, NJ: Jason Aronson Inc.

Rivera, M. (1991). *Multiple personality: An outcome of child abuse.* Toronto: Education/Dissociation.

Roberts, A. R. (1981). *Sheltering battered women.* New York: Springer.

Roberts, A. R. (1990). *Contemporary perspectives on crisis intervention.* Englewood Cliffs, NJ: Prentice-Hall.

Roberts, A. R. (1998). Crisis intervention: A practical guide to immediate help for victims families. In A. Horton & J. Williamson (Eds.), *Abuse and religion* (p. 606). Lexington, MA: D. C. Heath.

Roberts, A. R. (Ed.). (2000a). *Crisis intervention handbook: Assessment, treatment, and research.* Oxford, UK: Oxford University Press.

Roberts, A. R. (2000b). An overview of crisis theory and crisis intervention. In A. R. Roberts (Ed.), *Crisis intervention handbook: Assessment, treatment and research* (pp. 3–30). New York: Oxford University Press.

Robinson, R., Perry, V., & Carey, B. (1995). African Americans. In U.S. DHHS, PHS, SAMHSA, & CSAT, *Implementing cultural competence in the treatment of racial/ethnic substance abusers.* (pp. 1–21). Rockville, MD: Technical Resources.

Rogers, C. (1951). *Client-centered therapy: Its current practice, implications, and theory.* Boston: Houghton-Mifflin.

Romeo, F. (2000). The educator's role in reporting the emotional abuse of children. *Journal of Instructional Psychology, 27*, 315–322.

Rosewater, L. B. (1982). An MMPI profile for battered women (Doctoral dissertation, Union Graduate School, Ann Arbor, 1982). *Dissertation Abstracts International.*

Rosewater, L. B. (1985a). Schizophrenic or battered? In L. B. Rosewater & L. E. A. Walker (Eds.), *Handbook on feminist therapy: Psychotherapy with women* (pp. 24–43). New York: Springer.

Rosewater, L. B. (1985b). Feminist interpretations of traditional testing. In L. B. Rosewater & L. E. A. Walker (Eds.), *Handbook on feminist therapy: Psychotherapy with women* (pp. 57–71). New York: Springer.

Rothbaum, B. O. & Foa, E. B. (1992). Exposure therapy for rape victims with post-traumatic stress disorder. *The Behavior Therapist, 15*, 219–222.

Rouse, B. A. (1995). *Substance abuse and mental health statistics sourcebook.* DHHS

Publication No. (SMA) 95–3064. Washington, DC: Government Printing Office.

Russell, D. E., & Bolen, R. M. (2000). *The epidemic of rape and child sexual abuse in the United States.* Thousand Oaks, CA: Sage Publications.

Saunders, D. G., & Hanusa, D. (1986). Cognitive-behavioral treatment of men who batter: The short term effects of group therapy. *Journal of Family Violence, 1,* 357–372.

Schmookler, E. (1996). *Trauma treatment manual.* Albany, CA. Available from http://trauma-pages.com

Schneider, J. (1984). *Stress, loss and grief.* New York: Aspen Publishers, Inc.

Schneidman, E. (1985). *Definition of suicide.* New York: John Wiley & Sons.

Schreder, C. (Producer), & Greenwald, R. (Director). (1995). *The burning bed* [Motion picture]. United States: Anchor Bay Entertainment.

Schuckit, M. A. (1995). Alcohol related disorders. In H. I. Kaplan & B. J. Sadock (Eds.), *Comprehensive textbook of psychiatry* (6th ed., pp. 120–138). Baltimore: Williams & Wilkins.

Schuerger, J. M., & Reigle, N. (1988). Personality and biographic data that characterize men who abuse their wives. *Journal of Clinical Psychology, 44,* 75–81.

Scully, D. (1990). *Understanding sexual violence: A study of convicted rapists.* Boston: Unwin Hyman, Inc.

Seligman, M. (1990, 1998). *Learned optimism.* New York: Pocket Books.

Shaffer, D. A., Gould, M. S., & Hicks, R. C. (1994). Worsening suicide rates in black teenagers. *American Journal of Psychiatry, 151,* 1810–1812.

Silverman, A. B., Reinherz, H. Z., & Giaconia, R. M. (1996). The long-term sequalae of child and adolescent abuse: A longitudinal community study. *Child Abuse and Neglect, 20,* 709–723.

Simpson, J. A., & Rholes, W. S. (1998). *Attachment theory and close relationships.* New York: Guilford Press.

Slaikeu, K.A. (1984). *Crisis Intervention: A handbook for practice and research.* Newton, MA: Allyn & Bacon.

Slaikeu, K. A. (1990). *Crisis intervention: A handbook for practice and research* (2nd ed.). Boston: Allyn & Bacon.

Slovic, P., & Monahan, J. (1995). Probability, danger and coercion: A study of risk perception and decision making in mental health law. *Professional Psychology: Research & Practice, 26,* 499–506.

Smith, J., & Williams, J. (1992). From abusive household to dating violence. *Journal of Family Violence, 7,* 153–165.

Sonkin, D. J., & Durphy, M. (1993). *Learning to live without violence* (3rd ed.). San Francisco, CA: Volcano Press.

Sontag, D. (2002, April 28). Who was responsible for Elizabeth Shin? *New York Times,* Section 6, pp. 57, 61.

Stark, E. (1996). Mandatory arrests of batterers: A reply to critics. In E. S. Buzawa & C. G. Buzawa (Eds.), *Do arrests and restraining orders work?* (pp. 115–149). Thousand Oaks, CA: Sage Publications.

Steffens, D. C., & Blazer, D. G. (1999). Suicide in the elderly. In D. G. Jacobs (Ed.), *The Harvard Medical School guide to suicide assessment and intervention* (pp. 443–462). San Francisco: Jossey-Bass.

Stern, E. (2001, July). Tarasoff cases weight patients' confidentiality rights with society's protection needs. *Massachusetts Psychologist, masspsy.com, 11.*

Stone, O., & Ho, A. K. (Producers); Stone, O. (Director) (1989) *Born on the Fourth of July,* Universal Pictures.

Stordeur, R. A., & Stille, R. (1989). *Ending men's violence against their partners: One road to peace.* Thousand Oaks, CA: Sage Publications.

Stosny, S. (1995). *Treating attachment abuse: A compassionate approach.* New York: Springer Publishing Company.

Straus, M., & Smith, C. (1990). Family patterns and child abuse. In M. Straus & R. Gelles (Eds.), *Physical violence in American families: Risk factors and adaptations to violence in 8,145 families.* New Brunswick, NJ: Transaction Publishing.

Straus, M., & Stewart, J. (1999). Corporal punishment by American parents: National data on prevalence, chronicity, severity, and duration, in relation to child and family characteristics. *Clinical Child and Family Psychology Review, 2,* 55–70.

Strong, B., & DeVault, C. (1994). *Human sexuality.* Mountain View, CA: Mayfield.

Styron, W. (1990). *Darkness visible: A memoir of madness.* New York: Random House.

Substance Abuse & Mental Health Services Administration, Office of Applied Statistics. (2002). 2001 National Household Survey on Drug Abuse. Retrieved from http://www.samhsa.gov.

Sue, D., Sue, D. W., & Sue, S. (2003). *Understanding abnormal behavior*. Boston: Houghton Mifflin Co.

Tarasoff v. Board of Regents of the University of California, 551 P.2d 334 (1976).

Tetreault, P. A., & Barnett, M. A. (1987). Reactions to stranger and acquaintance rape. *Psychology of Women Quarterly, 11,* 353–358.

Tobolowsky, P. M. (2000). *Understanding victimology*. Cincinnati: Anderson Publishing.

Tolman, R. M. (1989). The development of a measure of psychological maltreatment of women by their male partners. *Violence & Victims, 4,* 159–177.

Tomasulo, D. (1998). *Action methods in group psychotherapy: Practical aspects*. Ann Arbor, MI: Braun-Brumfield, Inc.

Tower, C. (1999). *Understanding child abuse and neglect*. Needham Heights, MA: Allyn & Bacon.

Toynbee, A. (1969). *Man's concern with death.* New York: McGraw-Hill.

Trovato, F. (1986). The relationship between marital dissolution and suicide: The Canadian case. *Journal of Marriage and the Family, 48,* 341–348.

Truscott, D., Evens, J., & Mansell, S. (1995). Outpatient psychotherapy with dangerous clients: A model for decision making. *Professional Psychology: Research & Practice, 26,* 484–490.

Tsuang, M. T., Fleming, J. A., & Simpson, J. C. (1999). Suicide and schizophrenia. In D.G. Jacobs (Ed.), *The Harvard Medical School guide to suicide assessment and intervention* (pp. 287–299). San Francisco: Jossey-Bass.

Understanding violent children: Hearing before the Subcommittee on Early Childhood, Youth, and Families, of the House Committee on Education and the Workforce, 105th Cong., (1998) (testimony of Scott Poland).

Underwood, M., & Dunne-Maxim, K. (1997). *Managing sudden traumatic loss in the schools*: New Jersey adolescent suicide prevention project. Piscataway, NJ: University Behavioral Healthcare.

United Nations Secretariat. (1996). *Demographics yearbook.* New York: Department for Economic and Social Information and Policy Analysis, Statistical Division, United Nations.

U.S. Department of Health and Human Services, National Mental Health Information Center. (2000). *Training manual for mental health and human service workers in major disasters.* Retrieved October 24, 2002, from http://www.mentalhealth.org/publications/allpubs/ADM90–538/tmsection2.asp

U.S. Department of Justice. (1998). *Violence by Intimates: Analysis of Data on Crime by Current or Former Spouses, Boyfriends and Girlfriends.* Bureau of Justice Statistics, NJS-167237, Washington, DC.

U.S. Department of Justice. (2000). *Violence by intimates: Analysis of data on crime by current or former spouses, boyfriends and girlfriends.* Bureau of Justice Statistics, Washington, DC.

van der Kolk, B., McFarlane, A., and Weisaeth, L. (Eds.). (1996). *Traumatic stress: The effects of overwhelming experience on mind, body and society.* New York: Guilford Press.

van Emmerick, A., Kamphuis, J., Hulsbosch, A., & Emmelkamp, P. (2002). Single session debriefing after psychological trauma: A meta-analysis. *Lancet, 360,* 741–742.

Varia, R., Abidin, R.R., & Dass, P. (1996). Perceptions of abuse: Effects on adult psychological and social adjustment. *Child Abuse and Neglect, 18,* 11–25.

Walker, L. (1980). *The battered woman.* New York: Harper & Row.

Walker, L. (1994b). *The abused woman: A survivor therapy approach* (manual & video). New York: Newbridge Communications Inc.

Walker, L. (2000). *The battered woman syndrome* (2nd ed.). New York: Springer Publishing Co.

Walsh, F. (1998). *Strengthening family resilience.* New York: Guilford.

Warner, E. A. (1993). Cocaine abuse. *Annals of Internal Medicine, 119,* 226–235.

Webster, L. & Browning, J. (2002). Child maltreatment. In S.E. Brock & P. Lazarus (Eds.), *Best practices in crisis intervention.* National Association of School Psychologists: Washington, DC.

Weiche, V. R., & Richards, A. L. (1995). *Intimate betrayal: Understanding and responding to the trauma of acquaintance rape.* Thousand Oaks, CA: Sage.

Weishaar, M., & Beck, A. (1990). The suicidal patient: How should the therapist respond? In K. Hawton, et al. (Eds.), *Dilemmas and difficulties in the management of psychiatric patients* (pp. 65–76). Oxford, UK: Oxford University Press.

Weiss, A. (2001). The no-suicide contract: Possibilities and pitfalls. *American Journal of Psychotherapy, 55*(3), 414–416.

Weiss, R. D., & Hufford, M. R. (1999). Substance abuse and suicide. In D. G. Jacob

(Ed.), *The Harvard Medical School guide to suicide assessment and intervention* (pp. 300–310). San Francisco: Jossey-Bass.

Weissman, M. M., Bruce, M., Leaf, P., Florio, L., & Holzer, C. (1991). Affective disorders. In L. Robins & E. Reiger (Eds.), *Psychiatric disorders in America* (pp. 53–80). New York: Free Press.

Weitzman, J. (1985). Engaging the severely dysfunctional family in treatment: Basic considerations. *Family Process, 24*, 473–485.

Weller, S. (1992). Why is date rape so hard to prove? *Health, 6*, 62–64.

Wilhelm, R. (1967). *The book of changes or The I Ching*. Princeton, NJ: Princeton University Press.

Wilson, K., & Sigman, P. (1996, February). *Guide to disaster recovery program design and implementation: The Missouri model*. Jefferson City, MO: Missouri Department of Mental Health.

Wolfe, D. A. (1987). *Child abuse: Implications for child development and psychopathology*.

Beverly Hills, CA: Sage.

Worden, J. W. (1982). *Grief counseling and grief therapy: A handbook for the mental health practitioner*. New York: Springer.

Yost, D. A. (1996). Alcohol withdrawal syndrome. *American Family Physician, 54*, 657–664.

Young, M. (2001). *Victim assistance: Frontiers and fundamentals*. Washington, DC: National Organization for Victim Assistance.

Young, M. E., & Long, L. L. (1998). *Counseling and therapy for couples*. Pacific Grove, CA: Brooks/Cole Co.

Zenere, F. (1998, November). NASP/NEAT community crisis response. *NASP Communique, 27*, 38–39.

Zisook, S., Shuchter, S. R., & Lyons, L. E. (1987). Predictors of psychological reactions during the early stage of widowhood. *Psychiatric Clinics of North America, 10*, 355–368.

NAME INDEX

271

SUBJECT INDEX

Page numbers in *italics* indicate figures or tables.

A.A. (Alcoholics Anonymous), 102, 118, 119, *120, 121*
abortion, 195–196
abuse, defined, 75
  See also child abuse and neglect; emotional abuse; physical abuse; sexual abuse; verbal abuse
abusive sexual contact, defined, 156–157
acceptance, in counseling, 31, 86
acceptance stage of grief, 184
acquaintance rape, 155–156, 158, 168–170
Acting Out Person (Level III), 144
active listening, 37, 148
acute battering phase, in cycle of violence, 82
acute grief, 183
acute stress disorder, 12, *13*
adjustment disorder, 12, *14*
Administration for Children and Families, 62
adolescents and young adults, 101, 126, *127, 129,* 181
Adoption Assistance and Child Welfare Act (1980), 55–56
Adult Children of Alcoholics, *120*
adventuresomeness, in counselors, 29
African Americans
  child abuse and neglect, 52
  grief reactions, 181
  homicide as cause of death, 141
  spirituality, 16
  substance abuse, 101
  suicide, 126, *127*
aggravated sexual abuse, defined, 156
agitated depression, and suicide risk, 130, 134
Al-Anon, 119, *120,* 121
Alateen, *120*
alcohol, physiological effects of, 106
alcohol and drug crises, 99–123
  crisis intervention and case management, 107–118, *112*
  defining substance use disorders, 101–107
  organizations, 122–123
  scope of drug and alcohol problems, 100–101
  treatment options, 118–121, *119, 120–121*
Alcohol & Drug Abuse Commission, 123

Alcoholics Anonymous (A.A.), 102, 118, 119, *120, 121*
alcoholism
  inpatient treatment programs, 118
  and intimate partner violence, 81, 115–116
  risk factors and protective factors, *112*
  See also substance dependence
ambiguity, tolerance for, 28
American Academy of Experts in Traumatic Stress, 18
American Association of Suicidology, 152, 230
American Counseling Association, 46, 149, 150–151, 242, 249
American Foundation for Suicide Prevention, 152
American Medical Association, 74
American Psychiatric Association
  acute stress disorder symptoms, *13*
  adjustment disorder symptoms, *14*
  diagnosis, 10
  Posttraumatic Stress Disorder, *12,* 161–162
  substance abuse disorders, 99, 102, 103, 103n, 105n, 106n
American Psychological Association, 46, 149, 242, 248–249
American Red Cross, 241, 242, 248, 249–250, 251, 256
American School Counselor Association, 46, 231
AmeriCorps, 240
anger, as stage of grief, 183
anger management training, 88
anger styles, 80–81
anticipatory grief, 182
Antisocial Personality Disorder, 80, 142, 161
Anxiety Level (Level I), 143
Asian Americans, 16, *127*
assault, defined, 75
assertiveness training, 88
assessment step, in LAPC model, 42–43
attending, 35–37

bargaining stage of grief, 183
battered women, 76–78, 86–87, 94, 96–97
batterers
  assessing, 89–91, *90–91*